Practical Pharmacology

AF530682

Practical Pharmacology

As per the Competency-based Medical Education Curriculum (NMC)

Sixth Edition

Pramila V Yadav MBBS MD (Pharmacology)
Professor and Head, Department of Pharmacology
MGM Medical College Vashi
Navi Mumbai, Maharashtra, India

Pradnya Deolekar MBBS MD (Pharmacology)
Professor, Department of Pharmacology
Dr DY Patil Medical College
Navi Mumbai, Maharashtra, India

Kavitha Dongerkery MBBS MD (Pharmacology)
Associate Professor, Department of Pharmacology
Dr DY Patil Medical College
Navi Mumbai, Maharashtra, India

Mayakalyani Srivathsan MBBS MD (Pharmacology)
Senior Resident, Department of Pharmacology
Dr DY Patil Medical College
Navi Mumbai, Maharashtra, India

JAYPEE

JAYPEE BROTHERS MEDICAL PUBLISHERS
The Health Sciences Publisher
New Delhi | London

Jaypee Brothers Medical Publishers (P) Ltd

Headquarters
Jaypee Brothers Medical Publishers (P) Ltd
EMCA House
23/23-B, Ansari Road, Daryaganj
New Delhi - 110 002, India
Landline: +91-11-23272143, +91-11-23272703
+91-11-23282021, +91-11-23245672
Email: jaypee@jaypeebrothers.com

Corporate Office
Jaypee Brothers Medical Publishers (P) Ltd
4838/24, Ansari Road, Daryaganj
New Delhi 110 002, India
Phone: +91-11-43574357
Fax: +91-11-43574314
Email: jaypee@jaypeebrothers.com

Overseas Office
J.P. Medical Ltd
83 Victoria Street, London
SW1H 0HW (UK)
Phone: +44 20 3170 8910
Fax: +44 (0)20 3008 6180
Email: info@jpmedpub.com

Website: www.jaypeebrothers.com

Website: www.jaypeedigital.com

© 2024, Jaypee Brothers Medical Publishers

The views and opinions expressed in this book are solely those of the original contributor(s)/author(s) and do not necessarily represent those of editor(s) and publisher of the book.

All rights reserved. No part of this publication may be reproduced, stored or transmitted in any form or by any means, electronic, mechanical, photocopying, recording or otherwise, without the prior permission in writing of the publishers.

All brand names and product names used in this book are trade names, service marks, trademarks or registered trademarks of their respective owners. The publisher is not associated with any product or vendor mentioned in this book.

Medical knowledge and practice change constantly. This book is designed to provide accurate, authoritative information about the subject matter in question. However, readers are advised to check the most current information available on procedures included and check information from the manufacturer of each product to be administered, to verify the recommended dose, formula, method and duration of administration, adverse effects and contraindications. It is the responsibility of the practitioner to take all appropriate safety precautions. Neither the publisher nor the author(s)/editor(s) assume any liability for any injury and/or damage to persons or property arising from or related to use of material in this book.

This book is sold on the understanding that the publisher is not engaged in providing professional medical services. If such advice or services are required, the services of a competent medical professional should be sought.

Every effort has been made where necessary to contact holders of copyright to obtain permission to reproduce copyright material. If any have been inadvertently overlooked, the publisher will be pleased to make the necessary arrangements at the first opportunity.

Inquiries for bulk sales may be solicited at: jaypee@jaypeebrothers.com

Practical Pharmacology

Fifth Edition: 2017
Sixth Edition: **2024**

ISBN: 978-93-5696-489-1

Printed in India at Sterling Graphics Pvt. Ltd.

Dedicated to

My parents—Mr Shriram and Mrs Kalavati Yadav
My lovely daughters—Akanksha and Neha

Preface

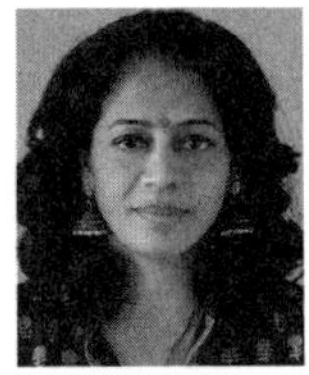

Pramila V Yadav

Recently, the National Medical Council (NMC) restructured the curriculum and introduced Competency-Based Medical Education (CBME) as a way to incorporate knowledge, skills and attitude in the undergraduate training program. While innovative, CBME poses a challenge to students and teachers as they adapt to this new system of education.

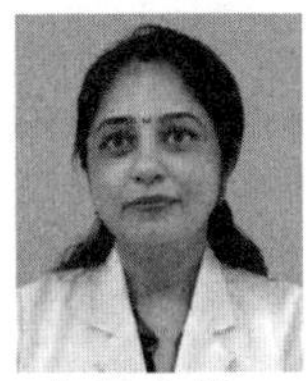

Pradnya Deolekar

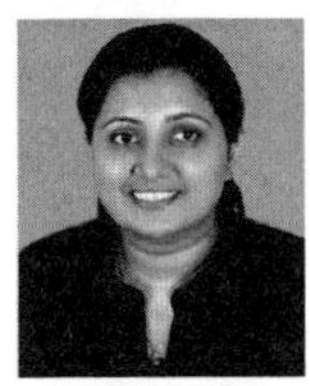

Kavitha Dongerkery

Pharmacology is an integral part of the MBBS course and is at the core of all clinical subjects that a student learns. Undoubtedly, the subject is expansive. This book is an earnest effort to make the key topics in practical pharmacology as comprehensive and concise as possible. Information is presented as flowcharts, tables, diagrams, photographs and checklists wherever appropriate so that a student is able to revise the subject matter quickly. Sufficient examples are provided to explain each concept. Filled adverse drug reaction (ADR) forms are provided to inculcate the habit of reporting ADRs in future physicians. Dose calculations are also explained with solved examples. This book will be useful in giving the student a proper orientation of what is expected in the practical examinations as well as practical skills essential to clinical practice.

"Change is inevitable. Growth is optional."—**John Maxwell**

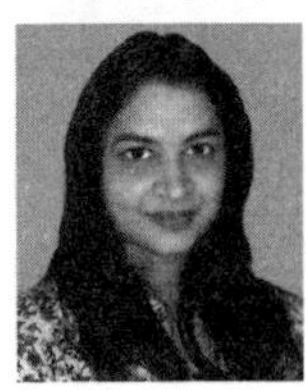

Mayakalyani Shrivathsan

As we navigate this new era of medical education, our intentions remain to help students develop all the expertise necessary to become competent physicians. We also seek to continually improve our own skills in teaching the ever-evolving subject which is pharmacology. We are always open to productive feedback that will improve how we deliver information in the best possible way. We hope our purposeful attempt will help students and teachers alike in their future endeavor and learning. For any feedback, write to drpramilayadav10@gmail.com, phone no. 9820792968.

As Brian Gallant once said, "Education is something we have to keep pursuing day after day".

We wish the students all the very best in all their future endeavors and hope this book guides them in their journey.

Pramila Yadav
Pradnya Deolekar
Kavitha Dongerkery
Mayakalyani Shrivathsan

Acknowledgments

I sincerely wish to thank the following:

- Our family members for their support and encouragement
- My publisher M/s Jaypee Brothers Medical Publishers (P) Ltd, New Delhi, India, who helped and guided me, Shri Jitendar P Vij (Group Chairman), Mr Ankit Vij (Managing Director), Mr MS Mani (Group President), Dr Madhu Choudhary (Director-Educational Publishing), Ms Pooja Bhandari [Director-Production (Books and Journals)], Ms Sunita Katla (EA to Group Chairman and Publishing Manager), Ms Samina Khan (EA to Director-Educational Publishing), Dr Sangeeta Yadav (Development Editor), Mr Ajay Kumar Sharma [Deputy General Manager (Books and Journals)], Mr Rajesh Sharma (Production Coordinator), Ms Seema Dogra (Cover Visualizer), Mr Vakil Khan (Proofreader), Mr Kapil Dev Sharma (Typesetter), Mr Nitesh Jain (Graphic Designer) and their team members, for all their support to work in this project and make it a success. Without their cooperation, I could not have completed this project.

Contents

Syllabus

List of Practical/Tutorials/Integrated Learning/Seminars/Small group teaching Topics

Number	*COMPETENCY The student should be able to*	*Practical/tutorials/integrated learning/seminars/small group teaching topics*	*Hours*
	Practical's		
PHI.10	Describe parts of a correct, complete and legible generic prescription. Identify errors in prescription and correct appropriately	Prescription writing	2
PH5.7	Demonstrate an understanding of the legal and ethical aspects of prescribing drugs		
	Practical's Clinical Pharmacy		
PH2.1	Demonstrate understanding of the use of various dosage forms (oral/local/parenteral; solid/liquid)	Introduction to practical pharmacology	2
		Route of administration—oral	2
		Introduction to pharmacy Pharmacy preparations (solution, suspension, emulsion)	6
		Route of administration-topical	2
		Pharmacy preparations (lotion, liniment, ointment)	6
		Route of administration-parental	2
PH2.3	Demonstrate the appropriate setting up of an intravenous drip in a simulated environment	Skill lab	2
PH2.2	Prepare oral rehydration solution from ORS packet and explain its use	Pharmacy preparation (ORS powder)	2

PH2.4	Demonstrate the correct method of calculation of drug dosage in patients including those used in special situations	PK-I	2
		PK-II	2
Clinical Pharmacology			
PH3.1	Write a rational, correct and legible generic prescription for a given condition and communicate the same to the patient	Single drug therapy	2
		Multiple drug therapy	4
		Fixed drug combination	2
PH3.2	Perform and interpret a critical appraisal (audit) of a given prescription	Criticism of prescription	4
PH3.3	Perform a critical evaluation of the drug promotional literature	Sources of drug information including scrutiny of promotional literature	4
PH3.6	Demonstrate how to optimize interaction with pharmaceutical representative to get authentic information on drugs	Skill lab	
PH3.4	To recognize and report an adverse drug reaction	ADR-I	2
		ADR-II	2
		ADR reporting system and forms	2
		Subjective and objective effects of drugs	
PH3.5	To prepare and explain a list of P-drugs for a given case/ condition	Rational pharmacotherapy I	2
		Case study-I	2
		Case study-II	2
		Rational pharmacotherapy	2
PH3.7	Prepare a list of essential medicines for a healthcare facility	National essential drug list	2
PH3.8	Communicate effectively with a patient on the proper use of prescribed medication	Skill station: Steps for durg delivery (topical and inhalational)	2

Experimental Pharmacology			
PH4.1	Administer drugs through various routes in a simulated environment using mannequins	Skill lab-parenteral routes	2
PH4.2	Demonstrate the effects of drugs on blood pressure (vasopressor and vaso-depressors with appropriate blockers) using computer aided learning	Screening techniques for new drugs	2
		PD-I	2
		PD-II	2
		CAL based learning	2
		CAL based learning	2
		CAL based learning	2

1 CHAPTER

Introduction to Routes of Administration and Oral Dosage Forms

ROUTES OF DRUG ADMINISTRATION (FIG. 1.1)

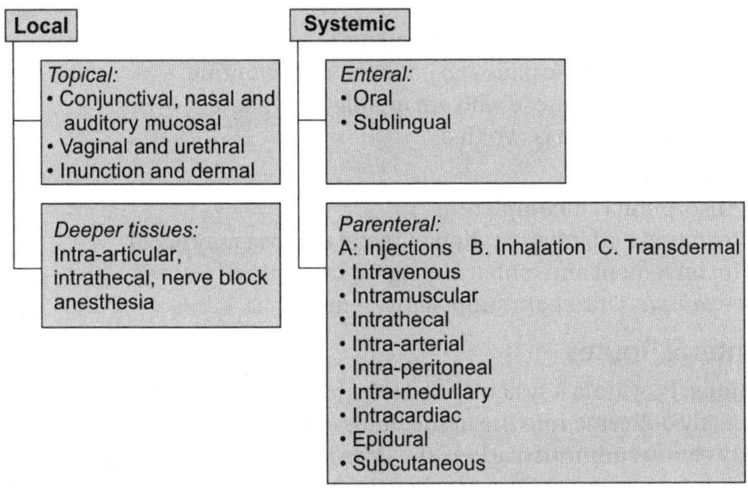

Fig. 1.1: Classification of routes of drug administration.

Enteral Routes

a. **Oral administration:** Most convenient route. The drug is simply swallowed through the mouth.

   Advantages:
   - Painless
   - Cheap
   - Safe
   - Self-administered

   Disadvantages:
   - Delayed onset, not used in emergency
   - Not suitable for unconscious, uncooperative patient
   - Cannot be given in patients with severe vomiting and diarrhea
   - Drugs that are destroyed by digestive juices (insulin) cannot be given.

b. **Sublingual administration:** The drug is kept under the tongue or sometimes crushed and spread over the buccal mucous membranes.

Advantages:
- The quick onset of action.
- Bypasses the first-pass metabolism
- The effect can be terminated by spitting out the tablet.
- Self-administered

Disadvantages:
- Irritant drugs cannot be used.
- Not suitable for drugs with bad taste.

For example, glyceryl trinitrate, isosorbide dinitrate, nifedipine.

c. **Rectal administration:** The rectal mucous membrane has a rich blood supply.

Advantages:
- Can be used in unconscious patient
- Useful in geriatric patients; patients with vomiting
- Can be used in those who are unable to swallow
- Gastric irritation is avoided

Disadvantages:
- Absorption is incomplete
- Irritation and inflammation of rectal mucosa may occur
- Inconvenient and embarrassing for the patient

For example, Diazepam suppository, enema.

Parenteral Routes

Injections: Provide fast systemic effects bypassing first-pass inactivation. Drugs are directly delivered into the tissue fluids or blood.

a. **Intravenous administration:** The drug may be administered as a bolus or as an infusion and the drug is given in superficial veins.
Site: Through the lumen of veins, mainly the antecubital vein.

Advantages:
- The quick onset of action
- The most useful route in emergencies
- Provides 100% bioavailability
- A large volume of solutions can be given.
- Can be used in unconscious, uncooperative patients
- GIT irritant drugs can also be infused by this route.

Disadvantages:
- Strict aseptic conditions are needed.
- Assistance is required for the administration of drug
- Painful
- Irritation of the veins may cause thrombophlebitis.
- The introduction of air may produce an embolism.

For example, glucose, dopamine and norepinephrine drip for IV infusion. Antibiotics, heparin, diazepam.

b. **Intramuscular injection:**

Site: Deltoid muscle or gluteal mass of left or right buttock. Vastus muscle underlying the lateral surface of the thigh.

Advantages:

- Vascularity of muscle is good so absorption of drug is rapid than by SC route.
- The absorption is reliable, predictable.
- Mild irritant drugs can be given.
- Depot preparations can be used: Depot medroxyprogesterone acetate (DMPA).

Disadvantages:

- Aseptic precaution is required.
- Painful
- Chances of nerve damage and paralysis, if injected into nerve.
- Large volume cannot be given (maximum of 5–10 mL).

For example, various antibiotics, antiemetics, non-steroidal anti-inflammatory drugs (NSAIDs),, adrenaline.

Intraperitoneal Administration

Site: Into the peritoneal space

Advantages:

Rapid absorption due to larger surface area.

Disadvantages:

- Aseptic conditions are required.
- Painful, risky due to chances of adhesions and infections in peritoneal cavity (peritonitis).

For example, administering dialyzing fluids for peritoneal dialysis in cases of poisoning and renal failure.

Intrathecal (Intraspinal) Administration

Site: Into the subarachnoid space

Advantages:

- The drug after diffusing from the lumbar sac passes into the subarachnoid space. Thus, significant CSF levels are produced.
- The drug acts directly on the meninges and the spinal cord.

Disadvantages:

- Strict aseptic conditions are needed.
- Great expertise is required to give such injections.
- Painful and risky procedure

For example, xylocaine injection for providing spinal anesthesia, radiopaque contrast media for myelography (Visualize spinal cord)

Intramedullary Administration

Site: Injection into the tibial or sternal bone marrow.

Advantages:

The onset of action is very fast.

Disadvantages:

- Risky procedure
- Painful
- Strict aseptic conditions are needed and skill is also required to give such injections.

For example, bone marrow transplantation

Intra-arterial Administration

Site: Into the lumen of the desired artery.

Advantages:

Greater concentration of the drug can be delivered at the desired site of action

Disadvantages:

- Strict aseptic conditions are needed.
- Great expertise is required.

For example, radiopaque contrast media for coronary angiography and cerebral angiography. Many anticancer drugs.

Subcutaneous Administration

Site: The drug is injected in the subcutaneous tissue under the skin.

Advantages:

- Effect is uniform and sustained.
- Highly suitable for depot preparations and implants
- Suspensions, colloids and oily preparations can be administered.
- Self-administration is possible.

Disadvantages:

- Absorption is slow and so is the onset of action.
- Cannot be used for emergency situation
- Only non-irritant drugs can be given
- Only small volume of drug can be administered (maximum 1 mL).

For example, lignocaine, insulin, vaccines

Intradermal (Intracutaneous Route)

Site: Drug is injected into the outer layers of skin raising a bleb.

Advantages:

- Since very small amount of drug produces the effect it is used for the sensitivity test.
- Useful for the administration of vaccines

Disadvantages:
- Absorption is slow.
- Very small amount (0.5 mL) can be administered.

For example, diagnostic tests, allergy testing, vaccines, such as BCG, measles.

Epidural Injection

The drug is injected through a vertebral interspace between the dura of the spinal cord and the lining of the spinal canal.

For example, lidocaine injection to provide the epidural nerve block.

Intracardiac Injection

This injection is given by a long needle into the heart muscle through the left fourth intercostal space close to the sternum.

For example, injection of adrenaline to restart the heart beat in cases of sudden cardiac arrest.

Inhalational Administration

Site: Inspiration through nose or mouth.

Advantages:
- Faster absorption and hence quick onset of action due to larger surface area of alveoli.
- Dose required is very less, so systemic toxicity is minimized.
- Self-administered

Disadvantages:
Bronchial irritation leading to increased bronchial and salivary secretions.

For example, oxygen, general anesthetics.

Transdermal Administration

Site: Adhesive patch applied to chest, upper abdomen or mastoid region.

Advantages:
- Slow but sustained release of the drug for several days.
- Duration of action is prolonged.
- Bypasses first-pass metabolism
- Systemic side effects are reduced.

Disadvantages:
- Nil; if irritation occurs, the site of application can be changed.
- Expensive

For example, nitroglycerine, scopolamine, nicotine transdermal patches

Local Routes

Topical

- Conjunctival, nasal and auditory mucosal
- Ointments or aqueous solution of drugs are applied or instilled onto the conjunctiva for local effects, e.g., gentamicin and ciprofloxacin.
- **Nasal:** Drugs can be administered through the nasal route for systemic absorption and for local effects.

For example, decongestant nasal drops (oxymetazoline), and budesonide nasal spray for allergic rhinitis.

- Ear drops
- Vaginal and urethral
- Solutions, ointments, emulsions, foams, tablets, suppositories and pessaries of various antifungal agents (clotrimazole) and metronidazole. Drug solutions and pencil-shaped bougies for urethral use.
- *Inunction and dermal:*
  Site: Rubbing the drug preparation onto the skin (inunction-liniment for pain relief) or can be dusted or sprayed over the surface of the skin (dermal -neomycin powder).

Advantages:
Safe and convenient

Disadvantages:
- Difficulty in ascertaining the amount of the drug absorbed.
- Systemic absorption may take place if the skin has abrasions.

Deeper tissues: Certain deep areas can be approached by using a syringe and needle.
For example, intra-articular injection: Hydrocortisone in knee joint.

Intra-articular Administration

Site: Injection directly into the joint space.

Advantages:
Ensures higher concentration of drug in a localized area.

Disadvantages:
- Strict aseptic conditions are needed.
- Repeated administration into the joint space may further damage the joint
- Painful procedure

For example, hydrocortisone injection for the treatment of rheumatoid arthritis.

ORAL DOSAGE FORMS

Figure 1.2 depicts the classification of oral dosage forms.

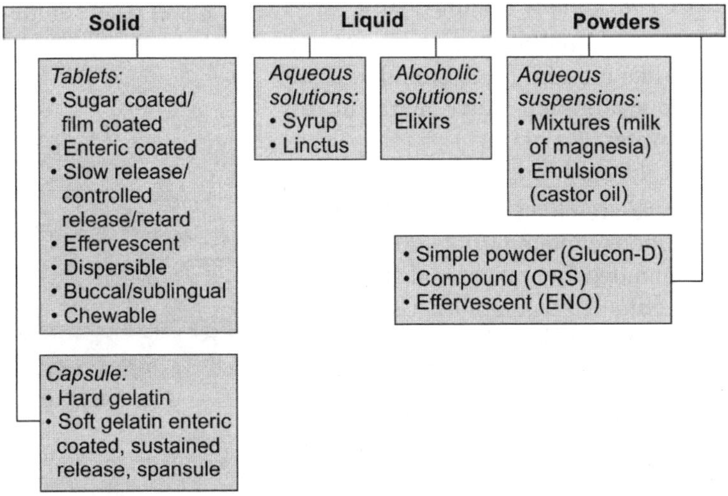

Fig. 1.2: Classification of oral dosage forms.

LIQUID DOSAGE FORMS (MIXTURES) (FIG. 1.3)

Solution: Absorb rapidly because they do not need to be dissolved.

Suspension: One or more substances dispersed in water using a suspending agent. Must be shaken before use.

Emulsion: Suspensions of fats/oils in water using an emulsifying agent—cod liver oil emulsion.

Gels: Colloidal aqueous suspension of hydrated inorganic substances—aluminum hydroxide gel.

Magma: Bulky suspensions—milk of magnesia.

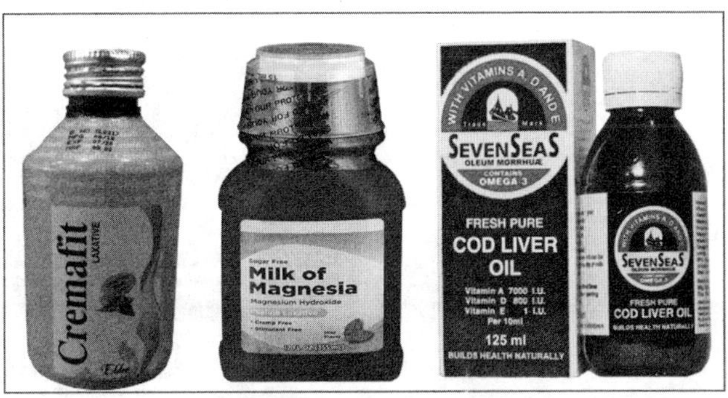

Fig. 1.3: Liquid dosage forms.

Syrups: These are concentrated aqueous preparations of a sugar or sugar substitute with/without flavoring agents and medicinal substances. *For example,* vitamin syrup.

Linctus: Viscous liquid syrup containing some demulcent-like menthol, It is intended to be sipped and swallowed slowly without the addition of water.
For example, Linctus codeine.

Elixirs: These are clear, sweetened hydroalcoholic solutions containing not > 20% alcohol. These are intended for oral use and are usually flavored to enhance palatability. Usually less sweet than syrups and less viscous.
For example, promethazine **(Fig. 1.4)**.

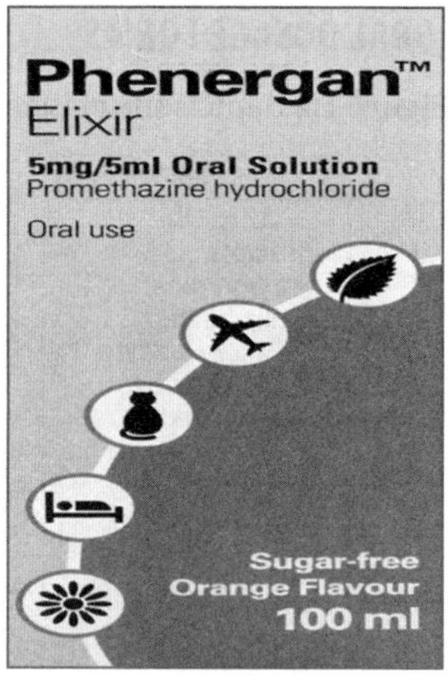

Fig. 1.4: Elixir.

Tincture: Alcoholic solution of the vegetable drugs. They usually contain 70–90% alcohol **(Fig. 1.5)**.

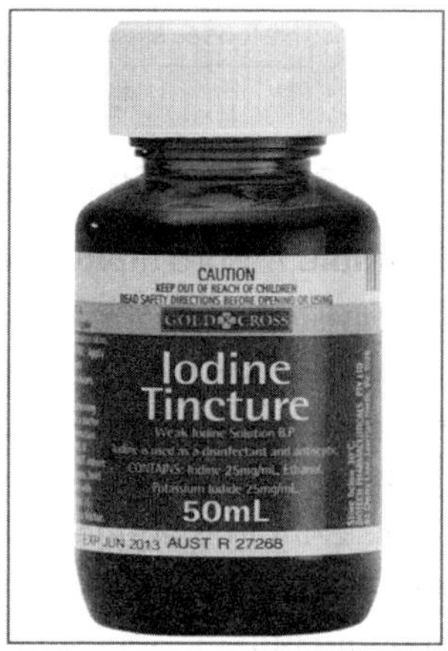

Fig. 1.5: Tincture.

Tablets (Figs. 1.6A to C)

Contains granulated/powdered drugs that are compressed into different shapes/sizes. Tablets can be SCORED (marked with an indented line across the surface) so they can be broken into smaller doses.

- Regular
- Chewable
- Sublingual
- Sugar coated/Film-coated tablet
- Enteric coated
- Extended release

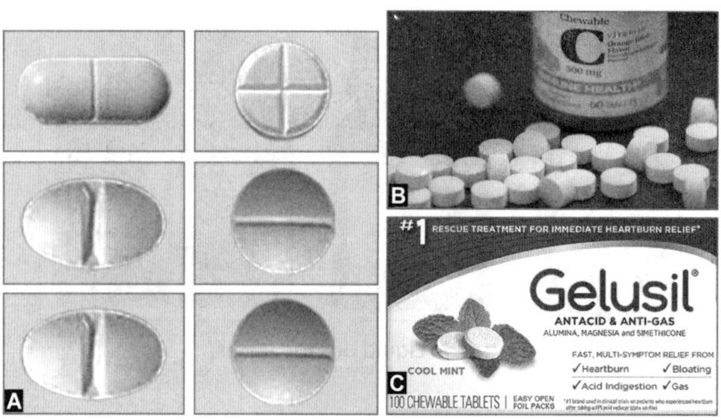

Figs. 1.6A to C: Tablets.

Buccal and Sublingual Tablets (Fig. 1.7)

Advantages:
- Quick onset of action
- Bypasses the first pass metabolism
- Effect can be terminated by spitting out the tablet
- Self-administered

Disadvantages:
- Irritant drugs cannot be used.
- Not suitable for drugs with bad taste

For example, glyceryl trinitrate, isosorbide dinitrate, nifedipine.

Sugar-coated/Film-coated tablet: Coating is done to mask bitter/unpleasant taste. They are coloured to provide an attractive appearance.

Enteric-coated:

Advantage:
This is done for drugs that get destroyed in the stomach (e.g., Pantoprazole) **Figure 1.8**, to achieve a desired concentration of the drug in the small intestine, to get absorbed from here.

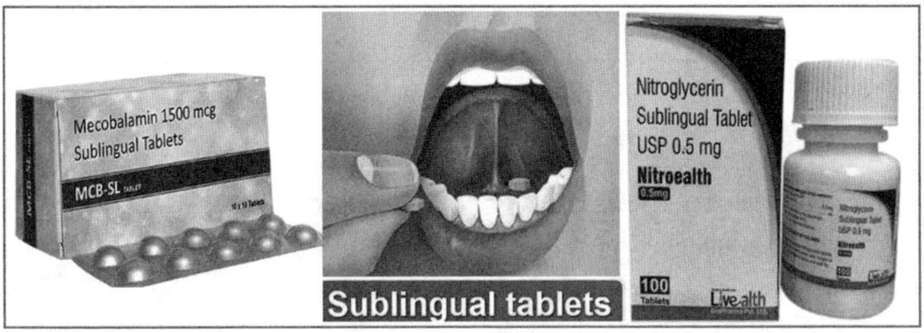

Fig. 1.7: Sublingual tablets.

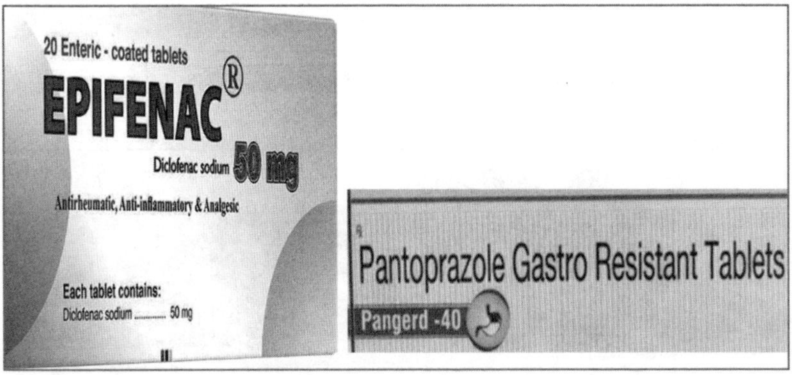

Fig. 1.8: Gastro-resistant tablets.

Extended-release/Slow/Sustained/Retard/Controlled Release Tablet (Fig. 1.9):

Large doses formulated for slow absorption-prolonged action and sustained effect.

Drug particles have an individual coating with different types of inert resins so that each type of coating dissolves at different time intervals.

Advantage:

- Slow-release tablets provide a uniform and sustained release of the drug over a period of 10–12 hours providing a longer duration of action.
- Controlled-release preparations are appropriate for drugs of a shorter half-life because of poor compliance could lead to therapeutic failure.
- Providing a uniform and sustained release also reduces the incidence of side effects

For example, metformin causes a lot git adverse when taken as a plain tablet, and a slow-release tablet of metformin reduces the incidence of diarrhea.

Compressed tablet: Drug is subjected to large mechanical pressure.

Capsules (Fig. 1.10)

Cylindrical envelopes of GELATIN in which the drug is enclosed. Hard/soft depending on the amount of glycerine in gelatin.

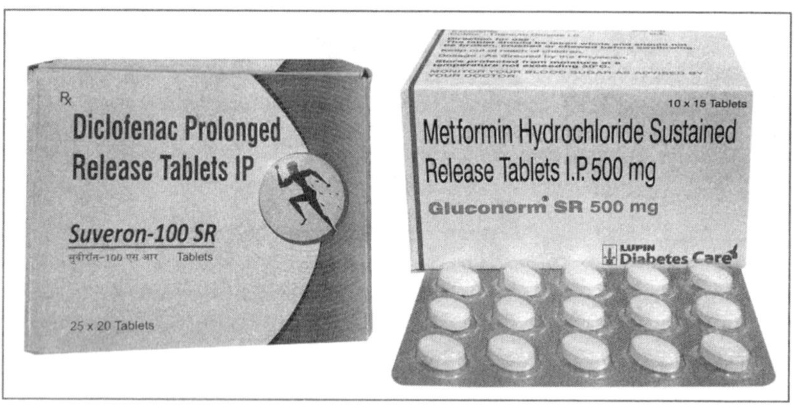

Fig. 1.9: Prolonged/sustained release tablets.

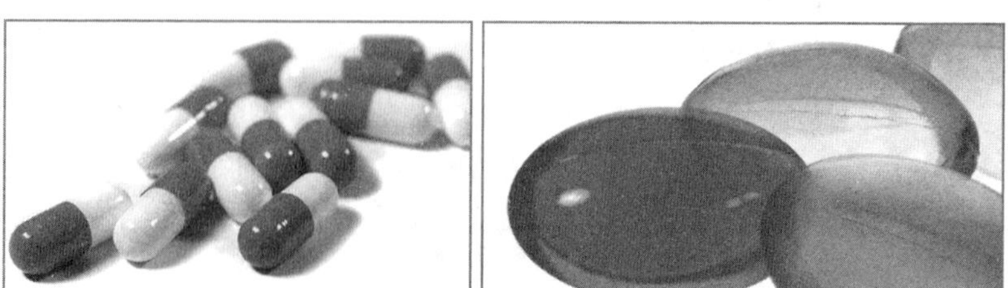

Fig. 1.10: Capsules.

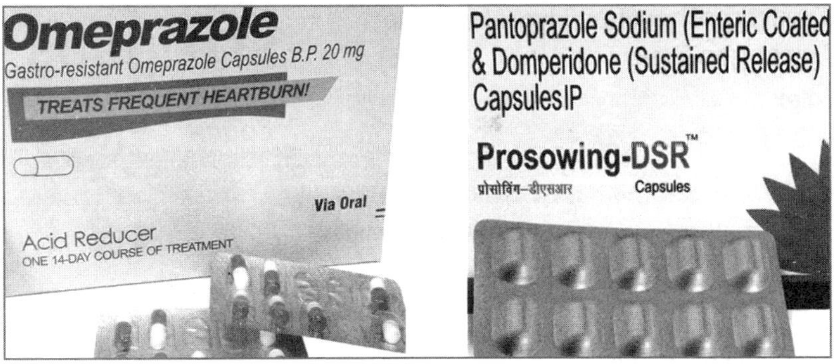

Fig. 1.11: Modified capsules.

Modified release capsules (Fig. 1.11): These are hard or soft gelatin capsules in which the contents or the shell or both are prepared by a special process to modify the rate of releasing the active ingredients of the capsule. It includes delayed-release capsules (gastro-resistant capsules) and sustained-release capsules (extended-release capsules).

Enteric capsules: These are hard or soft gelatin capsules that are resisted against the gastric fluid but dissolves in the intestinal fluid to release its contents.

Spansules (Fig. 1.12): Multidrug preparations can be delivered easily by spansules or granules in capsule technology. This type of delivery system is designed to release a drug or a medicament at two or more different rates or in different spans of time. A quick/slow release system provides an initial release of a drug followed by a constant rate of drug release over an extended period of time.

Lozenges/Troches (Fig. 1.13)

- Flat or round preparations kept in the mouth till they dissolve, liberating the drug.
- Temporarily produce high concentrations in the oral cavity—thus used to treat local conditions, such as cough, sore throat.

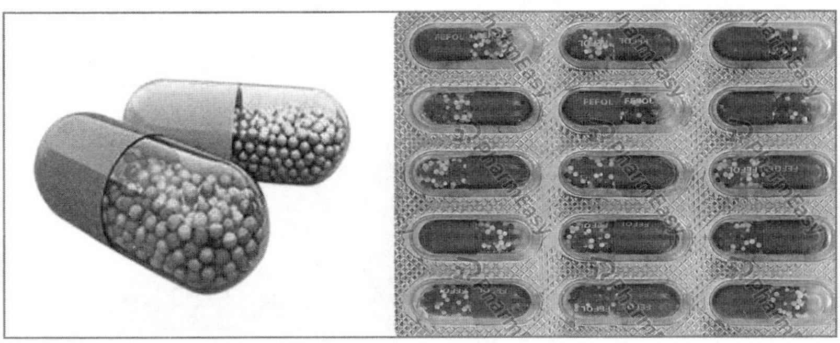

Fig. 1.12: Spansules.

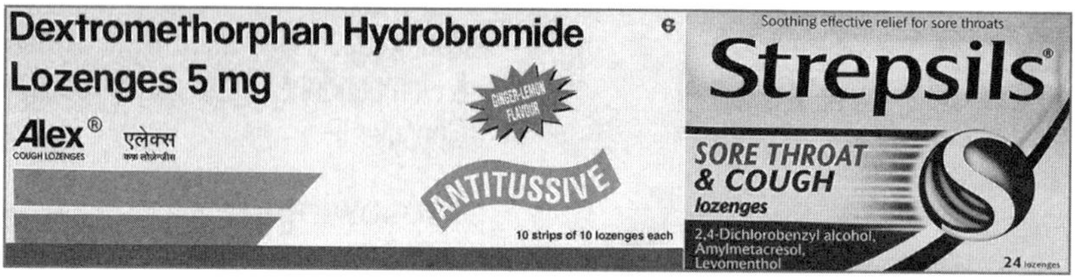

Fig. 1.13: Lozenges.

Powders (Fig. 1.14): One or more drugs in dry and finely divided state. Effervescent powders dissolve in water to release carbon dioxide, making the preparation palatable.

How to reconstitute suspension for oral use?

- Step 1: Determine the type and volume of diluent needed
- Step 2: Gently shake the bottle to loosen the powder. Open the cap of the bottle.
- Step 3: For antibiotic bottles with markings, carefully add cool boiled water to about half the height of the final marking on the bottle.
- Step 4: Replace the cap of the bottle. Shake the bottle until all the powder is thoroughly mixed.
- Step 5: Allow the suspension to stand for about 2–5 minutes to rid the air bubbles in the bottle.
- Step 6: Open the cap. Carefully add water till the final marking on the bottle.
- Step 7: Replace the cap of the bottle. Invert the bottle and shake the bottle vigorously for at least 5 seconds to get an even suspension. Make sure the medication has dispersed completely before administering it to the patient.
- Step 8: Shake the prepared suspension well before giving each dose. To make sure that you are giving the right dose, use the calibrated medication cup.

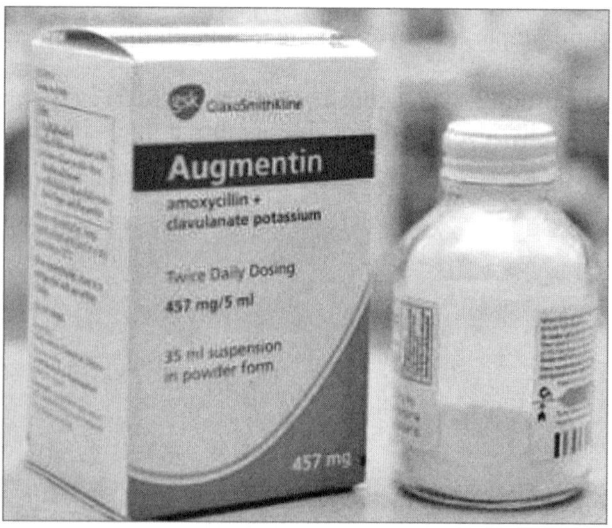

Fig. 1.14: Oral powder for reconstitution.

- Step 9: The suspension should either be stored in the refrigerator or kept at room temperature in a cool dry place below 25–30°C unless otherwise stated. Do not freeze the preparation.
- Step 10: Discard any remaining suspension upon expiry as advised after reconstitution.

Examples of oral suspension: Cefuroxime axetil, cephalexin, cefpodoxime proxetil, cefixime, azithromycin, amoxicillin.

2 CHAPTER

Topical Dosage Forms

TOPICAL DOSAGE FORMS

- **Skin, hair and nails:** Ointments, creams, gels/jellies, pastes, lotions, liniments, medicated dressings, powders, shampoos, and soaps.
- **Eye:** Eye drops, eye ointments, eye lotions, intraocular solutions, contact lens solutions, ophthalmic strips.
- **Ear:** Ear drops, ear ointments and otic irrigation solutions.
- **Nasal mucosa:** Nasal drops, nasal sprays and nasal packs.
- **Bronchi:** Solutions or powders given via inhalers, spacers, nebulisers.
- **Vaginal mucosa:** Suppositories/Pessaries, tablets, capsules, ointments, creams, douches, sprays, foams, sponges, and medicated vaginal rings.
- **Urethral mucosa:** Bougies, ointments and gels.
- **Specialized drug delivery systems:** Transdermal patch/Transdermal therapeutic system (though applied topically drug is absorbed into systemic circulation for action).

Examples

1. Ointment (Fig. 2.1): Semisolid greasy preparations, which may contain one or more active ingredients, uniformly incorporated in an hydrocarbon (oil base), e.g., Mupirocin ointment for bacterial skin infections. It is to be used on dry and scaly skin surface and mucous membranes. The drug is trapped under the dressing and, the layer of the skin is soften from sweating, enabling the drug to penetrate deeply into the tissues. Eye ointments are formulated to melt quickly so that vision.

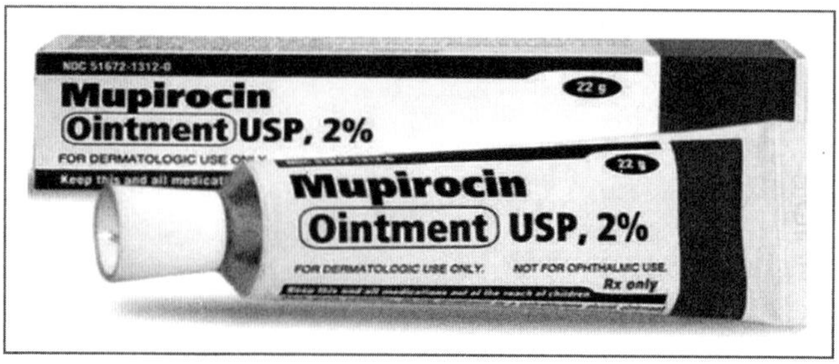

Fig. 2.1: Ointment.

Instructions

- **Consult a medical professional:** Consult a qualified medical practitioner to learn about the safety of the product and its possible side effects. Check expiry date of medication and that it is in good condition and not contaminated.
- **Clean and sanitize:** The affected area should be carefully cleaned with soap and dried before application. Hands should also be washed before and after application to avoid contamination or possible transmission of the infection.
- **Only apply to affected areas:** Topical medicine should only be applied to the affected areas gently in the direction of hair growth (Do not rub vigorously, unless the dosage form is liniment). Extra precaution should be taken when applying to areas that rub together, for example, the armpits or between the buttocks. Application should be done sparingly as these areas absorb more medication than other parts of the body. Steroid cream and ointment also need to apply sparingly in contrast to emollients, which can be use more plentifully.
- **Use as directed:** Instructions for the application on amount and duration is as stated by the practitioner. The amount will depend on the type of disease and the severity of the disease state. Never apply a cream that is prescribed for one service user to another person.
- **How to apply topical medication:** During application, take care to avoid coming into contact with the drug. Wearing gloves and cleaning hands after application can help.

If it is a liquid medicament (Suspension or emulsion) then shake the bottle before use. All dosage forms except liniments need to be applied without rubbing, on the affected part with the help of cotton swab.

2. Lotion (Fig. 2.2): Liquid preparations containing one or more active ingredients, intended for topical application to the skin and mucous membrane **without friction**, lotion invariably contains astringent, antiseptic and protectives. Lotions are used on wet and oozing surface. (weeping eczema, bullous diseases). These medications are preferably supplied in amber or blue coloured bottles to protect them from sunlight. *For example,* Calamine lotion.

*Uses of Calamine lotion***:** Sunburn, urticaria, itching, insect bite, cosmetic purpose. Calamine provides astringent, antipruritic, soothing and a protective effect on skin.

Advantage: Systemic side effects of drugs are avoided because of local application.

Disadvantage: Patient may experience a gritty feeling.

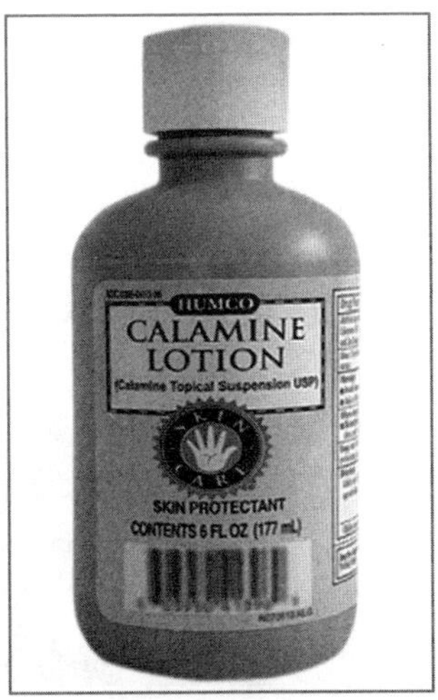

Fig. 2.2: Lotion.

3. Liniment (Fig. 2.3): Liquid preparations containing one or more active ingredients, generally with rubefacient, analgesic, counter irritant actions. It is used for external application **with friction**, e.g., Turpentine liniment.

Uses of Turpentine liniment: Applied temporarily for minor aches and pains of muscle, joints, sprains, backache, lumbago, stiff neck, torticolis.

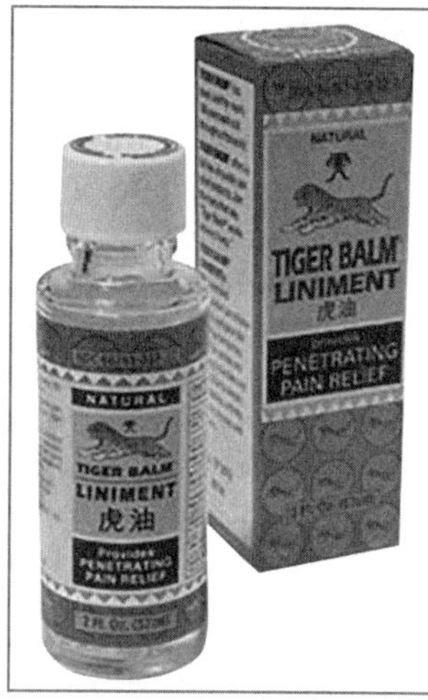

Fig. 2.3: Liniment.

4. Gels (Fig. 2.4): Transparent or translucent non-greasy rich in moisture, semisolid preparation meant for topical application. A gel rich in liquid is called as jelly.

5. Types of Suppositories:

- Rectal suppository
- Vaginal suppository
- Urethral suppository

Rectal suppositories (Fig. 2.5): are semisolid dosage forms intended for insertion into body orifices (rectum, vagina, urethra) where they melt, soften, or dissolve and exert a local or systemic effect.

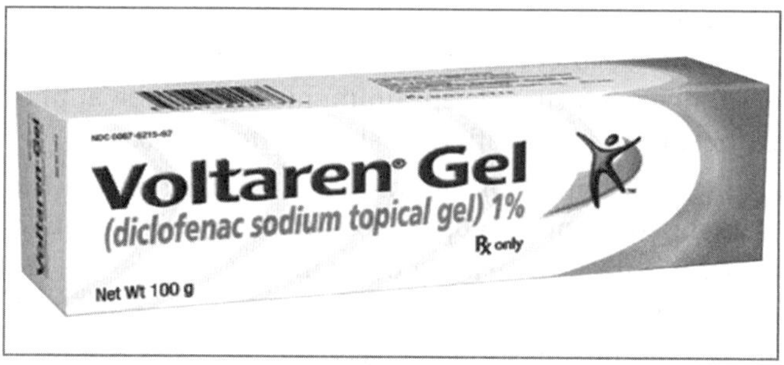

Fig. 2.4: Gels.

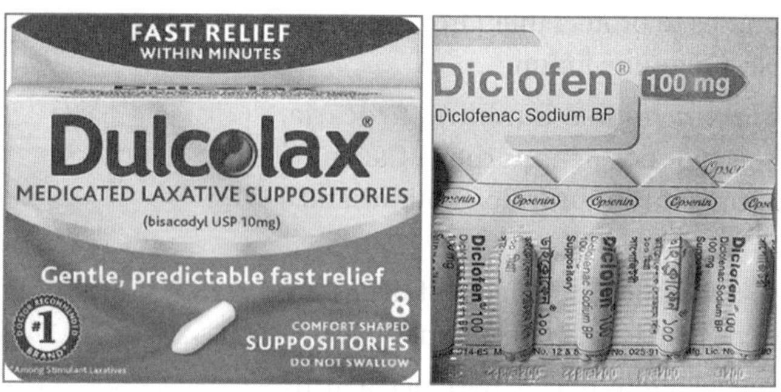

Fig. 2.5: Suppositories.

Advantages and disadvantages of rectal route:

Advantages

- ❖ Can be used in unconscious patient
- ❖ Useful in geriatric patients; patients with vomiting
- ❖ Can be used for those who are unable to swallow
- ❖ Gastric irritation is avoided.

Disadvantages:

- ❖ Absorption is incomplete.
- ❖ Irritation and inflammation of rectal mucosa may occur.
- ❖ Inconvenient and embarrassing for patient

Local action: Rectal suppositories relieve constipation.

For example, dulcolax (Bisacodyl), diclofenac suppositories relieve pain in hemorrhoids, and hydrocortisone suppositories for piles.

Systemic action: Diazepam suppositories in febrile convulsions in children, acetaminophen (Paracetamol) for fever, ergotamine + caffeine suppositories for migraine, morphine suppositories for pain.

6. Pessary (Fig. 2.6): Pessary is a vaginal suppository, similar to rectal suppository. It is ovoid shaped with a rounded apex. Vaginal inserts can be used as antifungal in vaginal candidiasis. *For example,* clotrimazole, miconazole, metronidazole for vaginal candidiasis.

7. Bougies/urethral inserts (Fig. 2.7): These are solid pencil-shaped body meant for urethral administration.

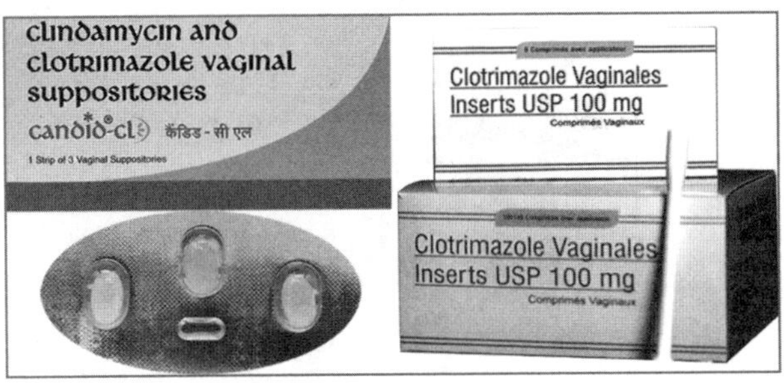

Fig. 2.6: Pessary.

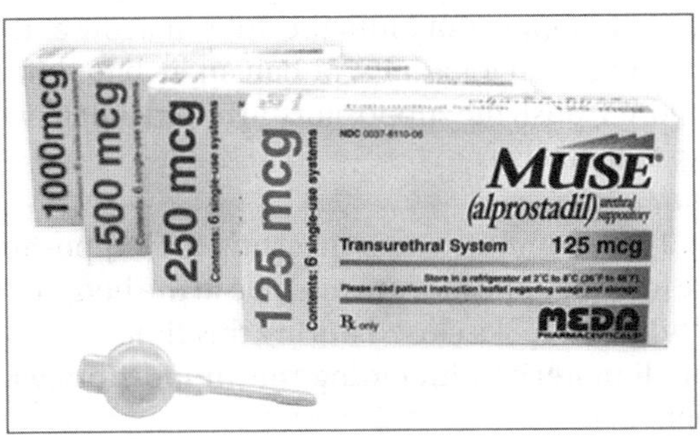

Fig. 2.7: Bougies.

How to insert a rectal suppository

Check the expiry date of the medication and that it is in good condition and not contaminated.

Anyone using a rectal suppository may want to refer to the following steps for guidance:

a. *Get prepared:*
   - The patient will be instructed to pass stool to empty the colon, as suppository medication is most effective when the bowel is empty.
   - He/she will be told to wash hands thoroughly with soap and warm water or use a hand sanitiser. Dry the hands thoroughly on a clean towel or paper towel.
   - The patient may use a disposable glove if desired.

b. *Get ready to insert the suppository:*
   - Dip the tip of the suppository in water, or apply a small amount of water-based lubricant, such as K-Y. A lubricant helps the suppository more easily slide into the rectum.
   - Remove clothing from the lower half of the body.
   - Find the correct position. Either stand up with one foot on a chair or lie down on one side with the top leg bent slightly toward the stomach.
   - Caregivers giving the suppository to another person often find it easier if the person is lying down.

c. *Insert the suppository:*

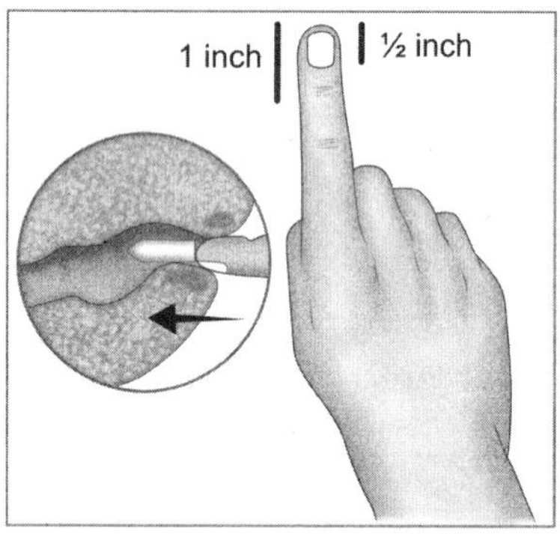

   - Relax the muscles of the buttocks and open the cheeks.
   - Gently insert the suppository into the anus, narrow end first.
   - Push it in about 1 inch for adults, or half an inch for infants.
   - In older children, push the suppository in approximately half to one inch, depending on their size.

d. *Relax and clean up:*
   - Sit or lie still for 10 minutes after inserting the suppository. Staying still allows time for the suppository to dissolve in the body. Parents may need to hold a child's buttocks closed during this time.
   - Dispose of all materials, including the suppository wrapper and any tissue paper.
   - Wash the hands thoroughly with soap and warm water.

- Try to avoid passing stool for up to 60 minutes after inserting the suppository, unless it is a laxative. Not passing stool gives the medication enough time to enter the bloodstream and start working.

How to insert a vaginal suppository

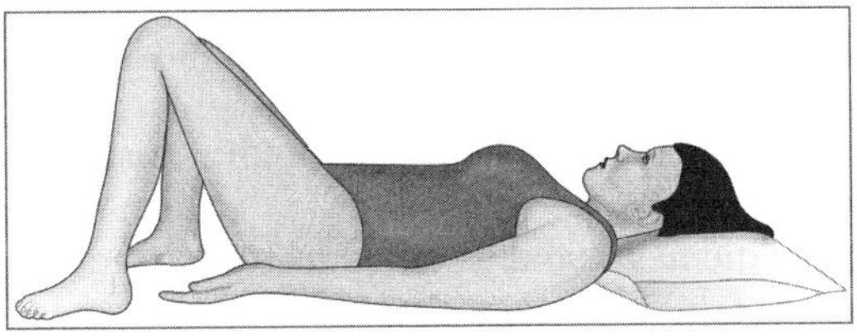

To place a suppository into the vagina, follow these tips:

a. *Get prepared:*
   - Wash hands with soap and warm water, or use a hand sanitizer if these are not available. Dry the hands well on a clean towel or paper towel.
   - Unwrap the suppository, and place it in the accompanying applicator.
   - Either stand with the knees bent and feet apart or lie down with the knees bent toward the chest.

b. *Insert the suppository:*

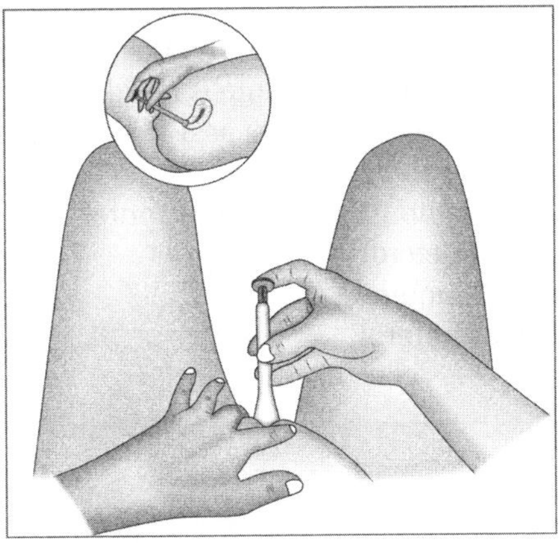

   - Place the applicator into the vagina, as far as possible, without causing discomfort.
   - Press down on the plunger to push in the suppository.
   - Remove the applicator from the vagina, and dispose of it.

c. *Relax and clean up:*
   - Lie down for 10 minutes to allow the medicine to enter the body.
   - Wash the hands once more with soap and warm water.

Informing and educating the patient regarding the use and storage:

❖ The following tips may help people who need to use suppositories:

❖ Avoid exercise or vigorous movement for 60 minutes after inserting the medication.

❖ Do not use petroleum jelly, such as vaseline, to lubricate the suppository. This stops it from melting. Only use water, or a water-based lubricant.

- Store suppositories in the refrigerator or another cool place, so they do not melt. Always follow the storage directions on the label.
- Trim fingernails before inserting suppositories. This prevents cuts and scrapes. Alternatively, wear a latex glove.
- Some people may notice the suppository falls out. This can occur because they have not pushed it far enough into the rectum. Push the medication in about 1 inch.
- Those who struggle to use suppositories should consider asking a partner or caregiver for help.
- As with other medicines, avoid missing doses. Missed doses may reduce the effectiveness of the treatment.

8. Inhalation delivery systems: Inhalation dosage forms **(Fig. 2.8)** contain drug particles or solutions administered by the respiratory route for local or systemic effect. Aerosols are formed as drug solution or micro-ionized drug powder is converted into mist/dust respectively. Particle size in the range of 3 to 5 μm will reach in central and small airways.

- Identify the parts of an inhaler (As shown in the figure)
- How to use it? and what instructions will you give the patient?
  (See procedure for correct use for MDI)
- What is the mechanism/rationale of this instrument/route?
  - MDI delivers a specific amount of medication directly to the lungs. Advantages of using inhalation route is rapid onset, avoiding first pass metabolism, lesser adverse effects as a lower dose is given and dose titration as per need can be done.
- What are the drugs commonly given by this route?
  - Fluticasone and salmeterol
  - Budesonide and formoterol
  - Fluticasone and formoterol
  - Salbutamol

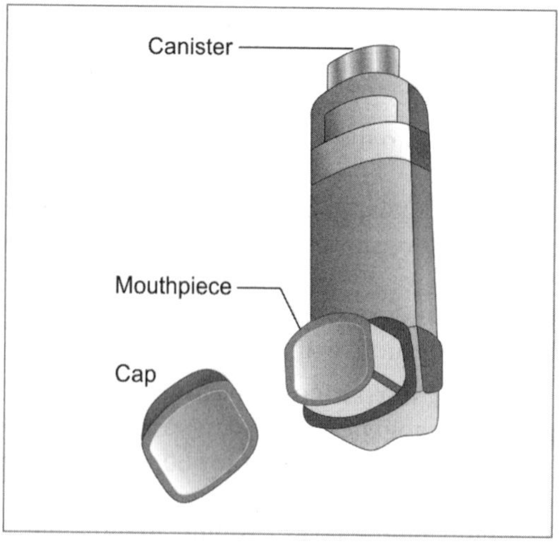

Fig. 2.8: Inhaler.

Metered dose inhaler (MDI): It is a device used to deliver a specific amount of medication to the lungs. A metered dose inhaler has a pressurized container of medication that fits into a mouthpiece. The standard metered dose inhaler (MDI) on activating releases a fixed dose of medicine in aerosol form.

Procedure for correct use (For MDI)

i. Cough up as much sputum as possible
ii. Shake the inhaler before use
iii. Hold the inhaler as indicated in the manufacturer's instructions (this is held usually upside down)
iv. Fully exhale
v. Place the lips tightly around the mouthpiece
vi. Tilt the head backwards slightly
vii. Breathe out slowly, emptying the lungs
viii. Breathe in deeply and activate the inhaler (press the metallic bottle), keeping the tongue down. The coordination between activating the inhaler and breathing in is critical for effective delivery of the drug into the lungs
ix. The aerosolized drug is drawn into the lungs by continuing to inhale deeply before holding the breath for 10 seconds to allow absorption into the bronchial walls.
x. Hold your breath for ten to fifteen seconds
xi. Breathe out through the nose
xii. Rinse the mouth with warm water

Spacer: Use of MDI requires proper hand breath coordination. The patient has to first breathe in slowly through the mouth. At the same time, when he presses the canister, to release the drug he has to continue to breathe in slowly and steadily. This is difficult for the elderly and children. Spacer overcomes this problem. The drug comes into the spacer so the velocity of the aerosolized drug slows down, and the patient can breathe from the spacer on its own accord. The need for hand-to-breathe coordination is reduced **(Fig. 2.9)**.

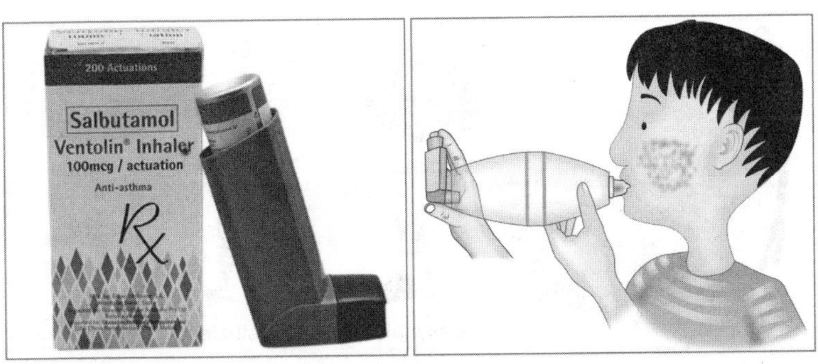

Fig. 2.9: Salbutamol inhaler.

Rotahaler

Procedure of the rotahaler

i. Check the mouthpiece for foreign objects
ii. Twist the barrel in either direction until it stops
iii. Take a capsule (designed for a rotahaler) and insert the clear (thinner/white) end into the raised hole of the rotahaler. Push this new capsule in until it is level with the top of the hole
iv. Hold the rotahaler vertically, and turn the lower end as far as it will go in the opposite direction. This will open the capsule
v. Cough up as much sputum as possible and gently breathe out
vi. Place the lips tightly around the mouthpiece
vii. Tilt the head backwards slightly
viii. Breathe in through your mouth as quickly and deeply as possible. Continue to take a full, deep breath
ix. Hold your breath for up to ten seconds. This allows the medication time to deposit in the airway
x. Breathe out through the nose then resume normal breathing
xi. After each use, pull the two halves of the rotahaler apart and throw away the loose capsule shell
xii. Reassemble the rotahaler

Repeat steps 1–7 when more than one rotacap is prescribed.

Care of the rotahaler
Clean the rotahaler **(Fig. 2.10)** once every two weeks or sooner if needed. Regular cleaning will prevent powder accumulation inside the rotahaler. Remove the empty capsule shell before washing the rotahaler. Rinse the two halves of your rotahaler in warm water. Shake off any excess water.

Nebulizer: A device which converts drug solution into an aerosol for direct inhalation via a mask or mouthpiece. The droplets which are sufficiently fine and uniform in size reach the bronchioles.

9. Otic solution (Ear drops): This is an aqueous or a viscous solution meant to be administered to the external ear and dispensed in a dropper bottle.

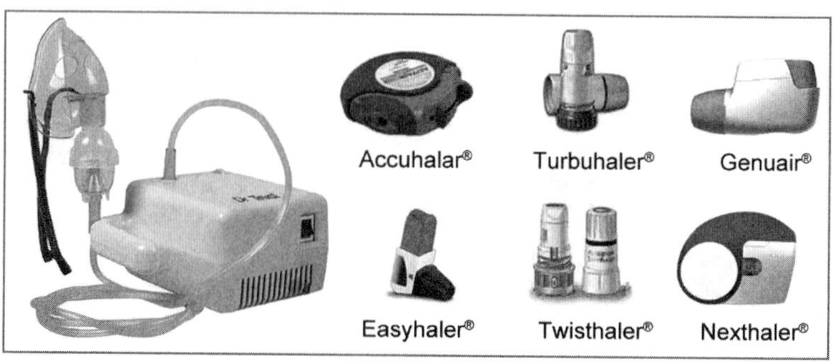

Fig. 2.10: Rotahaler.

Generally analgesics, antimicrobials and anti-inflammatory agents are administered as ear drops.

Procedure

i. Lie on one side with the ear upward
ii. Gently pull the lobe to expose the ear canal
iii. Instill the amount (usually 4–5) of drops
iv. Wait for five minutes before turning to the other ear
v. Use cotton wool to close the ear canal after applying the drops only if the manufacturer explicitly recommends this
vi. Ear drops should not burn or sting longer than a few minutes

Ophthalmic solutions (Eye drops): These are sterile solutions that may contain one or more active pharmaceutical ingredients intended for application to the conjunctiva, the conjunctival sac or the eyelids.

Procedure

i. Wash your hands
ii. Do not touch the dropper opening
iii. Ask the patient to look upward
iv. Pull the lower eyelid down to make a 'gutter' or pouch
v. Bring the dropper as close to the 'gutter' as possible without touching it or the eye
vi. Instill the prescribed number of drops (usually 1 or 2) in the 'gutter'
vii. Close the eye for about two minutes. Do not shut the eye too tight
viii. Excess fluid can be removed with a tissue. Do not rub
ix. If more than one kind of eye drop is used, wait at least five minutes before instilling the next drops. Eye drops may cause a burning feeling but this should not last for more than a few minutes. If it does last longer, consult a doctor or pharmacist.

When giving eye drops to children

- Let the child lie back in head lowered position
- Eyes should be closed.
- Gently retract lower eyelid and instil the drug into the corner of conjunctival sac
- Keep the head straight
- Remove the excess fluid

10. **Oral drops:** These are liquid preparations for oral use that are intended to be administered in small volumes with the aid of a suitable measuring device **(Fig. 2.11)**.
11. **Dusting powder:** These are locally applied non-toxic preparations that are intended to have no

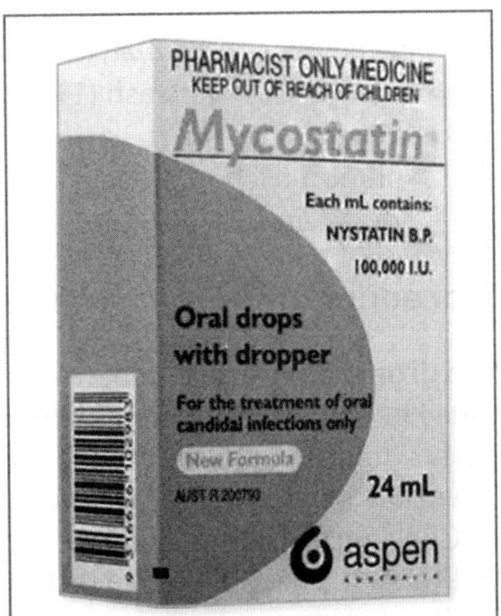

Fig. 2.11: Oral drops.

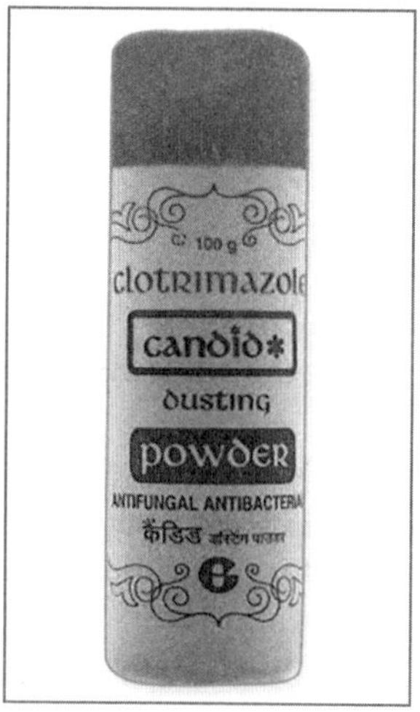

Fig. 2.12: Clotrimazole powder.

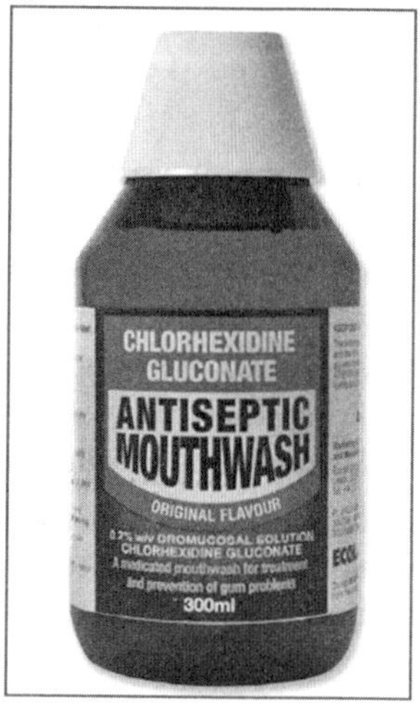

Fig. 2.13: Mouthwash.

systemic action. They are dispensed in a very fine state to enhance effectiveness and minimize irritation. *For example,* Neomycin, clotrimazole **(Fig. 2.12)**.

12. **Mouthwash:** It is an aqueous solution which is most often used for its deodorant, cleansing and antiseptic effect. Mouthwashes are also used for the relief of pain from ulcerative lesions of the mouth and for the treatment of oropharyngeal infections. *For example,* chlorhexidine antiseptic mouthwash **(Fig. 2.13)**.

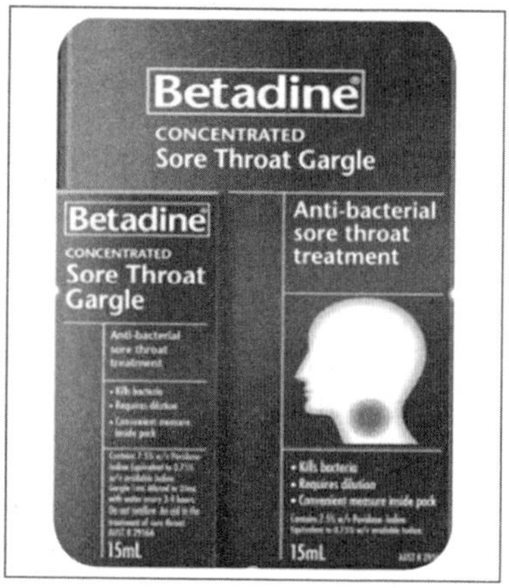

Fig. 2.14: Betadine gargle.

13. **Mouth gargle:** It is an aqueous solution used to prevent or treat throat infections. *For example,* saline gargle for sore throat **(Fig. 2.14)**.

Procedure for Administration

Eye drops: They are aqueous or oily solutions for instilling into conjunctival sac. They are used as anaesthetics, anti-infective or anti-inflammatory agents, miotics, mydriatics and artificial tears. For example, atropine sulfate (mydriatics), pilocarpine nitrate (miotic), timolol maleate.

1. Checking for expiry date and correct drug.
2. Proper instructions given to the patients on the correct method of using the dosage form:
   - Wash your hands

- Do not touch the dropper opening
- Look upward
- Pull the lower eyelid down to make a 'gutter' or pouch
- Bring the dropper as close to the 'gutter' as possible without touching it or the eye
- Instill the prescribed number of drops (usually 1 or 2) in the 'gutter'
- Close the eye for about two minutes. Do not shut the eye too tight
- Excess fluid can be removed with a tissue. Do not rub

3. Proper caution regarding methods/side effects given to the patients.
   - If more than one kind of eye drop is used, wait at least five minutes before instilling the next drops. Eye drops may cause a burning feeling but this should not last for more than a few minutes. If it does last longer, consult a doctor or pharmacist.
   - Discard eye drops 4 weeks after opening bottle.
4. Attitude (tone of voice, gesture, audibility) while giving instructions.

Administration of eye drops to children:

- ❖ Let the child lie down in head lowered position
- ❖ Gently pull down the lower eyelid to form a pocket into which the eye drop is instil
- ❖ Hold for 30 sec

Eye ointment (Oculentum): They are semisolid preparations with a greasy base, to be applied in the eye, e.g., neomycin eye ointment, chloramphenicol eye ointment, tetracycline eye ointment.

Procedure

i. Wash your hands
ii. Do not touch anything with the tip of the tube
iii. Tilt the head backwards a little
iv. Take the tube in one hand and pull down the lower eyelid with the other hand, to make a 'gutter'
v. Bring the tip of the tube as close to the "gutter" as possible
vi. Apply the amount (usually 1 cm length) of ointment
vii. Close the eye for two minutes
viii. Remove excess ointment with a tissue
ix. Clean the tip of the tube with other tissue

Ear drops: They are aqueous or oily solutions instilled in the ear, e.g., wax softeners, sodium bicarbonate.

Procedure

i. Lie on one side with the ear upward.
ii. Gently pull the lobe to expose the ear canal.
iii. Instil the amount (usually 4-5) of drops.
iv. Wait for five minutes before turning to the other ear.
v. Use cotton wool to close the ear canal after applying the drops only if the manufacturer explicitly recommends this.
vi. Ear drops should not burn or sting longer than a few minutes.

Nasal drops: They are aqueous solutions of drugs instilled into the nose with a dropper, e.g., xylometazoline, ephedrine, etc.

Procedure

i. Blow the nose
ii. Sit down and tilt head backward strongly or lie down with a pillow under the shoulders; keep head straight
iii. Insert the dropper one centimeter into the nostril
iv. Instill the number of drops prescribed (usually 3–4 drops)
v. Sit up after a few seconds, the drops will then drip into the pharynx
vi. Repeat the producer for the other nostril, if necessary
vii. Rinse the dropper with boiled water

Nasal sprays: These are drugs or combinations of drugs which by virtue of their high vapor pressure, can be carried by an air current into nasal passage and exert their effect.

For example, beclomethasone, calcitonin, vasopressin, etc.

Procedure

i. Blow the nose
ii. Sit with the head slightly tilted forward
iii. Shake the spray. Insert the tip in one nostril
iv. Close the other nostril and mouth
v. Spray by squeezing the vial (flask, container) and sniff slowly
vi. Remove the tip form the nose and bend the head forward strongly (head between the knees)
vii. Sit up after a few seconds; the spray will drip down the pharynx
viii. Breath through the mouth
ix. Repeat the procedure for the other nostril, if necessary
x. Rinse the tip with boiled water

Suppositories: A suppository is a drug delivery system that is inserted either into the rectum (rectal suppository), vagina (vaginal suppository) or urethra (urethral suppository) where it dissolves. They are used to deliver both systemically acting and locally acting medications. They are solid, uniformly medicated masses of medicaments, e.g., glycerine, bisacodyl.

Transdermal patch

The term topical medication generally refers to medications applied to the skin that move through passive diffusion into the skin itself, creating a local effect.

Transdermal medications **(Fig. 2.15)** are applied to the skin, cross the skin barrier, drug enter the systemic circulation and exert effects in areas other than the site of application. Though applied topically on the skin effects are seen in the system.

Site: Adhesive patch applied to chest, upper abdomen or mastoid region **(Fig. 2.16)**.

Advantages

- Slow but sustained release of the drug for several days
- Duration of action is prolonged

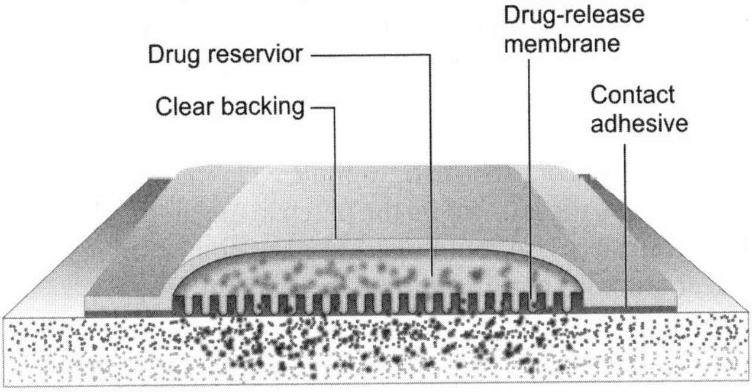

Fig. 2.15: Parts of the transdermal patch.

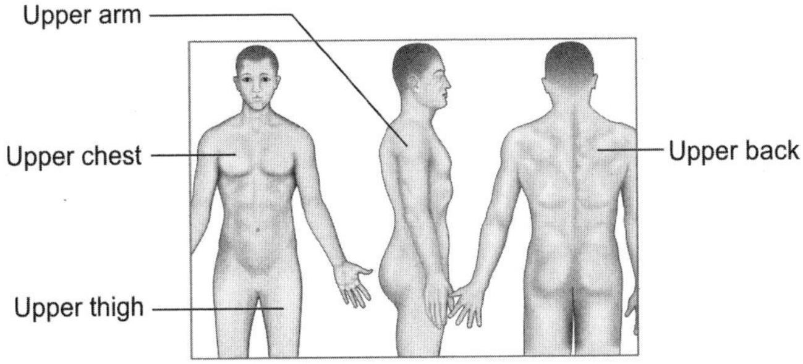

Fig. 2.16: Sites of application.

- Bypasses first pass metabolism
- Systemic side effects are reduced

Disadvantages

- Nil; if irritation occurs, the site of application can be changed.
- Expensive
- Only lipid soluble drugs can be given by this route
  For example, Nitroglycerine (NTG)—angina
  - Scopolamine (Hyoscine—motion sickness)
  - Nicotine—smoking cessation
  - Estrogen—Hormone replacement therapy
  - Fentanyl—cancer pain.

Method of use of transdermal patch:

- Read all instructions that come with your patch. The instructions will tell you where to place the patch, how long to wear it, and when to remove and replace it.
- Wash your hands with soap and water. If water is not available, you can use hand sanitizer instead.
- Decide where you will place the new patch. Your doctor's instructions and the drug's label or package insert should give information on where to put it. When placing a patch, choose a spot where the patch will attach well. Avoid skin that—has open cuts or sores, is sweaty, and has lots of hair.

- Prepare and clean the skin to remove any dirt, lotions, oils, or powders.
- Take the patch out of the packaging. Remove the protective liner on the patch as directed by the patch instructions. Be careful not to touch the sticky side of the patch.
- Place the patch, sticky side down, onto the clean area of skin. Using the palm of your hand, press down on the patch to make sure the patch is firmly attached to your skin. Use your fingers to press along the edges of the patch. The patch should be smooth, with no bumps or folds.

3 CHAPTER

Parenteral Dosage Forms

- Ampules
- Vials
- Pouches

DIFFERENCE BETWEEN AMPULES AND VIALS

Table 3.1 depicts the difference between ampoules and vials.

Table 3.1: Ampules and vials.

Ampules	*Vials*
It is a sealed vial that contains drug solution	It is a small cylindrical container made of glass typically for holding liquid medications
Thin-walled glass containers sealed by fusion of glass after filling	Thick-walled glass containers sealed after filling by a stopper made up of cork
Odd shaped	Flat shaped
Ampules cannot be reused	They can be sterilized and used again
Temporary storage vehicle	Content can be stored for a longer period
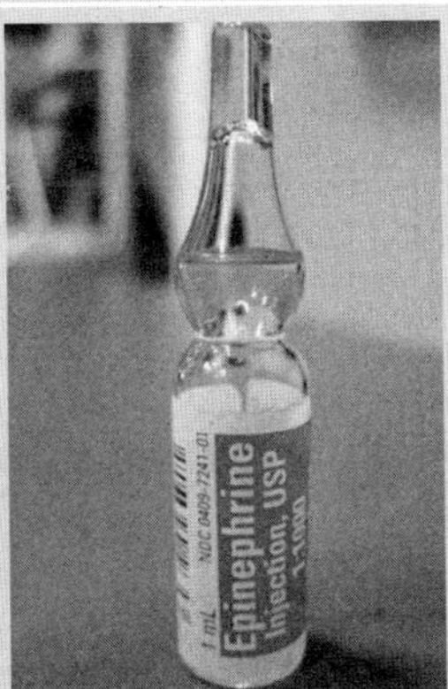	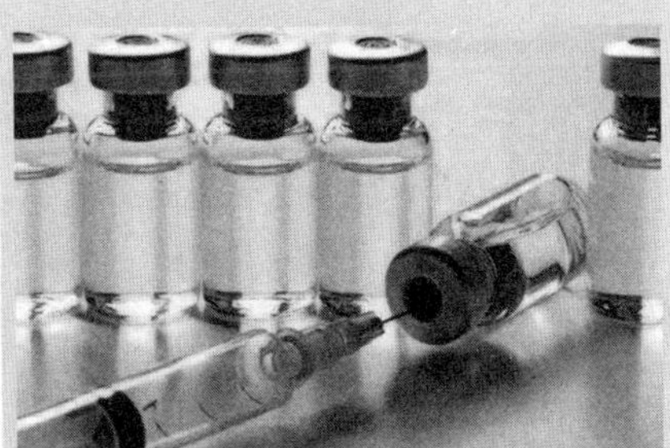

Technique of aspirating drug from ampule into syringe:

1. Wash your hands properly with soap and water.
2. Take out syringe and needle from disposable pack taking care not to touch naked end of syringe.
3. Put the needle on the syringe.
4. Remove the liquid from the neck of the ampule by flicking or tapping it or swinging it fast in a downward-spiralling movement.
5. File around the neck of the ampule.
6. Carefully break off the top of the ampule. Protect your fingers with gauze if ampule is made of glass **(Fig. 3.1).**
7. For a plastic ampule twist the top.
8. Remove cover from needle.
9. Aspirate the fluid from the ampule.
10. Remove any air from the syringe.
11. Clean up, dispose of working needle safely and wash your hands.

Technique of aspirating drug from vial into syringe:

1. Wash your hands properly with soap and water.
2. Take out syringe and needle from disposable pack taking care not to touch naked end of syringe. Use a syringe with at least twice the required amount of drug or solution.
3. Put the needle on the syringe.
4. Remove protective covering from vial cap. Disinfect the top of the vial with a cotton swab soaked in disinfectant
5. Remove cover from needle.
6. Suck up as much air as the amount of solution needed to aspirate.
7. Insert needle into vial through rubber cap and push down and then mix.
8. Pump air into vial (creating pressure).
9. Aspirate the required amount of solution and 0.1 mL extra. Make sure the tip of the needle is below the fluid surface
10. Pull the needle out of the vial.
11. Remove the air from the syringe **(Fig. 3.2)**
12. Clean up, dispose of waste safely and wash your hands.

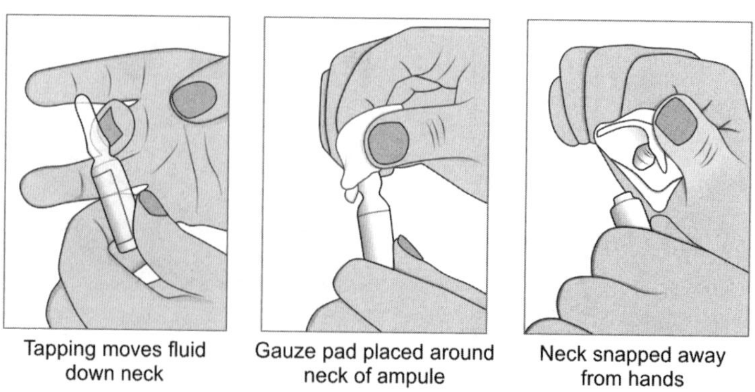

Fig. 3.1: Technique of aspirating drug from vial into syringe.

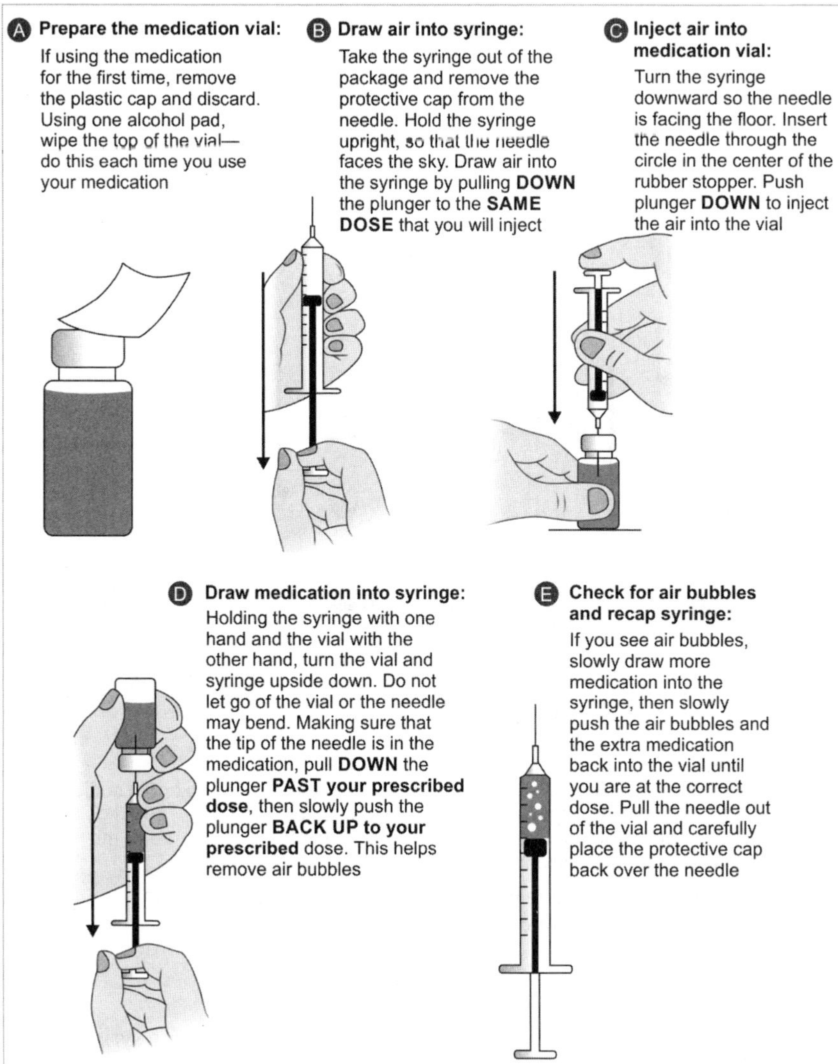

Fig. 3.2: Technique of aspirating drug from vial into syringe.

Technique to dissolve the dry medicine in vial and aspirate drug solution into syringe:

1. Wash your hands properly with soap and water.
2. Take out syringe and needle from disposable pack taking care not to touch naked end of syringe.
3. Put the needle on the syringe.
4. Aspirate solvent into syringe from the ampule.
5. Remove protective covering from cap of vial. Disinfect the rubber cap (top) of the vial containing the dry/powdered medicine.
6. Insert the needle into the vial, hold the whole unit upright.

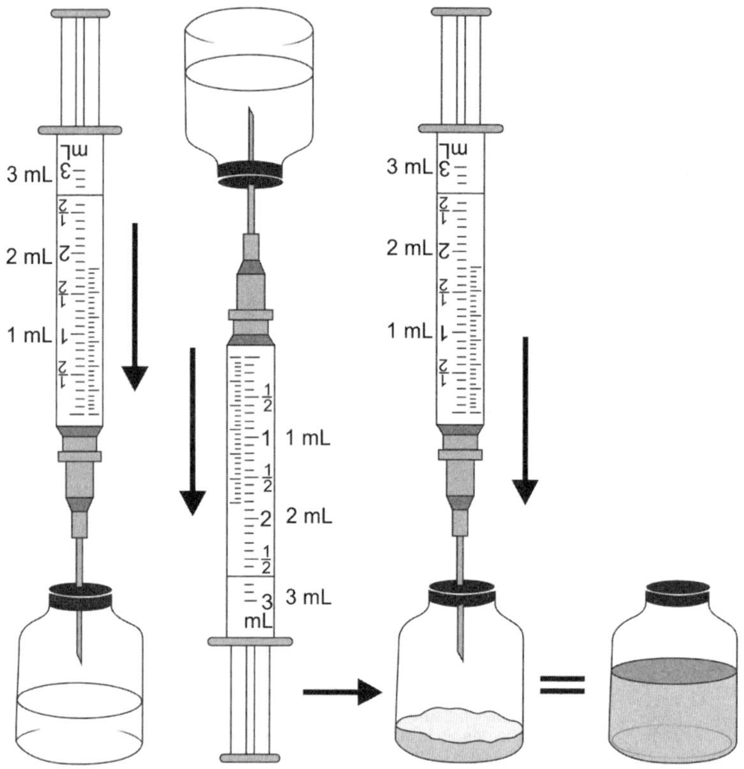

Fig. 3.3: Technique to dissolve the dry medicine in vial and aspirate drug solution into syringe.

7. Suck up as much air as the amount of solvent already in the syringe.
8. Inject only the fluid into the vial, not the air **(Fig. 3.3)**.
9. Shake well.
10. Turn the vial upside-down.
11. Inject the air into the vial (creating the pressure).
12. Aspirate the total amount of solution.
13. Remove any air from the syringe.
14. Clean up, dispose of waste safely and wash hands.

It is recommended that all antibiotics that are reconstituted and are to be used later should be labeled in the following way (*see* example): (1) Hour and date reconstituted. (2) Strength of reconstituted antibiotic. (3) Initials of the preparer.

TYPES OF SYRINGES (FIGURES 3.4 TO 3.7)

Syringes are used to administer parenteral medications. A syringe consists of a plunger, a barrel, and a needle hub. Syringes are made of glass or plastic material. Glass syringes can be reused after sterilization but currently not used.

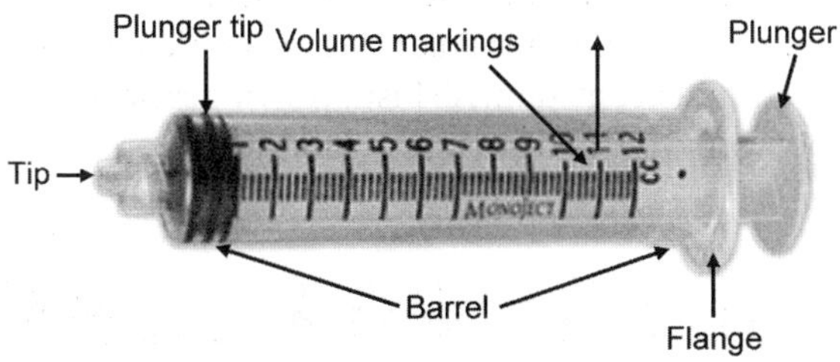

Fig. 3.4: Hypodermic syringe (Hypo: under, Dermic: skin).

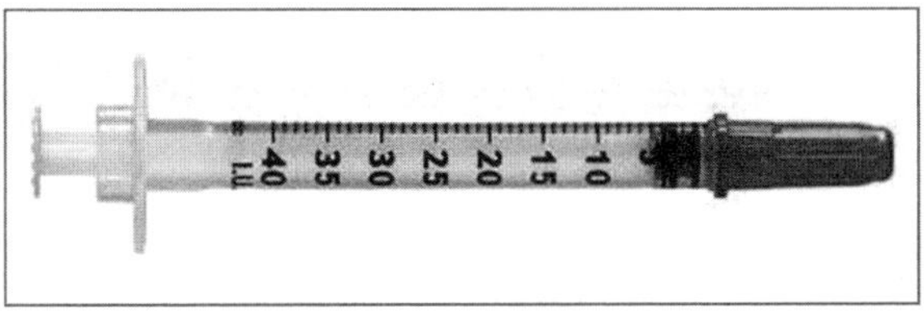

Fig. 3.5: Insulin syringe.

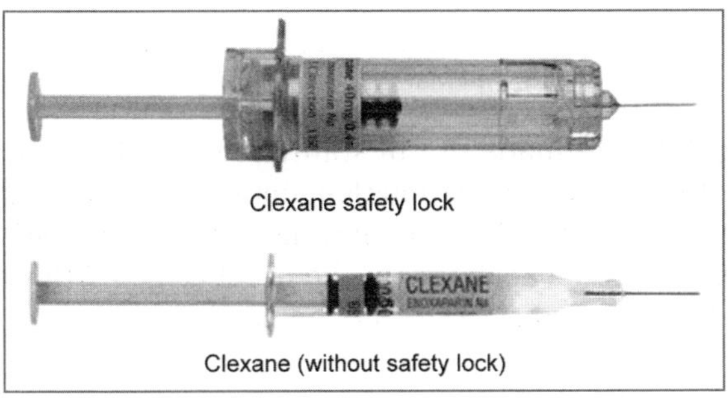

Fig. 3.6: Prefilled syringe.

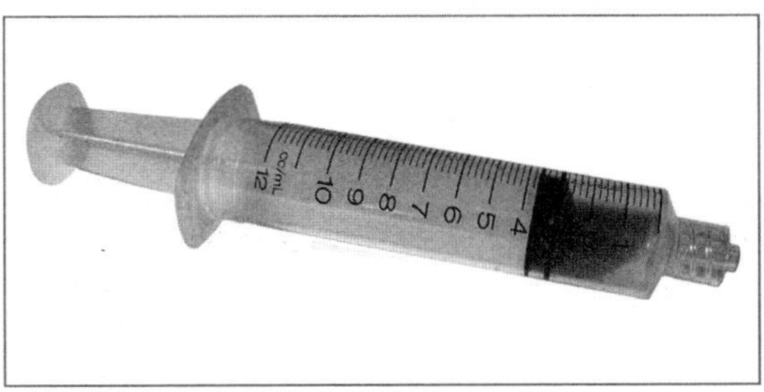

Fig. 3.7: Luer lock syringe.

Disposable syringes are made of plastic, and are used with disposable needles and used for single use.

Luer lock syringes have threads in the needle hub that provide a secure connection of needles, tubing, or other devices.

Insulin is administered using a specific insulin syringe. Insulin syringes are marked in units **(Fig. 3.8)**, not milliliters (mL), because insulin is prescribed by providers in units, not mLs. A regular syringe marked in milliliters should never be used to administer insulin. All insulin syringes have red caps for quick identification, but verify the markings are in units to prevent a medication error.

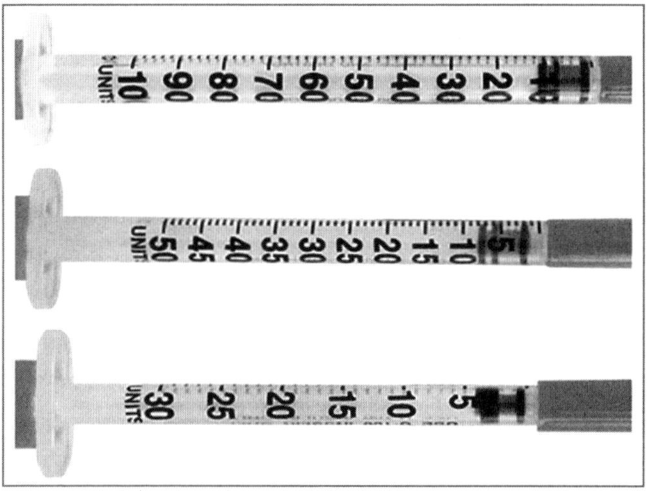

Fig. 3.8: Markings on a syringe.

Needles **(Fig. 3.9)** are made out of stainless steel. They are sterile and disposable and are available in various lengths and sizes. A needle is made up of the hub, shaft, and bevel. The hub fits onto the tip of the syringe. All three parts must remain sterile at all times. The bevel **(Fig. 3.10)** is the tip of the needle that is slanted to create a slit into the skin.

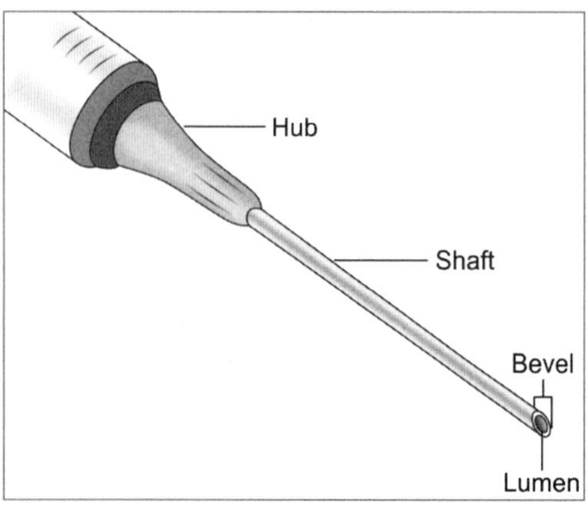

Fig. 3.9: Parts of a needle.

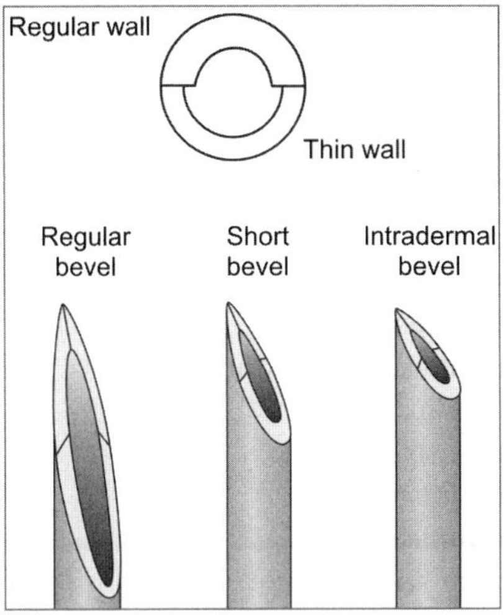

Fig. 3.10: Bevel.

Regular/long bevel is meant for subcutaneous, intramuscular and short bevel is for Intravenous.

GAUGE AND LENGTH

The gauge of a needle refers to its diameter. Needles range in various sized gauges from small diameter (25 to 29 gauge) to large diameter (18 to 22 gauge). Note that the larger the diameter of a needle, the smaller the gauge number. Larger diameter needles (18 to 22 gauge) are typically used to administer thicker medications or blood products.

21-gauge needle (green color) is the largest commonly used needle for Intramuscular injection.

Needle Length (Fig. 3.11)

Needle length can range from 3/8" to 3-1/2". A 3/8" to 3/4" needle is recommended for intradermal injection where needles between 7/8" to 1-1/2" are designed for intramuscular injections. 1/2" to 5/8" needles are made for

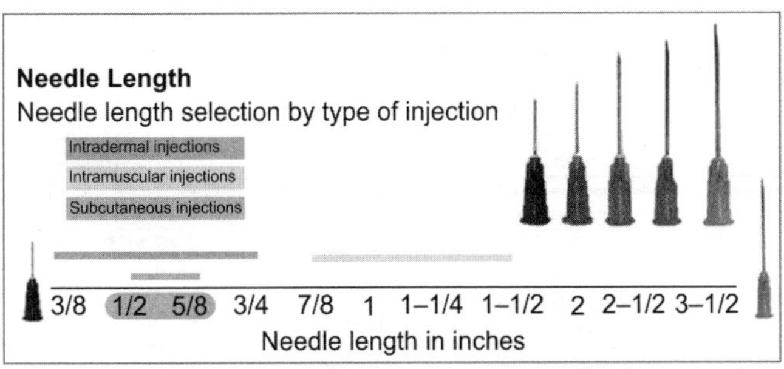

Fig. 3.11: Summarized injection information.

subcutaneous injections and may be overlapped for use with intradermal injections as well.

PARENTERAL ROUTES (FIG. 3.12)

1. Intravenous administration
2. Intramuscular injection
3. Intraperitoneal administration
4. Intrathecal (intraspinal) administration
5. Intramedullary administration
6. Intra-arterial administration
7. Intra-articular administration
8. Subcutaneous administration
9. Intradermal (intracutaneous route)
10. Epidural injection
11. Intracardiac injection

Advantages and Disadvantages of IM Route (Fig. 3.13)

Advantages

- Vascularity of muscle is good, so absorption of drug is rapid than by SC route
- The absorption is reliable, predictable
- Mild irritant drugs can be given
- Depot preparations can be used

Disadvantages

- Aseptic precaution is required
- Painful

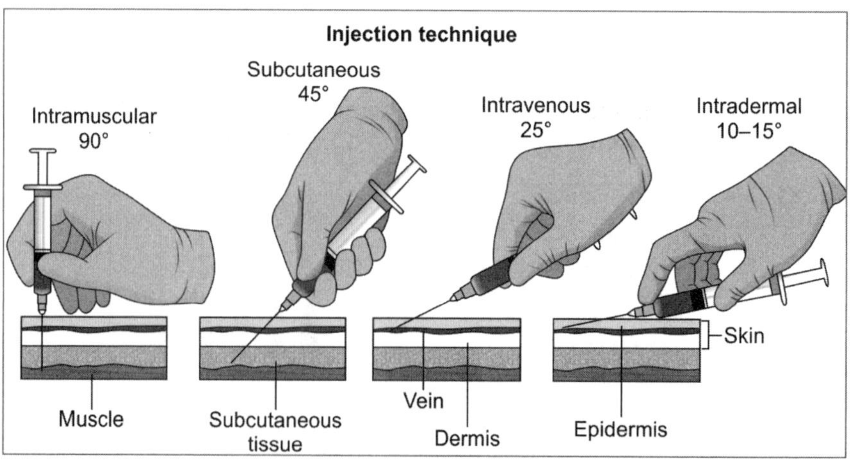

Fig. 3.12: Angles for administration of injections.

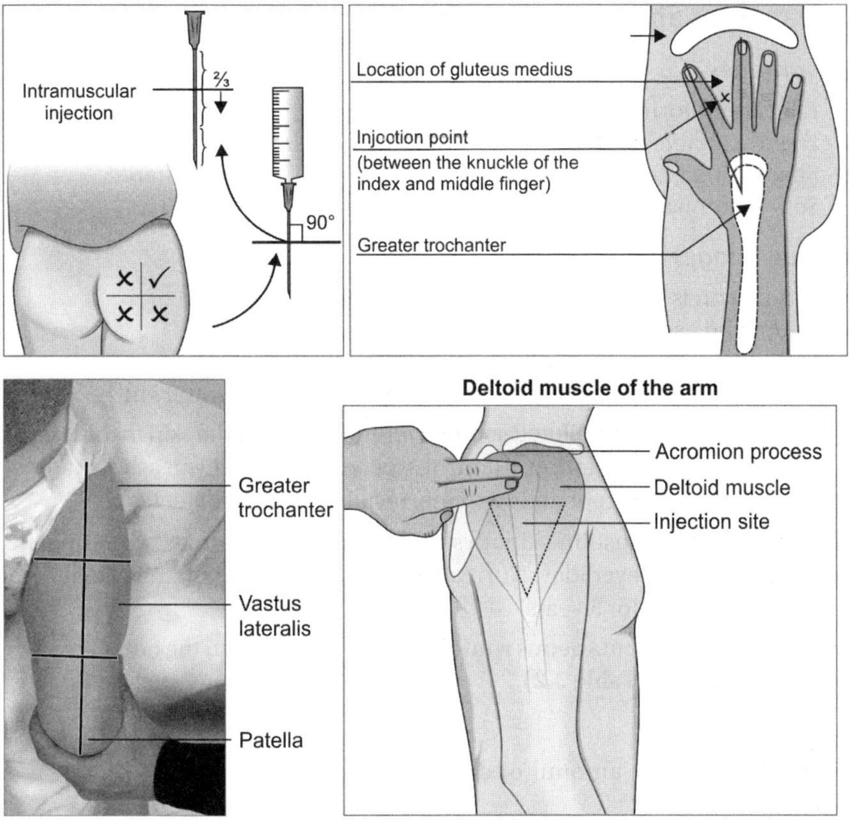

Fig. 3.13: Intramuscular route of administration.

- Chances of nerve damage and paralysis, if injected into nerve
- Large volume cannot be given (maximum of 5–10 mL)

For example, various antibiotics, antiemetics, diclofenac 70 mg deep IM for pain, adrenaline (0.5 mg or 0.5 mL 1:1000 solution), iron dextran (Z track technique), amikacin 10–15 mg/kg IM daily for MDR TB

Vaccines: Hepatitis B, tetanus toxoid, DPT, gamma globulin, antirabies serum, Covid vaccine (Covishield).

Depot formulation:

- Inj benzathine penicillin G 2.4 mu/monthly in rheumatic heart disease
- Inj haloperidol decanoate (every 2–4 weeks) and Inj penfluridol decanoate (once in week) for prolonged treatment and improved patient compliance in schizophrenia.
- Depot medroxyprogesterone acetate (DMPA) 150 mg 3 monthly interval.

Note: Drugs not used by IM route—heparin (Hematoma), benzodiazepines because of erratic absorption.

Advantages and Disadvantages of SC Route

Advantages

- Effect is uniform and sustained
- Highly suitable for depot preparations and implants
- Suspensions, colloids and oily preparations can be administered
- Self- administration is possible

Disadvantages

- Absorption is slow and so is the onset of action
- Cannot be used for emergency situation
- Only non-irritant drugs can be given
- Only small volume of drug can be administered (maximum 1ml)

For example, lignocaine diluted solution infiltrated under the skin in the area of minor operations (incision, excision, hydrocoele), vaccines (measles, mumps, rubella), Japanese encephalitis vaccine, insulin (given in diabetes).

Note: Side effect of insulin—lipodystrophy can be minimized by rotating the site of SC injection everyday. Norplant 6 capsules (each containing 36 mg) of levonorgestrel acts for 5 years,

Intradermal (intracutaneous route): Drug is injected into the outer layers of skin raising a bleb **(Table 3.2)**.

Advantages

- Since very small amount of drug produces the effect it is used for the sensitivity test.
- Useful for the administration of vaccines.

Disadvantages

- Absorption is slow
- Very small amount (0.5 mL) can be administered.

For example, diagnostic tests, allergy testing, vaccines, such as BCG, measles.

Intravenous Injections (IV) (Fig 3.14)

An intravenous infusion is a liquid administered directly into the bloodstream via a vein. Drug is given in one of the superficial veins.

Drug is either given as (Table 3.3):

1. Bolus IV injection, e.g., adenosine in PSVT (immediate action is required), furosemide in acute pulmonary edema.
2. Slow IV injections over 5–10 minutes, e.g., calcium gluconate (to avoid toxicity of calcium on heart).
3. Slow IV infusion, e.g., oxytocin in induction of labour (slow and sustained action is required) this is done by dissolving drug in 50–100 mL of isotonic glucose or saline.
4. Rapid IV infusion is sometimes used, e.g., fluids in shock. Drug is usually in aqueous form. It should be non-irritant to vascular endothelium.

Table 3.2: Difference between types of injections.

Injection types	*Locations*	*Needle gauge and length*	*Total amount of injectable fluid*	*Degree of angle when injecting*	*Considerations*
Intradermal 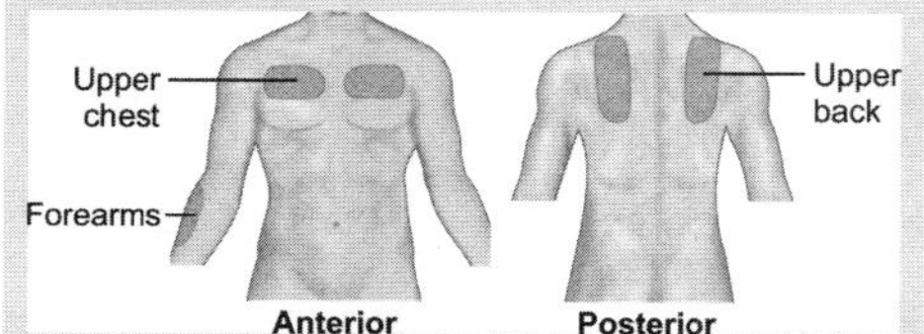 	• Upper third of the forearm 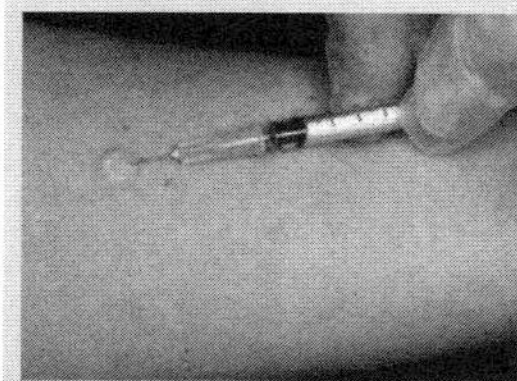 • Outer aspects upper arms • Between scapula	• 25–27G • 3/8″ to 5/8″	0.1 mL	5–15 degrees	Forearm: Tuberculosis (TB) testing Allergy testing. Local anesthesia BCG vaccine
Subcutaneous 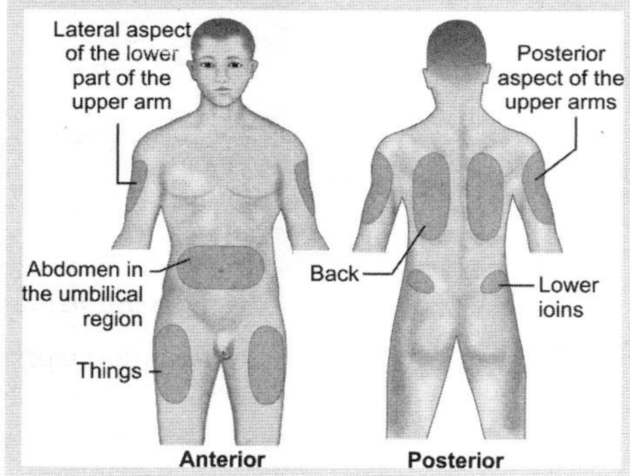 	• Outer upper arms • Anterior thighs • Upper outer gluteal Area • Upper back • Abdomen	• 25–31G • 1/2″ to 5/8″	Up to 1 mL Up to 0.5 mL in infants and small children	45–90 degrees	The older patient's skin is less elastic, and subcutaneous tissue may be reduced in the skinfolds. The upper abdomen should be used for patients with less subcutaneous tissue

Contd...

Contd...

Injection types	*Locations*	*Needle gauge and length*	*Total amount of injectable fluid*	*Degree of angle when injecting*	*Considerations*
Intramuscular 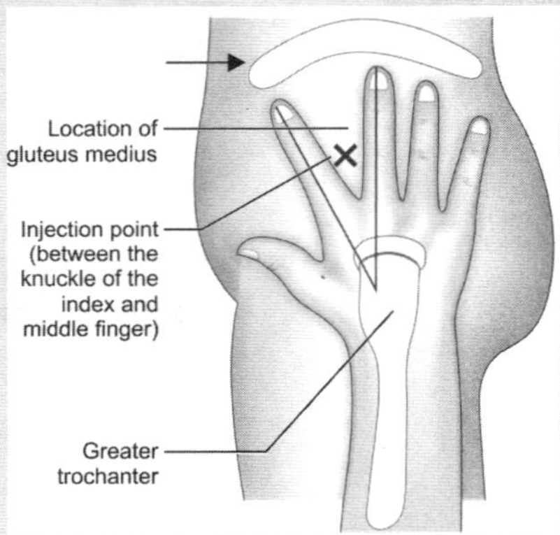 	**Ventrogluteal** • Vastus lateralis • Deltoid	• 18 to 25G • 1/2″ to 1 1/2″ (based on age/size of patient and site used)	0.5–1 mL (infants and children) 2–5 mL (adults)	90 degrees	The vastus lateralis site is preferred for infants because that muscle is most developed. The ventrogluteal site is recommended

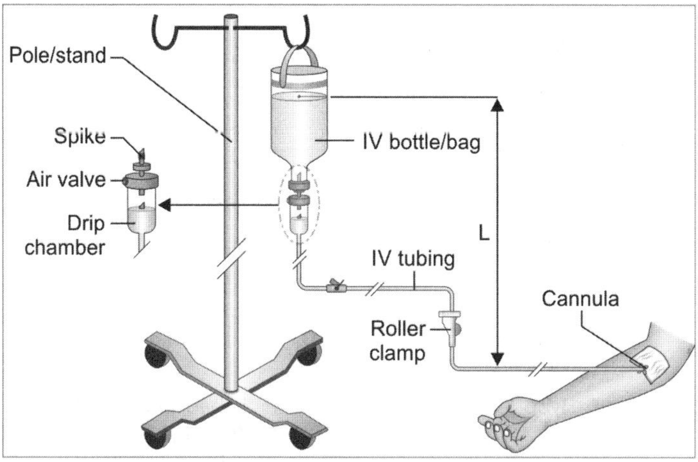

Fig. 3.14: Intravenous route of administration.

Table 3.3: Difference between IV bolus and IV infusion.

Features	***IV bolus***	***IV infusion***
Definition	When a sterile, single, discrete amount dose of drug product, medication, or solution is administered all at once over a short period of time generally within a short time 1–30 minutes by using a hypodermic needle and a syringe is called IV bolus	When a sterile, large volume of drug product, medication, or solution is administered through a vein into the blood slowly and continuously at a constant or zero-order rate over a long period of time generally more than 30 minutes to several hours is called IV infusion
Administration time	Within 1–30 minutes	More than 30 minutes to several hours
Administration rate	Inconstant rate and express by mg/min	Constant rate and express by mg/hr
Fashion of administration	Rapid	Slow and continuous
Onset of action	Rapid	Slow
Duration of action	Short	Prolonged
Purpose of use	For an emergency and to achieve the desired plasma level rapidly	For continuous and prolonged plasma drug concentration and control of plasma drug levels more precisely
Volume	Small	Large
Control of drug delivery	No precise control	Precise control

Contd...

Contd...

Features	***IV bolus***	***IV infusion***
Adverse effect	Chance of anaphylaxis or adverse effect is more	Chance of anaphylaxis or adverse effect is less
Discomfort	Less	More
Precaution	More precaution	Less precaution
Operation	Easier	Less easier than IV bolus
Types of IV bolus vs IV infusion	A. Intermittent IV infusion and B. Continuous IV infusion A. High rate of infusion and B. Low rate of infusion	A. Single IV bolus and B. Multiple IV bolus
Equipment	Hypodermic needle and syringe	IV bag, peripheral cannula, Tourniquet, drip set (insertion spike, drip chamber, screw clamp, extension tube with secondary port, hollow needle, Y-Set/T-Set/V connector sets)
Examples	Edrophonium IV bolus injection Morphine IV bolus injections	**IV infusion,** e.g., due to short t ½ dopamine, dobutamine (for cardiogenic shock), oxytocin (for induction of labor), Noradrenaline (for septic shock), sodium nitroprusside for hypertensive emergencies **To reduce toxicity**: Vancomycin (to prevent red man syndrome) Aminophylline (to prevent cardiac arrest)

Important Note: IV bolus dose, e.g., thiopentone sodium.

Syringe of appropriate size, ampule with required drug or solution, needle of right size, disinfectant, gauze.

Traditional intravenous (IV) infusion therapy set—1-pole/stand, 2-IV bottle/bag, 3-spike, 4-air valve, 5-drip chamber, 7—IV tubing, 8-roller clamp, and 9-cannula.

Intravenous bolus:

The following steps have to be followed during administration of drug by intravenous bolus:

1. **Expiry date and correct drug:** Check the expiry date of the drug and ensure that the vial or ampule contains the right drug in the right strength.
2. **Sterility:** During the preparation procedure, materials should be kept sterile. Wash your hands prior to preparing the injection and also after the procedure. Disinfect the injection site with appropriate antiseptic. Take care not to prick yourself or somebody else during the procedure.
3. **Technique:** Dissolve dry medicine and aspirate the drug into syringe

4. **Administration of drug:** Reassure the patient and explain the procedure. Uncover the arm completely. Apply tourniquet and look for a suitable vein and wait for the vein to swell. Disinfect the skin and stabilize the vein by pulling the skin taut in the longitudinal direction of the vein with another hand. Insert the needle at an angle of around 45° with keeping the beveling of the needle up. Aspirate and if blood appears, loosen the tourniquet and inject the drug slowly. Withdraw the needle swiftly and press the sterile cotton onto the opening and secure with adhesive tape.
5. **Disposal of waste:** Make sure that the contaminated wastes including the needle and syringe are disposed safely.

Step 01: Introduce yourself to the patient and clarify the patient's identity. Explain the procedure to the patient and gain informed consent to continue. Inform that cannulation may cause some discomfort but that it will be short lived.

Step 02: Ensure that you have all of your equipment ready as follows—spirit, gloves, alcohol wipe, disposable tourniquet, IV cannula, suitable plaster, syringe, saline.

Step 03: Sanitize your hands using alcohol cleanser.

Step 04: Position the arm so that it is comfortable for the patient and identify a vein.

Step 05: Apply the tourniquet and re-check the vein

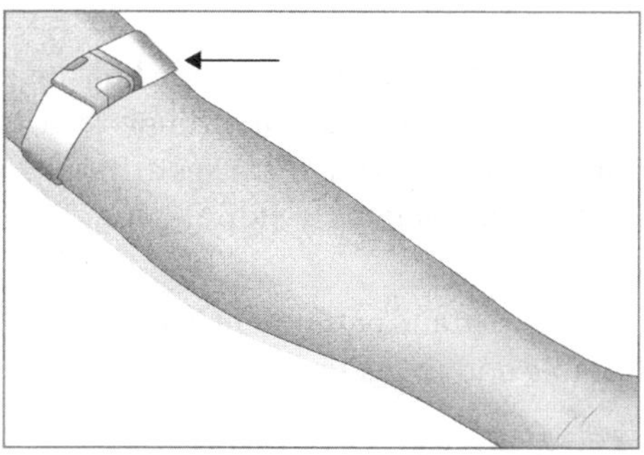

Step 06: Put on your gloves, clean the patient's skin with the alcohol wipe and let it dry.

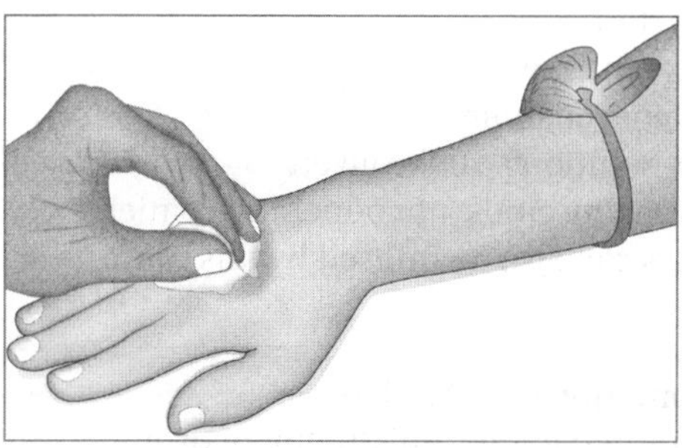

Step 07: Remove the cannula from its packaging and remove the needle cover ensuring not to touch the needle.

Step 08: Stretch the skin distally and inform the patient that they should expect a sharp scratch.

Step 09: Insert the needle, bevel upwards at about 30°. Advance the needle until a flashback of blood is seen in the hub at the back of the cannula

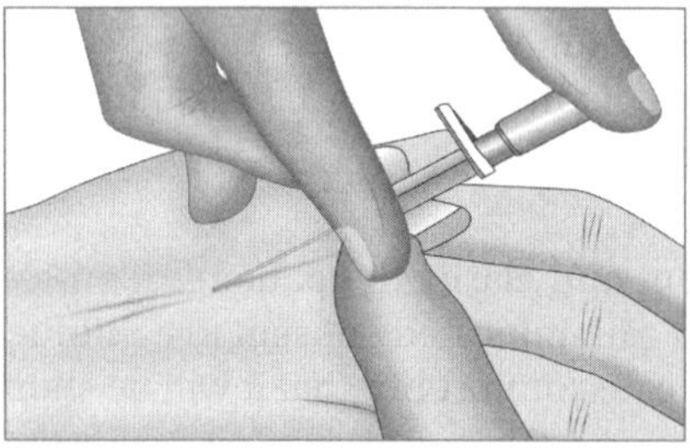

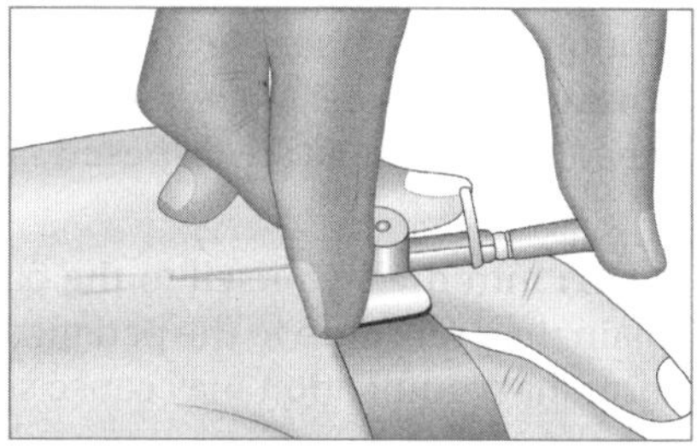

Step 10: Once the flashback of blood is seen, progress the entire cannula a further 2 mm, then fix the needle, advancing the rest of the cannula into the vein.

Step 11: Release the tourniquet, apply pressure to the vein at the tip of the cannula and remove the needle fully. Remove the cap from the needle and put this on the end of the cannula.

Step 12: Carefully dispose of the needle into the sharps bin.

Step 13: Apply the dressing to the cannula to fix it in place and ensure that the date sticker has been completed and applied.

Step 14: Check that the use-by date on the saline has not passed. If the date is ok, fill the syringe with saline and flush it through the cannula to check for patency. If there is any resistance, or if it causes any pain, or you notice any localized tissue swelling—immediately stop flushing, remove the cannula and start again.

Step 15: Dispose of your gloves and equipment in the clinical waste bin, ensure the patient is comfortable and thank them.

Advantages and Disadvantages of IV Route

Advantages

- Quick onset of action
- Most useful route in emergencies
- Provides 100% bioavailability
- Large volume of solutions can be given
- Can be used in unconscious, uncooperative patients
- GIT irritant drugs can also be infused by this route

Disadvantages

- Strict aseptic conditions are needed
- Assistance is required for administration of drug

- ❖ Painful
- ❖ Irritation of the veins may cause thrombophlebitis
- ❖ Introduction of air may produce embolism

Two types of administration sets are available—macrodrip (the standard type) and microdrip **(Fig. 3.15)**.

A standard macrodrip set delivers 10, 12, 15, or 20 drops/mL (gtt/mL), depending on the manufacturer; Macrodrip tubing is typically used to infuse fluids at a rapid rate.

Microdrip set usually delivers 50 to 60 drops/mL(gtt/mL). It is often used to infuse fluids to pediatric and neonatal patients or medications requiring a precise flow rate. Gtt comes from Latin noun gutta ("drop").

Based on the drip factor, rate of the infusion can be adjusted by tightening or loosening the roller clamp and by counting the drops in the drip chamber each minute. For example, for macrodrip tubing with a drip factor of 20 gtt/mL, 20 drops is equivalent one mL. If you set the rate at 20 drops per minute, one mL is infusing per minute, or 60 mL per hour. If you double the rate to 40 drops per minute, you increase the rate to 120 mL per hour.

Macrodrip

- ❖ 10 gtt/mL—divide the infusion rate by 6
- ❖ 15 gtt/mL—divide the infusion rate by 4
- ❖ 20 gtt/mL—divide the infusion rate by 3

Microdrip: 60 gtt/mL divided by 60 is 1. Therefore, the drip rate is the same as the flow rate (drip rate = flow rate).

For example, administer 1 liter of lactated Ringer's solution IV over 10 hours. There are no electronic infusion pumps available and the only IV tubing set in stock has a drip factor of 20 drops/mL. How many drops per minute (gtt/min) will you run the infusion?

Step 1: Convert liters to mL

1 liter = 1000 mL

Step 2: Determine the hourly rate of the infusion. Take total volume (1000 mL) and divide by time (10 hours).

$$\frac{1000\text{ mL}}{10\text{ hr}} = 100\text{ mL/hour}$$

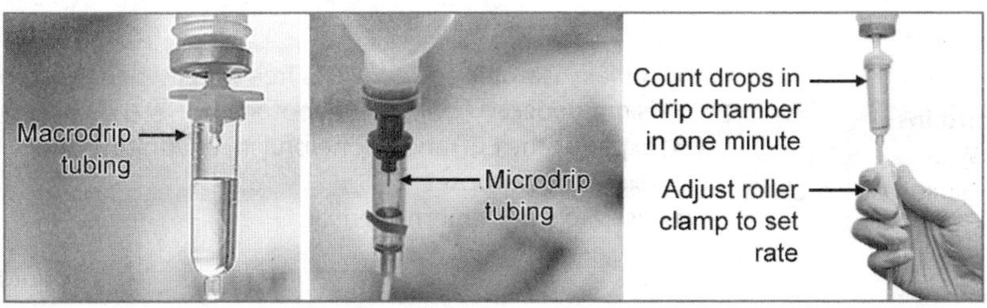

Fig. 3.15: Macrodrip and microdrip tubing.

Step 3: Divide the hourly infusion rate by the drip factor. Our tubing drip factor is 20 gtts/mL so we divide the hourly rate by 3.

$$\frac{100}{3 \text{ gtt/min}} = 100 \text{ mL/hour}$$

Ans: 33 gtt/min

Supplemental fluids used in intravenous therapy to restore or maintain normal fluid volume and electrolyte balance when the oral route is impossible.

IV fluid therapy is an efficient and effective way of supplying fluids directly into the intravascular fluid compartment, replacing electrolyte losses, and administering medications and blood products.

Types of IV Fluids (Table 3.4)

1. **Crystalloids:** Isotonic saline
2. **Colloids:** Hydroxyethyl starch, albumin, dextran
3. **Blood and blood products**

5 R's in the use of IV fluids: Resuscitation, routine maintenance, replacement, redistribution and reassessment

- **Resuscitation:** For initial stabilization and overlaps with further replacement therapy
- **Replacement:** To correct body fluid deficit
- **Routine maintenance:** Insensible fluid losses are replaced
- **Redistribution:** To correct fluid and electrolyte redistribution imbalance
- **Reassessment**

Table 3.4: Commonly use crystalloids.

Isotonic solutions	
Normal saline solution (NSS) (0.9 and NaCl)	
Osmolality 308 mOsm/L **Contains** • Water • Sodium (154 mEq/L) • Chloride (154 mEq/L)	**Uses** • Isotonic solution of choice for expanding ECF volume • Infused to correct extracellular fluid volume deficit • Used alongside administration of blood products • Used to replace large sodium losses such as burn injuries and trauma **Caution** Should not be used with heart failure, pulmonary edema, and renal impairment
Dextrose 5% in water (D5W)	
Osmolality 252 mOsm/L **Contains** • Water • Glucose (50 g/L)	**Uses** • Initially isotonic and provides free water when dextrose is metabolized (making it hypotonic) • Expands the ECF and ICF, helpful in rehydrating and excretory purposes • Used to treat hypernatremia

Contd...

Contd...

<table>
<tr><th colspan="2">Isotonic solutions</th></tr>
<tr><td colspan="2">Dextrose 5% in water (D5W)</td></tr>
<tr><td></td><td>Caution
Should NOT be used for fluid resuscitation because hyperglycemia can result. Should be avoided in clients at risk for increased intracranial pressure</td></tr>
<tr><td colspan="2">Lactated Ringer's solution in 5% dextrose</td></tr>
<tr><td>Other names
• OSLRS
• LR
• Ringer's lactate
• Hartmann solution
Osmolality
273 mOsm/L
Contains
• Water
• Sodium (130 mEq/L)
• Potassium (4 mEq/L)
• Calcium (3 mEq/L)
• Chloride (109 mEq/L)
• lactate (28 mEq/L)</td><td>Uses
• Used to correct dehydration, sodium depletion, and replace GI tract fluid losses
• Also used in fluid losses caused by burns, fistula drainage, and trauma
• Often administered for patients with metabolic acidosis because it is an alkalizing solution
Caution
• Should not be given to patients who cannot metabolize lactate (e.g., liver disease, lactic acidosis)
• Used in caution for patients with heart failure and renal failure</td></tr>
<tr><td colspan="2">Ringer's solution</td></tr>
<tr><td>Osmolality
• 273 mOsm/L
• Similar composition with lactated Ringer's but without the lactate</td><td>Uses
Similar indications for lactated Ringer's solution but without the contraindications related to lactate</td></tr>
</table>

4 CHAPTER

Preparation of Oral Rehydration Solution from an ORS Packet and Deliberating its Application in Clinical Practice

PRINCIPLES OF MANAGEMENT IN DIARRHEA

Rational management of diarrhea depends on establishing the underlying cause and instituting specific therapy (only if necessary), since most diarrheas are self-limiting.

Therapeutic measures may be grouped into:

a. Treatment of fluid depletion, shock and acidosis
b. Maintenance of nutrition
c. Drug therapy

ORS: ORAL REHYDRATION SALT

Goal is to

- To **correct** existing deficits of fluid and electrolytes rapidly (termed "rehydration therapy").
- To **replace** further losses as they occur until diarrhea stops (termed "maintenance therapy").

Fluid losses can be replaced either orally or intravenously; the latter route is usually needed only for initial rehydration of patients who are severely dehydrated.

Indication of ORS

- There is loss of water and electrolytes from the body in liquid stools, from vomiting, also increased by fever. These losses cause dehydration (due to the loss of water and sodium chloride), base-deficit acidosis (due to the loss of bicarbonate), and potassium depletion. Dehydration can cause decreased blood volume (hypovolaemia), cardiovascular collapse, and death if not treated promptly. **Aim** of ORS is to **REPLENISH** the lost electrolytes during dehydration. When a balanced isotonic solution of glucose and salt is given, glucose-linked sodium absorption occurs along with water and other electrolytes.

- The intestinal absorption of sodium, is enhanced by the active absorption of certain food molecules such as glucose (which is derived from the breakdown of sucrose or cooked starches) or L-amino acids (which are derived from the breakdown of proteins.

Composition of ORS

Balanced mixture of **glucose and electrolytes** for use in treating and preventing dehydration, potassium depletion, and base deficit. So potassium and citrate (or bicarbonate) salts have been included, in addition to sodium chloride. This mixture of salts and glucose is termed *oral rehydration salts* (ORS); when ORS is dissolved in water, the mixture is called *ORS solution.*

Types of ORS

1. Original WHO formula
2. Citrate based ORS/low osmolality ORS **(Table 4.1)**
3. Rice-based ORS
4. Super ORS
5. Super super ORS/Super ORS with nutrients—zinc, magnesium, selenium, vitamin A
6. Home available ORS

Original WHO Formula

In 1984, ORS was based on the composition of cholera stools in children. Standard ORS formula from WHO and UNICEF has been replaced by low osmolarity ORS which was launched in 2003 with decrease in sodium and glucose concentration and hence decrease in osmolarity from 311 to 245.

It contained Na bicarbonate which reacted with glucose to produce furfural compound which shortened the shelf life of ORS.

- The glucose helps the absorption of sodium and not as a source of fuel.
- The inclusion of trisodium citrate in place of sodium bicarbonate has made the product more stable, no discoloration and shelf life 2–3 years.

Table 4.1: Citrate-based ORS/low osmolality ORS.

Reduced osmolarity ORS	*Grams/L*	*Reduced osmo. ORS*	*mmoL/L*
Sodium chloride	2.6	Sodium	75
Glucose, anhydrous	13.5	Chloride	65
Potassium chloride	1.5	Glucose, anhydrous	75
Trisodium citrate	2.9	Potassium	20
		Citrate	10
		Total osmolality	245

- The new ORS contains lesser amount of sodium and glucose thereby resulting in a lower osmolarity. The reduced osmolarity reduces the stool output by 25% in comparison to the original formula.
- Trisodium citrate has direct effect in promoting glucose and sodium and in treating acidosis.
- It reduces vomiting by 30%.
- It has been demonstrated to reduce the need for IV therapy by > 30%.

Rice-based ORS

- Contains starches, such as rice, wheat flour and maize provides more substrate in the lumen without increasing osmolarity and hence more glucose mediated absorption
- Better taste, provides more calories than glucose based ORS.
- Culturally acceptable, reduces stool volume (40%) and shortens the duration of diarrhea.

Super ORS

Special types of ORS which instead of mono sugars contain more complex sugars or amino acids.

- They are complex sugar based, such as rice or amino acids (glycine or alanine) based and provide more calories (180 kcal/L) apart from rehydration.
- Reduce stool output, frequency of stools and duration, furnishes increase amount of calories (180 kcal/L)
- With gradual release of glucose, prevents secondary disaccharide intolerance.
- Contributes to weight gain, as it provides additional nutrition (especially malnourished).
- The disadvantages are short self-life (not more than 10 hours) and should be frequently prepared 2–3 times a day.

Super Super ORS/Super ORS with Nutrients—Zinc, Magnesium, Selenium, Vitamin A

Addition of zinc to super ORS

Advantages:

- Improved absorption of water and electrolytes by the intestine
- Faster regeneration of gut epithelium
- Increase levels of enterocyte brush border enzymes
- Enhanced immune response leading to increased clearance of the pathogens

Home Available ORS

Home prepared solutions are recommended for use by parents to give to their child immediately after an attack of diarrhea or vomiting starts before any signs of dehydration occur.

- Basically, it prevents dehydration and preserves good nutritional status by maintaining fluid and food intake
- Costless and easy to prepare at home and less need of hospitalization.

How to Prepare ORS at Home (Fig. 4.1)

Home ORS solution is easy to prepare, effective and can be used in emergency but be careful to mix the exact amounts. Too much sugar can make diarrhea worse and too much salt can be dangerous because of hypernatremia due to excess sodium.

How to Prepare ORS from Sachet

1. Put the contents of ORS in a clean container. Add the exact amount of clean water as indicated on the packet, usually one liter.
2. Add water only, never add fruit juice, coke, milk or soup etc.
3. Ready made ORS preparations **(Table 4.2)** are also available in various flavors and acceptance is very good in children.

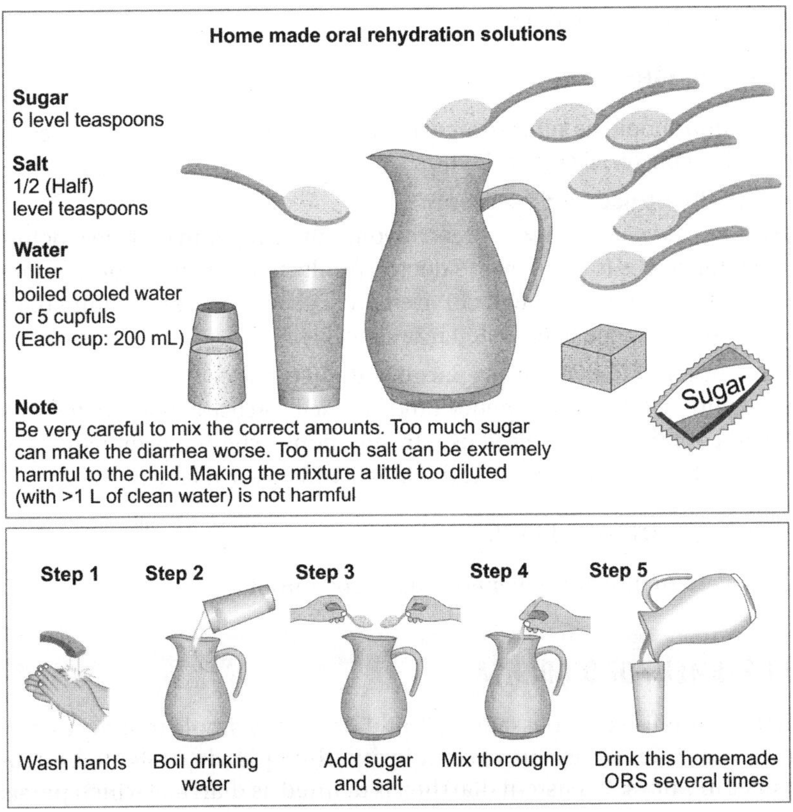

Fig. 4.1: Steps for ORS preparation.

Table 4.2: ORS preparation.

Ingredient	*QTY*	*QTY*
Clean boiled drinking water	1 liter	250 mL
Sugar	6 Levels tea spoon (1 teaspoon = 5 g)	1 level tea spoon
Salt	Half level tea spoon	One pinch
Stir the mixture till sugar dissolves		

How to Administer ORS

1. Should be given immediately
2. Can be given by spoon, dropper, cup, tumbler, syringe or nasogastric tube.
3. A child < 2 years: Give 1–2 teaspoon every 2–3 minutes.
4. A child > 2 years or older give half to one cup (250 mL) with each loose stool.
5. If the child vomits, wait for 10 minutes. Then give the solution more slowly (for example, a spoonful every 2–3 minutes).
6. If diarrhea continues after the ORS packets are used up, tell the mother to give other fluids as described in the first rule above or return for more ORS.
7. Breastfeeding to continue

Storage of ORS

The solution should be kept covered and not used more than 24 hours because of the risk of bacterial contamination.

Can the ORS be used for everyone?
ORS is safe and can be used to treat anyone suffering from diarrhea, before a detailed diagnosis is done by the doctor. Adults need rehydration treatment as much as children, although children must always be treated immediately because they become dehydrated more quickly.

What happens if the ORS is prepared with dirty water?
The benefits of fluid replacement would be lost if you use contaminated water. Boil and cool the water before use. In situations, where it is difficult to boil water, use the filtered water/portable water which is available.

Contraindications of ORS

Intussusception unconsciousness, high stool output.

MANAGEMENT OF DIARRHEA

Diarrhea is defined as passage of liquid or watery stools that occur more than three times a day. In vast majority, the episode of acute diarrhea subsides in 7 days. Persistent diarrhea is defined as diarrhea which persists > 2 weeks.

Causes

- **Bacterial:** *Escherichia coli*
- **Viral:** Rotavirus
- **Parasitic:** *Giardia lamblia, Entamoeba histolytica*

Cause of Acute Diarrhea (Table 4.3)

Table 4.3: Symptoms associated with dehydration.

Symptoms	*No dehydration*	*Some dehydration*	*Severe dehydration*
Mental status	Well; alert	Normal, fatigued or restless, **irritable**	Apathetic, **lethargic unconscious**
Thirst	Drink normally, might refuse liquids	**Thirsty, eager to drink**	**Drink poorly, unable to drink**
Eyes	Normal	**Slight sunken**	**Deeply sunken**
Skin fold/skin pinch	**Instant recoil**	**Recoil in <2 Sec**	**Recoil in >2 Sec**
Capillary refill	Normal	Prolonged	Prolonged; minimal
Extremities	Warm	Cool	Cold; mottled; cyanotic
Tears	Present	Decreased	Absent
Mouth and tongue	Moist	Dry	Parched
Heart rate	Normal	Normal to increase	Tachycardia/bradycardia
Quality of pulse	Normal	Normal to decrease	Weak, tready or impalpable
Breathing	Normal	Normal/fast	Deep

Management of No Dehydration (Table 4.4)

A. **Give the child more fluids than usual:** Use recommended home fluids. ORS solution, food-based fluids (such as soup, rice water, and yoghurt drinks) and plain water. Give as much of these fluids as the child will take. Use the amounts shown below for ORS as a guide. Continue giving these fluids until the diarrhea stops.
   - ORS is given as *replacement therapy for ongoing stool losses* only. Amount of ORS to be given.

Table 4.4: Replacement therapy in NO dehydration.

	Replacement therapy		
Age	*Infants (<2 Yr)*	*Children (2–10 Yr)*	*Children (>10 Yr)*
ORS is given after each loose stool	50–100 mL	100–200 mL	Add Lib
Total quantity	500 mL/Day	1000 mL/Day	2000 mL/Day

B. **Give the child plenty of food to prevent malnutrition:**
Continue to breast-feed frequently
If the child is 6 months or older, or already taking solid food
- Give starchy food mixed with pulses,vegetables.
- Give fresh fruit juice or mashed banana to provide potassium
- Give freshly prepared foods cook and mash or grind food well

C. Take the child to the health worker if the child does not get better in 3 days or develops any of the following: Many watery stools, eating or drinking poorly, repeated vomiting, fever, marked thirst, blood in stools **(Table 4.5)**.

ORS is given to prevent dehydration along with normal diet, breastfeeding to continue along with complimentary foods.

Some Dehydration

A. **How much ORS solution should be given?** Rehydration therapy includes ORS 50–100 mL/kg over 3–4 hours, continue breastfeeding. If ORS cannot be taken orally use nasogastric tube, If after 4 hours while assessment child has still some dehydration ORT is repeated as above for 4 hours **OR** according to the following **Table 4.6**.

B. **Observe the child carefully and help the mother give ORS solution:** Show her how much solution to give her child. Show her how to give it—a

Table 4.5: Difficulties encountered in home therapy for diarrhea.

Difficulty	*Possible solution*
• The mother is disappointed because she is not given a prescription for drugs or the child does not receive an injection	Explain that the diarrhea will stop by itself after a few days also, explain that drugs do not help to stop diarrhea, but that fluid replacement and continued feeding will help to shorten the illness and also maintain her child's strength and growth
• The mother believes that food should not be given during diarrhea	Ask her to explain her beliefs about how diarrhea should be treated. Discuss with her the importance of feeding in order to keep her child strong and support normal growth, even during diarrhea
• The mother does not know what fluids to give her child at home	Ask her what fluids she can prepare at home and reach agreement on appropriate fluids for her child
• The mother does not have the ingredients to make a recommended fluid	Ask her if she can obtain the ingredients easily if she cannot, suggest another home fluid
• The child vomits after drinking ORS solution or other fluids	Explain that more fluid is usually kept down than is vomited. Tell the mother to wart 10 minutes and then start giving fluid again, but more slowly

Contd...

Contd...

Difficulty	***Possible solution***
• The child refuses to drink	A child who has lost fluid will usually be thirsty and want to drink, even when there are no signs of dehydration if the child is not familiar with the taste of ORS solution, some persuasion may be needed at first. When a child drinks well to begin with, then loses interest in drinking, it usually means that sufficient fluid has been given
• The mother is given some packets of ORS for use at home but is afraid they will be used up before the diarrhea slops	Explain that after the ORS has been used up. She should give a recommended home fluid (such as rice water) or water, or she could return to the health facility for more packets of ORS in any event, she should continue to give extra fluid until the diarrhea stops

Table 4.6: Approximate amount of ORS solution to be given in first four Hours.

Age:*	***<4 months***	***4–11 months***	***12–23 months***	***2–4 years***	***5–14 years***	***15 years or older***
Weight:	<5 kg	5–7.9 kg	8–10.9 kg	11–15.9 kg	16–29.0 kg	30 kg or more
In mL	200–400	400–600	600–800	800–1200	1200–2200	2200–4000
In local measure						

* Use the patient's age only when you do not know the weight. The approximate amount of ORS required (in mL) can also be calculated by multiplying the patient's weight (in kg) times 75.

teaspoonful every 1–2 minutes for a child under 2 years, frequent sips from a cup for an older child. Check from time to time to see if there are problems. If the child vomits, wait 10 minutes and then continue giving ORS, but more slowly, for example, a spoonful every 2–3 minutes. If the child's eyelids become puffy, stop ORS and give plain water or breast milk.

C. **After 4 hours, reassess the child using the assessment chart:** If there are **no signs of dehydration,** shift to plan (for NO dehydration). When dehydration has been corrected, the child usually passes urine and may also be tired and fall asleep.
   - If signs indicating **some dehydration** are still present, repeat the (same plan for some dehydrations) but start to offer food, milk and juice.
   - If signs indicating **severe dehydration** have appeared, shift to IV fluids.

D. **Replacement of losses**
   Infants and children <10 kg:
   - 50–100 mL ORS for each loose stool or vomiting episode up to 500 mL per day

> *10 kg body weight:*

– 100–200 mL ORS for each loose stool or vomiting episode up to 1 L per day.

Maintenance therapy should begin when signs of dehydration disappear, usually within 4 hours and ORS should be given equal to diarrhea losses usually to a maximum of 10 mL/kg per stool.

COMMUNICATION

To improve their communications with mothers, doctors (and other health workers) must learn:

- To listen to the mother and take her concerns seriously;
- To speak to her in terms she can understand;
- To be supportive and encouraging, giving her praise and help rather than criticism;
- To use teaching methods that require her active participation.

Methods Employed

- Using examples, demonstrations, and practice
- Asking checking questions
- Providing illustrated instruction leaflets
- Giving encouragement and assistance

Using examples, demonstrations, and practice (Box 4.1)

- Combining instruction with the use of examples, demonstrations, and practice can greatly facilitate the learning process.
- **Showing pictures:** Use a drawing or a poster of a mother breastfeeding while discussing the importance of this practice for an infant's health.

Box 4.1: Demonstrations and practice.

Demonstrating: 1. Health worker teaching a mother how to carry out ORT at home can make the message clearer by showing her a half-cup (100 mL) of ORS. Solution (with a line marking the appropriate level) while instructing her to give her child that amount after each loose stool	2. A mother could be encouraged to watch another mother giving an infant ORS solution with a spoon so that she can see how to hold her child and how frequently to give the spoonful's of fluid
3. She should then practice giving ORS solution to her own child, with guidance from the health worker. In this way, the health worker can see which parts of the task the mother finds difficult, and can explain or demonstrate how they should be done	

- **Using specific names or instructions** appropriate to local circumstances (instead of stating a general rule): advise the mother to give **"banana or green coconut water"** (which are rich in potassium**), instead of simply telling her to give her child "fruit";** explain that she should feed her child "six times a day" instead of "frequently" or "more often than usual".
- **Showing an object:** Show the mother an infant feeding bottle when explaining that this should not be used for giving milk or other fluids to her infant. Show a cup and spoon for comparison.

ASKING CHECKING QUESTIONS

- Asking simple checking questions is a very effective way of confirming what a mother has learned about home therapy. For example, after explaining how to treat the child's diarrhea at home, the doctor might ask: "Describe how you would prepare the drink for Ana" or "Tell me the symptoms that mean you should bring Ana back to me".
- Checking question should be phrased in such a way that the answer cannot be just "yes" or "no". For example, it is not effective to ask: "Do you understand the symptoms that mean you should bring Ana back to see me?" The mother is likely to answer "yes", whether she understands them or not.
- The doctor should not ask the mother, "Did the nurse explain to you how to mix ORS solution?", or "Do you know how to mix ORS solution?", since the mother would probably be reluctant to answer "no". Instead, the doctor should ask questions such as "How much water will you mix with that ORS packet?", "How much of the solution will you give to MO?",

Providing Illustrated Instruction Leaflets

Specifically prepared pamphlet (or card) can greatly improve communication with the mother. It should summarize the important elements of caring for a child with diarrhea at home, and should have words and pictures that illustrate these points.

Advantages

- The pamphlet will simplify the task of training health workers in the messages to tell mothers.
- When she is at home, the pamphlet will remind the mother of what she was taught at he treatment facility, and support her if other family members or friends should disagree with her treatment.
- If the mother keeps the pamphlet, the next time her child has diarrhea she can refer to it and remind herself what to do.

Giving Encouragement and Assistance

Home treatment may seem to be unrewarding—she may expect ORT to stop the diarrhea, and be discouraged when it does not;

Several approaches should be used:

- **Emphasize the positive:** Explain that ORT will make the child stronger and that continued feeding will help the child to grow. Encourage the mother to look at the whole child, not just the child's stools. The child should be less fussy and more contented after ORT and feeding.
- **Give praise:** Praise is essential in building up a mother's confidence that she can treat her child successfully at home. Opportunities to praise the mother occur when she answers a checking question correctly, performs a practical task correctly.
- **Show interest:** Discuss with the mother how she will practise home therapy. Ask, for example, "What foods will you give your child?" When the mother answers, confirm that the food is suitable, or suggest another choice. Also discuss how she will prepare the food.
- **Assist with problems:** Ask questions to determine whether the mother has the necessary items for home therapy, e.g., a container to measure water

Severe Dehydration

A. Intravenous isotonic saline/plain Ringer solutions the fluid of choice and never use 5% dextrose alone. 100 mL/kg of fluid is given over 6 hours in children <12 months and over 3 hours above 12 months as shown in the table below:

Age	*30 mL/kg*	*70 mL/kg*
<12 months	1 hour*	5 hours
>12 months	30 minutes*	2 hours and 30 min

*The above can be repeated if child continues to have feeble or non-palpable radial pulse.

If IV fluids can not be given due to any reason because of transport, IV access difficulties ORS can be given 20 mL/kg/hours for 6 hours (Total 120 mL/kg) by nasogastric tube but child requires frequent assessment every 1–2 hours and if no improvement in hydration after 3 hours or abdominal distension or vomiting occurs switch to IV fluids.

The child should be reassess every 15–30 minutes for pulses , oral mucosa, respiratory rate, urine output, stool water loss after the first bolus of 100 mL/ kg of intravenous fluid.

B. Further management after the 100 mL/kg of IV fluids has been given includes:
   1. *Persistence of severe dehydration:* Intravenous infusion is repeated
   2. *Hydration is improved but some dehydration is present:* IV fluids are discontinued and ORS is continued over 4 hours as in some dehydration
   3. *No dehydration:* IV fluids are discontinued and ORS continued as per plan in no dehydration.

C. Replacement of losses in severe dehydration is same as in child with some dehydration

1. *Infants and children:* <10 kg 50–100 mL for each loose stool or vomiting episode up to 500 mL per day More than 10 kg: 100 to 200 mL ORS for each loose stool or vomiting episode up to 1 L per day
2. *Adolescents and adults:* Add libitum up to 2 L per day. Replace the losses as long as diarrhea or vomiting continues.

NUTRITION IN DIARRHEA

- All infants to continue breast feeds even during rehydration therapy.
- Lactose free milk not mandatory unless child has established evidence of lactose intolerance. Home made cereals mix with milk can be given.
- Home made/seasonal foods can be given. The meals can be given immediately after rehydration therapy after around 4 hours.

FOODS TO AVOID

- Dairy products except for curd and buttermilk
- **Sweetened drinks or carbonated drinks like soda**
- All fruit juices
- **Dry fruits and nuts**
- High fiber foods
- **Sugar**
- Sweets
- **Raw salads and sprouts**

Use of Zinc in ORS

Advantages

- Reduces the duration of diarrhea episode by 25%
- Reduces the stool volume by 30%
- Reduces the likelihood of subsequent occurrence in next 2–3 months
- Dose for kids above 6 months—20 mg daily for 14 days
- Dose for kids below 6 months—10 mg daily for 14 days
- Physiological effect of zinc on intestinal ion transport has not yet been established thoroughly. Zinc inhibits cAMP-induced, chloride-dependent fluid secretion by inhibiting basolateral potassium (K) channels. Zinc also improves the absorption of water and electrolytes, improves regeneration of the intestinal epithelium, increases the levels of brush border enzymes, and enhances the immune response, allowing for a better clearance of the pathogens.

PREBIOTICS AND PROBIOTICS

Fructo-oligosaccharides (FOS), galacto-oligosaccharides (GOS), and trans-galacto-oligosaccharides (TOS) are the most common prebiotics.

Probiotics: *Lactobacillus rhamnosus GG, Saccharomyces boulardii, Bifidobacterium* are useful agents.

They help treat diarrhea by repopulating and maintaining beneficial gut bacteria and correcting an imbalance. Probiotics fight pathogenic bacteria by competing for nutrients, boosting the immune system.

Antibiotics

Say no to antibiotics: Majority of cases of diarrhea are due to viral etiology and self-limiting and ORS is must to prevent dehydration as it is the most important cause of mortality in children. Antibiotics themselves diminish gut flora.

Indications of Antibiotics Therapy (Table 4.7)

Child with bacillary dysentery is another indication of antibiotic. Preterm and young infants are at high risk of sepsis with diarrhea and antibiotics have definitely animportant role in this group. Ideally microbiologic (culture) confirmation should be sought prior to antibiotics therapy.

Antisecretory agents: Racecadotril is an antisecretory drug exerts anti-diarrheal effects by inhibiting intestinal enkephalinase. It reduces stool output and duration but more data on efficacy is needed before it can be recommended for routine use in children with acute Diarrhea.

Table 4.7: Indications of antibiotic therapy.

Clinical conditions and circumstances that may indicate antibiotic therapy		
Condition	***Putative bacterial agent***	***Suggested antibiotic***
Dysenteric diarrhea	*Shigella, Yersinia, Campylobacter*	Azithromycin, ciprofloxacin
Fever, increased inflammation markers	*Shigella*	Azithromycin, ceftriaxone
Prolonged diarrhea	Gram-negative enterobacteria, *Clostridium difficile*	Metronidazole, co-trimoxazole
SIBO	Gram-negative enterobacteria	Metronidazole, rifaximin, co-trimoxazole
Antibiotic-associated diarrhea	*Clostridium difficile,* others	Metronidazole, vancomycin (only if *Clostridium difficile* is detected)
Traveler's diarrhea	ETEC, EPEC	Azithromycin, ciprofloxacin
Toxic state	Gram-negative enterobacteria, *Clostridium difficile*	Ceftriaxone

(ETEC: Enterotoxigenic *E. coli*; EPEC: Enteropathogenic *E. coli*)

5 CHAPTER Dosage Calculations and Prescribing in Special Populations

EXERCISES

1. **A patient is prescribed 30 mg of furosemide intravenously. Injection is available as 10 mg in 1 milliliter of liquid for IV. How many milliliters will you administer?**

   Required: 30 mg
   Available: 10 mg
   Volume: 1 mL

   $$\text{Dose(mL)} = \frac{\text{Required dose} \times \text{volume}}{\text{Available dose}}$$

   $$= 30 \times 1/10 = \mathbf{3\ mL}$$

2. **A patient is prescribed 22 mg of gentamicin sulfate by intramuscular injection. Injection is available as 20 mg in 2 mL of liquid for IM. How many milliliters will you administer?**

   Required: 22 mg
   Available: 20 mg
   Volume: 2 mL

   $$\text{Dose(mL)} = \frac{\text{Required dose} \times \text{volume}}{\text{Available dose}}$$

   $$= 22 \times 2/20 = \mathbf{2.2\ mL}$$

3. **A patient is prescribed 15 mg of a drug (antiemetic). You have 2 mL of solution on hand which contains 25 mg. What volume of solution would you give?**

   Required: 15 mg
   Available: 25 mg
   Volume: 2 mL

   $$\text{Dose(mL)} = \frac{\text{Required dose} \times \text{volume}}{\text{Available dose}}$$

   $$= 15 \times 2/25 = \mathbf{1.2\ mL}$$

4. **Calculate the drip rate for 100 mL of IV fluids to be given over a half hour via a giving set which delivers 10 drops/mL.**

   Volume to be administered: 100 mL
   Time: 30 min
   Drip factor: 10 drops/mL

   $$\text{Drip rate} = \frac{\text{Volume} \times \text{drip factor}}{\text{time}}$$

   $= 100 \times 10/30 =$ **33 drops/min**

5. **Calculate the drip rate for 500 mL of normal saline to be given over 4.5 hours via a giving set which delivers 15 drops/mL.**

   Volume to be administered: 500 mL
   Time: 4.5×60 min = 270 min
   Drip factor: 15 drops/mL

   $$\text{Drip rate} = \frac{\text{Volume} \times \text{drip factor}}{\text{time}}$$

   $= 500 \times 15/270 =$ **28 drops/min**

6. **Calculate the drip rate for 500 mL of dextrose 5% in water to be given over 4 hours via a giving set which delivers 15 drops/mL.**

   Volume to be administered: 500 mL
   Time: 4×60 min = 240 min
   Drip factor: 15 drops/mL

   $$\text{Drip rate} = \frac{\text{Volume} \times \text{drip factor}}{\text{time}}$$

   $= 500 \times 15/240 =$ **31 drops/min**

7. **How much noradrenaline (in mg) is present in 4 mL of a 1:1000 solution?**

   Noradrenaline 1:1,000 solution = 1 g in 1,000 mL
   i.e., 1,000 mg in 1,000 mL
   1 mg in 1 mL
   4 mg in 4 mL
   Therefore, 4 mg of noradrenaline is present in 4 mL of a 1:1,000 solution.

8. **How many mg of lignocaine are present in a 10 mL ampoule of lignocaine 1%?**

   Lignocaine 1% = 1 g/100 mL = 1,000 mg/100 mL = 10 mg/mL
   Thus, 10 mL will contain $10 \times 10 =$ **100 mg**

9. **How many mmol of sodium bicarbonate are present in 100 mL of an 8.4% solution?**

   Sodium bicarbonate 8.4% = 8.4 g/100 mL = 8,400 mg/100 mL, i.e., 84 mg/mL
   1 mmol sodium bicarbonate = 84 mg
   Thus, 1 mL contains 1 mmol sodium bicarbonate.
   100 mL will contain 100 mmol

10. **How many mg of adrenaline are there in a 10 mL ampoule of 0.25% bupivacaine with adrenaline in a 1:200,000 solution?**

Adrenaline 1: 200,000 solution: 1 g in 200,000: 1000 mg in 200,000: 1 mg in 200 mL

Thus, 10 mL will contain 10 × 1/200 = **0.05 mg**

11. **How many mL of a 1:10,000 solution would you need to obtain 1 mg of adrenaline?**

Adrenaline 1:10,000 solution: 1 g in 10,000 mL

i.e., 1,000 mg in 10,000 mL

1 mg in 10 mL

Therefore, if we have to obtain a dose of 1 mg, we have to take 10 mL

12. **A child was prescribed 250 mg of a drug to be taken every 4 hours. The drug was available in an oral suspension of 25 mg/2 mL. How many teaspoons will the child need to take?**

2 mL of the drug contains 25 mg

Thus, 20 mL will contain 250 mg

5 mL = 1 teaspoon

Thus, **20 mL = 4 teaspoons**

13. **A patient was prescribed heparin 2,000 units SC BD. Heparin is available as 25,000 units/5 mL vial. It is to be administered in an insulin syringe. How many units will be required?**

25,000 units in 5 mL = 5,000 units in 1 mL

Therefore, 2,000 units in 2,000 × 1/5,000 = 0.4 mL

In an insulin syringe, 1 mL = 100 units

0.4 mL = 0.4 × 100/1= **40 units**

14. **Calculate the half life of a drug with a volume of distribution of 60 L and a clearance of 2.1 L/min.**

$$T_{1/2} = \frac{0.693 \times Vd}{CL}$$

Vd: Volume of distribution; CL: Clearance

$T_{1/2}$ = 0.693 × 60/2.1 ~ **20 min**

15. **Calculate the target steady-state plasma concentration for a drug with a maintenance dose of 60 mg/hr and a clearance of 50 mL/min.**

$MD = C_{pss} \times CL$

MD: maintenance dose; C_{pss}: steady-state concentration; CL: clearance

$C_{pss} = MD / CL$

$$C_{pss} = \frac{60\,mg/hr}{50 \times 60\,mL/hr}$$

= **0.2 mg/mL or 200 µg/mL**

16. **Calculate the loading dose for a drug with Vd of 30 L and C_{pss} of 20 mg/L. Bioavailability is 60%.**

$$LD = \frac{Vd \times C_{pss}}{F}$$

Where F is bioavailability

LD = 30 × 20/0.6

= 6,000/6 = 1,000 mg or 1 g

17. **What is the dosing frequency for a drug with clearance of 10 L/hr, C_{pss} = 5 mg/L? The dose to be given is 300 mg over 24 hours.**

MD = CL × C_{pss}

= 10 × 5

= 50 mg/hr

Total dose = 300 mg

Thus, 50 mg/hour is to be given every 300/50 = 6 hours

Thus, frequency = 24/6 which is **4 times, i.e., QID**

18. **An infusion of 2 L D5 was started at 8 AM at a rate of 150 mL/hr. At what time will the infusion finish?**

150 mL is given over 1 hr

2L, i.e., 2,000 mL will require 2,000 × 1/150 = 13.33 or **13 hours and 20 min**

Infusion started at 8 AM, so it will end at **9: 20 PM**

PEDIATRIC DOSE CALCULATION

Most drugs in children are dosed according to body weight (mg/kg) or body surface area (BSA) (mg/m^2)

Formulae

- Clark's formula (weight-based)
  - Pediatric dose = body weight/70 × adult dose
    - For example, adult dose = 280 mg and child's weight = 20 kg
      - Pediatric dose = 20/70 × 280 = 80 mg
- Young's formula (age-based)
  - Pediatric dose = [Age (years)/age (years) + 12] × adult dose
    - For example, adult dose = 280 mg and child's age = 8 years
      - Pediatric dose = [8/8+12] × 280
        = 8/20 × 280
        = 112 mg
- Diling's formula (age-based)
  - Pediatric dose = [Age (years)/20] × adult dose
    - For example, adult dose = 300 mg and child's age = 8 years
      - Pediatric dose = [8/20] × 300
        = 120 mg

20.1 Calculate the dose of ceftriaxone in mLs for meningitis for a 5-year-old weighing 18 kg. The dose required is 100 mg/kg/day given IV once daily and the drug comes prediluted in a concentration of 40 mg/mL.

Step 1	Calculate the total dose	18 kg × 100 mg/kg/day = 1800 mg/day
Step 2	Divide the dose by the frequency	1800 mg/day ÷ 1 (daily) = 1800 mg/dose
Step 3	Convert the mg dose to mL	1800 mg/dose ÷ 40 mg/mL = 45 mL once daily

Renal Disease

- Dose adjustment in renal disease depends on the glomerular filtration rate and the therapeutic index of the drug.
- The GFR estimation according to every formula is
  - **The Cockroft Gault formula**
    - » GFR = {((140–age) × weight)/(72 × Serum Creatinine)} × 0.85 (if female)
- The drug dose should be reduced proportionally to the predicted reduction in drug clearance.
- Drugs requiring dose adjustments in renal disease are

• Allopurinol • Lithium • Acyclovir • Amphotericin B • Fexofenadine • Gabapentin • Rivaroxaban	• *Antimicrobials:* ▪ Aminoglycosides ▪ Cephalexin ▪ Amoxicillin ▪ Cefuroxime ▪ Ciprofloxacin ▪ Vancomycin ▪ Piperacillin/Tazobactam

Hepatic Disease

- **Assessing hepatic function:**
  Child-Pugh classification and scoring of the severity of liver disease

Clinical/biochemical indicator	1 point	2 points	3 points
Serum bilirubin (mg/dL)	<2	2–3	>3
Serum albumin (g/dL)	>3.5	2.8–3.5	<2.8
Prothrombin time (s > control)	<4	4–6	>6
Encephalopathy (grade)	None	1 or 2	3 or 4
Ascites	Absent	Slight	Moderate

- Hepatic clearance of a drug is dependent on the hepatic blood flow and hepatic extraction ratio of the drug.
  - If the drug is a high clearance drug (hepatic blood flow dependent) the dose is reduced by 50%.

For example, lignocaine, propranolol, morphine, nitrates.
- If the drug is low clearance (flow independent) the dose is reduced by 25%.
For example, paracetamol, warfarin, anticonvulsants.

Drug Use in Pregnancy

- FDA classified various drugs used in pregnancy into five categories—categories A, B, C, D and X. Category A is considered the safest category and category X is absolutely contraindicated in pregnancy.

Category	*Description*	*Examples*
A	Adequate, well-controlled studies in pregnant women have not shown an increased risk of fetal abnormalities	Vitamins, calcium and levothyroxine
B	Animal studies have revealed no evidence of harm to the fetus; however, there are no adequate and well-controlled studies in pregnant women. OR Animal studies have shown an adverse effect, but adequate and well-controlled studies in pregnant women have failed to demonstrate a risk to the fetus	Acetaminophen and amoxicillin
C	Animal studies have shown an adverse effect and there are no adequate and well-controlled studies in pregnant women. OR No animal studies have been conducted and there are no adequate and well-controlled studies in pregnant women **Risk cannot be ruled out**	Diltiazem and spironolactone
D	Studies, adequate well-controlled or observational, in pregnant women have demonstrated a risk to the fetus. However, the **benefits of therapy may outweigh the potential risk**	Phenytoin and valproic acid
X	Studies, adequate well-controlled or observational, in animals or pregnant women have demonstrated positive evidence of fetal abnormalities. The use of the product is **contraindicated** in women who are or may become pregnant	Thalidomide and warfarin, isotretinoin, estrogen and androgens

- On June 30, 2015, the US Food and Drug Administration (FDA) began implementation of the Pregnancy and Lactation Labeling Rule (PLLR), which replaced the pregnancy letter category system:

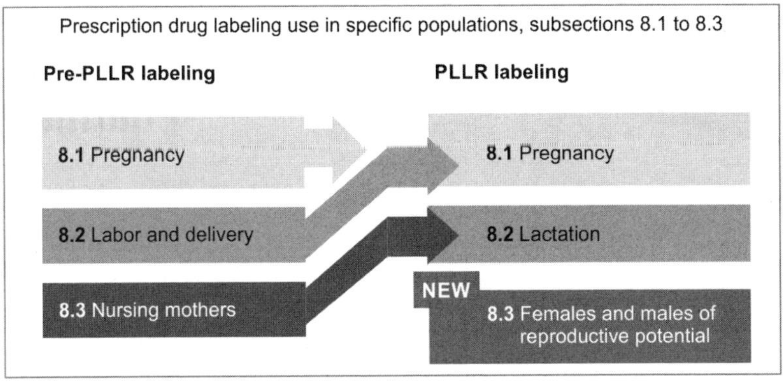

- **8.1: Pregnancy (including labor and delivery)**
  - Pregnancy exposure registry
  - Risk summary
  - Clinical considerations
  - Data
- **8.2: Lactation:**
  - Risk summary
  - Clinical considerations
  - Data
- **8.3: Females and males of reproductive potential:**
  - Pregnancy testing
  - Contraception
  - Infertility

Ganzoni Formula for Parenteral Iron Dosing

Description	***Result***
Ganzoni formula	Iron need (mg iron) = body weight (kg) × (target Hb – actual Hb) × 2.4 + depot iron need (mg iron)
Example patient	
50 kg patient Actual Hb = 11 10 mg/kg assumption for iron stores	Iron need = 50 × (15 – 11) × 2.4 + (10 × 50) Iron need = 980 mg

Dose for Parenteral Iron (FCM) in Anemia

Body weight	***Cumulative FCM dose (Ferric carboxymaltose) FCM***	
	Hb <10 g/dL	Hb 10–14 g/dL
<35 kg	500 mg	500 mg
35–<70 kg	1500 mg	1000 mg
>70 kg	2000 mg	1500 mg

Max tolerated dose: 1,000 mg of iron (20 mL) per dose per day. 1,000 mg of iron not to be administered more once a week.

6 CHAPTER

Pharmacy

The following points should be seen in a *commercial label:*

- The official (pharmacopoeial) nonproprietary name followed by recognized abbreviations of the respective official compendium (e.g., IP, BP, USP, etc.) has to be printed in a more conspicuous manner than the trade name.
- Net contents of all the active ingredients.
- Name and address or place of the manufacturer.
- Distinctive batch number, with the date of the manufacturer, and date of expiry.
- Alcoholic contents if > 3%.
- Schedule G, H, and X drugs. Label of drugs under this schedule have a conspicuous, at least 1 mm thick, line on the left side.
- **Symbol:** Rx for schedule H drugs
- N Rx in red for narcotic drugs
- X Rx for schedule X drugs
- The expiry date is applicable provided the drugs is stored under the specified conditions.
- Store in a cool place means between 10°C to 20°C.
- Store in a cold place means at a temperature not exceeding 8°C.

INDEX

(List of preparations included in this section)

- **Mixtures:**
  - *Solutions:* Salicylate mixture, carminative mixture
  - *Mixtures:* Suspensions: Mist alba
  - *Mixtures:* Emulsions—liquid paraffin, castor oil
- **Liniment:** Turpentine liniment
- **Lotion:** Calamine lotion
- **Ointment:** Antifungal ointment
- **Powder:** Oral rehydration salt

MIXTURES

Solutions

Definition

A mixture is a liquid medicament which contains dissolved, suspended or emulsified substances in a suitable vehicle and is meant for internal use. A single, effective dose of a mixture administered is called a draught.

Advantages

- Absorbed faster than solids preparations.
- Some drugs can be given only as mixtures, e.g., castor oil or liquid paraffin.
- Some substances are more effective if given in liquid form, e.g., antacids given in the form of a suspension for peptic ulcer.
- Some mixtures, e.g., potassium iodide are given in liquid form as they are irritant if taken in the dry state (powder or tablet) and may cause. They are often more palatable.
- They are easy to administer.

Methods to make mixtures more acceptable

Mixtures are less offensive and more elegant by altering or modifying their color, taste and flavor by addition of, correctives. Taste masked by adding sweet and/or sour agents or by making the mixture effervescent.

Disadvantages

- Increase in the incidence of dental caries
- Advisable to avoid them as far as possible

Agents used to mask taste

- **Sweetening agents:** These are commonly used in children and include sugar, glycerine, glycyrrhiza (incompatible with acids) and saccharine (1:2000 or 1:100000). These improve alkaline, sour or salty tastes. They do not improve astringent and bitter tastes.
- **Sour agents:** Citric acid and its preparations, e.g., lemon syrup. They improve salty, insipid and bitter tastes.

Agents for flavor

- The flavour is taste with smell. Flavoring agents include mild flavors—lemon, orange, cherry, raspberry, anise, and fennel. Strong flavors—cinnamon, clove, peppermint, cardamom or ginger (these are added to disagreeable substances).
- Other flavoring agents—oil of rose, oil of bitter almonds, lavender, vanillin and balsam.

Types of Mixtures

1. *Solutions (antipyretic mixture):*
   Solutions can be of two types:
   a. Simple solutions containing soluble solids, e.g., oral rehydration solution. The mixture is made my stirring the solid in the liquid.

b. Solutions containing insoluble solids made soluble with the use of other substances, e.g., mixture of Lugol's iodine (iodine in potassium iodide).

2. *Suspensions: (Mist Alba)*
   A suspension is a liquid medicament containing insoluble (diffusible or non-diffusible) substances which are homogeneously distributed throughout the vehicle with/without the help of a suspending agent.
   - Diffusible substances which do not dissolve in water but are mixed so that upon shaking the solids evenly diffuse throughout the liquid for sufficient time to ensure uniform distribution in each dose, e.g., Mist Alba.
   - Non-diffusible substances do not remain evenly distributed in the vehicle long enough to ensure uniformity of the measured dose, and hence a suspending agent has to be added. Often dry powders are dispensed so that the suspensions can be freshly prepared, e.g., ampicillin dry powder for suspension.

   Suspending agents help insoluble substances to stay uniformly distributed throughout the vehicle for a sufficient time after shaking, thereby ensuring that the same amount of ingredients are present in each dose.
3. *Emulsions: (Liquid paraffin)*
   An emulsion is defined as a system of two immiscible liquids, one of which is finely divided into small globules and dispersed into the other with the help of an emulsifying agent (emulgent).
   Thus, the three main components of an emulsion are:
   a. *Continuous/external phase:* The liquid that surrounds the globules of liquid in the dispersed phase.
      » Dispersed/internal phase: The liquid that is broken into fine globules.
      » Emulsions can be used for both internal and external administration and are of two types:
        i. Oil in water (o/w), i.e., oil as dispersed phase and water as continuous phase.
        ii. Water in oil (w/o), i.e., water as dispersed phase and oil as continuous phase.

Differences between o/w and w/o type emulsions:

Oil in water	*Water in oil*
Internal (since oil is better absorbed in a finely divided state, preparation is palatable when water is in the continuous phase) and external administration	Only external application
Milky white appearance	Waxy and translucent appearance
Free dilution by water	Free dilution by oil
Methylene blue imparts uniform blue color	Sudan III imparts uniform red color
Conducts electricity, e.g., Turpentine liniment	Does not conduct electricity, e.g., cold creams

Emulsifying Agents

These are substances, which concentrate as a film at the interface of the two immiscible liquids and thereby lower the interfacial tension. This helps the dispersion of the dispersed phase into fine globules and prevents it from separating into a different layer. There are many types of emulsifying agents and they can be classified into the following groups:

- **Gums :** Gum acacia, gum tragacanth
- **Soaps:** Monovalent, divalent alkalies
- **Proteins:** Casein, gelatin and egg yolk
- **Carbohydrates:** Maltose
- **Synthetic:** Carboxy-methyl-cellulose, Tween 80

Creaming or Sedimentation of an Emulsion

- It is well known that a layer of cream forms on the surface of milk when set aside for sometime.
- This creaming of an emulsion occurs when the oil or fat rises to the surface, but still remains in the form of globules which may be redistributed throughout the continuous phase by shaking. Hence, the instructions "SHAKE WELL BEFORE USE" should be written on the label. When the size of globules is larger, there is a tendency for the emulsion to cream faster.
- Creaming is undesirable since complete separation may take place and inaccurate dosage may result if shaking is not vigorous and prolonged.
- Creaming can be minimized by reducing the size of the fat globules and increasing the viscosity of the dispersion medium.

Cracking or Breaking of an Emulsion

- Unlike creaming which is a reversible process, cracking is an irreversible separation of the two phases, i.e., oil and water. It occurs due to faults in the process of preparing an emulsion.
- Reasons for the use of emulsion mixtures in pharmaceutics, i.e., they facilitate the administration of substances that are immiscible in water.

Pharmacy Preparations

- "Covering" properties of the emulgent mask the bad taste of liquids and make them palatable.
- In the case of an o/w emulsion, extremely small particles of the dispersed phase (oil) are more effective than if the oil is administered in an undivided state.

Examples of Naturally Occurring Emulsions

- **Latex:** It is the milky juice of certain plants and consists of an emulsion of rubber in water. The emulgent is the protein substance.
- **Egg yolk:** The yellow part of the egg is the oil emulsified by protein matter. Egg yolk itself is used as an emulgent under certain conditions.
- **Milk:** The most perfect and naturally occurring emulsion is milk. It contains fat emulsified by protein matter known as casein. It can be easily diluted

with water, without cracking and although it may cream, the fat readily diffuses again on shaking.

Examples:
- Antipyretic or salicylate mixture
- Carminative mixture
- Lugol's iodine

MIXTURES: SOLUTIONS

Antipyretic or Salicylate Mixture

Indications

- Used as antipyretic
- Also can be used as analgesic to relieve body aches and headaches.

Prescription of antipyretic mixture

Dr ABC
Address
Date:

For Mr XYZ
Age: Sex: Weight:
Address:

R_x:

	g/mL
Sodium salicylate	3/
Sodium bicarbonate	4/
Water (qs)	50/

Mix and prepare a mixture.
Divide into three equal doses.

Sign
Reg. No.:

LABEL:

ANTIPYRETIC MIXTURE

Name: ____________________ Age: ________ Sex: ________

Address· ____

Direction for use: One dose given thrice daily.

Date: ____________________ Sign of Pharmacist

TMC LABS

Actions of Ingredients

Sodium Salicylate

It has analgesic (at a dose of 600 mg) and antipyretic action. At higher doses (3–4 g/day), it has anti-inflammatory action. Fever is produced through the generation of IF, Ls, pyrogens, and interferons which induce prostaglandin production in the Hypothalamus. Sodium salicylate inhibits the production of Prostaglandins; therefore, resets the hypothalamic thermostat. It also rapidly reduces fever by promoting peripheral heat loss.

Sodium Bicarbonate

It acts as an antacid and therefore reduces gastric irritation produced by Sodium salicylate.

Water: It acts as a vehicle.

Questions

1. Define mixtures, and enumerate the type of mixtures.
2. Explain the advantages of mixtures.
3. Name agents used as correctives.

CARMINATIVE MIXTURE

Prescription for carminative mixture:

Dr ABC
Address
Date:

For Mr XYZ
Age: Sex: Weight:
Address
R_x:

	g/mL
Sodium bicarbonate	2/
Tincture cardamom compound	1/
Tinture belladonna	0/5
Water (to make)	2/5

Instructions:
Mix and make a solution.
The entire dose is to be taken after meal.

Sign
Reg. No.:
LABEL:

CARMINATIVE MIXTURE

Name: ____________________ Age: ________ Sex: ________
Address: ____
Whole dose to be taken after meal.
Date: __________________ Sign of Pharmacist

TMC LABS

Indications

Flatulence is abdominal discomfort because of increased accumulation of gas in the gastrointestinal tract. Drugs used in the treatment of these are called carminative.

The action of ingredients:

Sodium bicarbonate:
Systemic antacid reacts with gastric acid to liberate CO_2 and CO_2 increases peristalsis and relaxes the esophageal sphincter, Thereby decreasing abdominal discomfort.

Other uses of $NaHCO_3$:
- Acidosis
- Alkaline urine in barbiturate poisoning.

Tincture cardamom:

It is adjuvant, and has carminative, antispasmodic actions. It also acts as coloring and flavoring agent. It contains cardamom, cinnamon, cochined (red color), glycerine.

Tincture belladonna: Antispasmodic action.

Other drugs having carminative action: Peppermint oil, Spearmint oil tincture ginger, and sodium citrate. Dimethicone and simethicone decrease flatulence and act as antifoaming agents.

Tincture: It is an alcoholic solution of a non-volatile substance (70–90% alcohol).

MIXTURES: SUSPENSIONS

MIST ALBA

Liquid preparations containing insoluble (diffusible, or nondiffusible) substances dispersed homogenously throughout the vehicle with/without the aid of a suspending agent.

Two types: (a) Diffusible, e.g., Mist Alba, (b) Nondiffusible, e.g., chalk mixture.

Prescription of Mist Alba preparation:

Dr ABC
Address
Date:

For Mr XYZ
Age: Sex: Weight:
Address
Rx:

	g/mL
Magnesium sulfate	8/
Magnesium carbonate	1/
Water (qs)	25/

Mix and make a suspension.
The entire dose is to be taken early in the morning with plenty of water

Sign
Reg. No.:

LABEL:

MIST ALBA

Name: ____________________ Age:________ Sex:________
Address: ____

SHAKE WELL BEFORE USE

The entire dose is to be taken early in the morning with plenty of water.

Date: __________________ Sign of Pharmacist

TMC LABS

Indications

- It is used as saline or osmotic purgative in the following conditions: Preparation of bowel before surgery or radiological investigations of the abdomen
- In food/drug poisoning
- As an after purge in treatment of tapeworm infestation.

Actions of the Ingredients

Magnesium sulfate (Epsom salt)

- Magnesium sulfate is poorly absorbed from the intestine, and retains water by osmotic action, this distends the bowel and indirectly stimulates peristalsis.
- Magnesium in addition releases cholecystokinin secretion which also increases intestinal fluid secretion and gut motility.

Other uses of magnesium sulfate:

- Applied topically, it decreases edema of boils and carbuncles by its hygroscopic action.
- When given IV, it causes hypotension, therefore used in the treatment of eclampsia.

Adverse effects:

- Contraindicated in patients with renal insufficiency.
- Repeated use of saline purgatives can cause fluid and electrolyte imbalance.
- They are practically not used in treating constipation, because after constipation is common.

Antidote used overdosage of magnesium sulfate: Calcium gluconate IV

Magnesium carbonate:

- Acts as an adjuvant, potentiates the action of magnesium sulfate.
- Prevents the deposition of sulfates in the acidic urine so prevents the formation of stones.

Peppermint water:

- Acts as flavoring and carminative agent
- Used as a vehicle to distribute the above ingredients uniformly.

Important Points

- It is called Mist Alba because Alba means white.
- This mixture contains insoluble but diffusible substances, which do not dissolve in water, but are mixed upon shaking. Therefore, it is a suspension.
- Mist Alba mixture acts within 2 to 3 hours, therefore, it should be given early in the morning.
- It is an osmotic purgative leading to watery diarrhea and dehydration therefore it must be given with plenty of water to ensure that no loss of total body water occurs.
- It is given as draught preparation (single dose).

- Never used for treatment of functional constipation or in patients with piles, organic intestinal obstruction, appendicitis, or undiagnosed abdominal pain.
- **Other osmotic purgatives:** Magnesium hydroxide, sodium sulfate, (Glauber's salt), sodium potassium tartrate (Rochelle salt), lactulose.

Questions

1. Define mixture.
2. Enumerate types of mixtures.
3. Define suspension.
4. Define suspending agents.
5. Enumerate the properties of a good suspension.

MIXTURES: EMULSIONS

1. Liquid Paraffin

Emulsion is a liquid medicament containing two immiscible liquids, one of which is finely divided into small globules and dispersed into the other with the help of the emulsifying agent, e.g., liquid paraffin, castor oil.

Prescription for liquid paraffin emulsion:

Dr ABC
Address
Date:

For Mr XYZ
Age: Sex: Weight:
Address:
Rx:

	g/mL
Liquid paraffin	24/
Gum acacia	6/
Water (qs)	75/

Make an emulsion and dispense.
One dose at bedtime for three consecutive nights

Sign:
Reg. No.:

LABEL:

LIQUID PARAFFIN

Name: ____________________ Age: __________ Sex: __________
Address: ____

SHAKE WELL BEFORE USE

Directions: One dose at bedtime for three consecutive nights

Date: ___________________ Sign of Pharmacist

TMC LABS

Indications

It is used as a laxative in the following conditions:

- Bedridden patients (having myocardial infarction, postoperative fractures cases)
- In patients where straining at stools is to be avoided (patients with a hernia, piles, fissures, anal surgeries or post coronary artery bypass surgery (CABS). Here, it is important to keep stools soft.
- Used in constipation during pregnancy, and in old age.

Action of Ingredients

Liquid paraffin:

It is a mineral oil having lubricant action. It coats the stools and has softening action when taken for 2–3 days.

Disadvantages:

- Bland in taste.
- While swallowing, it can be aspirated into the lungs causing lipoid pneumonia
- From the intestinal mucosa, small amounts may go to the mesenteric lymph nodes causing granulomas.
- On chronic use, it interferes with the absorption of fat-soluble vitamins.
- May interfere with the healing near the anorectal region.
- May cross the anal sphincter and can cause embarrassment to the patient

Other uses of liquid Paraffin:

- Lubricant for insertion of catheters
- Skin emollient for various skin disorders, such as dry eczema.

Gum Acacia:

- Gummy exudates from Acacia arabica.
- It is a water-soluble emulsifying agent, used mainly to prepare o/w emulsions.

Important Points

Liquid paraffin takes 1–3 days to produce soft-formed feces—other emollient laxatives—docusates

CASTOR OIL EMULSION MIXTURE (EMULSION)

Prescription for castor oil emulsion:

Dr ABC
Address
Date:

For Mr XYZ
Age: Sex: Weight:
Address
Rx:

	g/mL
Castor oil	8/
(shake well before use)	
Gum acacia	2/
Water to make	25/

Instructions

Mix and make emulsion—shake well before use. Entire dose taken early in the morning before breakfast which plenty of fluids.

Sign:
Reg. No.:

LABEL:

CASTOR OIL EMULSION

Name: ____________ Age: ________ Sex: ________
Address: ____________________

A Whole dose taken early in the morning before breakfast with plenty of fluids

Date: ____________ Sign of Pharmacist

TMC LABS

Indications

It is used as saline or osmotic purgative in the following conditions:
- Preparation of bowel before surgery or radiological investigations of the abdomen
- In food/drug poisoning
- As an after purge in treatment of tapeworm infestation.

Action of Ingredients

Castor oil: Obtained from seeds of Ricinus communis. When taken orally, it acts in small intestine, hydrolyzed by pancreatic lipase to glycerol and ricinoleic acid. Ricinoleic acts as irritant and reduces absorption of electrolytes.

Disadvantages

- Structural damage to intestinal villi (long-term use)
- Dehydration
- After constipation

Gum Acacia: Suspending and emulsifying agent. Also helps to make emulsion palatable. Obtained from stems/branches of Acasia Arabica.

Other emulsifying agents: Gum tragacanth, casein, egg yolk carboxy methyl cellulose.

Questions

1. Define mixtures.
2. Enumerate types of mixtures.
3. Describe components of emulsions.
4. Types of emulsions.
5. Define emulsifying agents and give examples.
6. Explain cracking of emulsions.
7. Name two naturally occurring emulsions.

LOTIONS

Lotions are liquid preparations, containing one or more active ingredients, intended for topical application to skin or mucous membrane, without friction.

Types of lotions: For application on skin—the majority of lotions are for application to unbroken skin. However, some lotions, such as eye lotions, mouth washes, gargles or vaginal irrigation solutions can be applied to the mucosa.

Lotions are usually suspensions of solids in an aqueous medium, though some lotions may be solutions or emulsions.

Examples:
- **Suspensions:** Calamine lotion, hydrocortisone lotion
- **Solutions:** Povidone iodine solution, clotrimazole solution
- **Emulsions:** Benzyl benzoate lotion

Properties

- Lotions, usually have soothing and protective properties. Many lotions containing antiseptic, anesthetic, antihistaminic, antipruritic, astringent, anti-inflammatory or antimicrobial agents and other types of agents, such as sunscreens for the treatment or prevention of a variety of skin disorders.
- Lotions are also widely employed as cleansing preparations for mucosal surfaces as exemplified by eye lotions and mouthwashes. Lotions are stable preparations, lotions can be applied to hairy areas of the body, such as the scalp. However, they need to be used in relatively large quantities, especially for cleansing purposes.

Requirements of a good lotion:
- Though lotions are applied without friction, the insoluble matter they contain must be finely divided and made uniform so that an accurate amount of the dose is applied each time.
- Some particles having colloidal dimensions are more soothing to inflamed areas and more effective when applied to infected surfaces.
- If glycerine is added then it keeps the skin moist for long periods of time.
- Lotions which are meant to evaporate quickly from the skin surface, then the vehicle is alcoholic (e.g., salicylic acid lotion) and acetone may also be included.
- Lotions must be prepared and dispensed in an attractive manner, as the cosmetic aspect of lotions is of considerable importance.

Preparation of lotions:
Lotions are prepared by triturating the ingredients into a smooth paste and then adding the remaining vehicle with continuous trituration.

Dispensing and labeling:
- Lotions are preferably dispensed in oval bottles that are vertically ribbed (fluted) down the back. This characteristic of the lotion bottle warns the user (in the dark or if he has impaired eyesight) that the contents are not to be taken orally.

- The warning 'FOR EXTERNAL USE ONLY' should be put on the label. Patients should be told while dispensing, not to apply the lotion to broken skin and to keep inflammable products away from naked flames.

Examples:

Potassium permanganate lotion, tincture iodine lotion and calamine lotion.

Prescription for Calamine lotion:

Dr ABC
Address
Date:

For Mr XYZ
Age: Sex: Weight:
Address:
Rx:

	g/mL
Prepared calamine	7/5
Zinc oxide	2/5
Glycerine	2/5
Bentonite	1/5
Rose water (qs)	50/

Instructions:

Mix and prepare a lotion
To be applied over the affected part without friction.

Sign:
Reg. No.:

LABEL:

CALAMINE LOTION

Name: ____________________ Age: ________ Sex: ________
Address: ____
Mix and prepare a lotion
To be applied over the affected part without friction.
Date: ______________________ Sign of Pharmacist

TMC LABS

Calamine lotion has astringent, antipruritic and soothing action, so it is useful in dry eczema (not wet eczema), all forms of atopic allergies, sunburns, insect bites, pruritus and contact dermatitis.

Actions of Ingredients

- **Prepared calamine:** It is zinc carbonate (98%) tinted with ferric oxide (2%) which adds pink color to the lotion. It has astringent properties (astringent is a agent which causes precipitation of surface proteins, applied to skin or mucous forming a protective coating over the skin surface). It also has antipruritic action. It has a soothing and protective effect on the skin (protective are substances which prevent skin and mucous membrane from contact with irritant substances).

- **Zinc oxide:** It acts as an adjuvant. It has a mild astringent, and mild antiseptic action and an antiperspirant action.
- **Glycerine:** It is a hygroscopic solvent. It keeps the drug in contact with skin for longer time, prevents drying up of the lotion. It has demulcent and emollient actions. It also keeps the skin moist and soft.
- **Bentonite:** It is hydrated aluminum silicate. It is insoluble in water, and swells up to approximately 12 times its original volume to form a homogenous mass. It acts as an adsorbent increasing the viscosity of the lotion. It also acts as a suspending agent.
- **Rose water:** It has a cooling and soothing effect. It is used as a vehicle.

Important Points

- Calamine lotion is to be applied over the affected part twice or thrice a day but is not to be applied over mucous membrane.
- Other agents, such as sodium citrate and liquefied phenol are also added in some lotions. Sodium citrate acts as suspending agent for calamine and zinc oxide. It also helps to keep the product homogenous and also prevents frothing. Liquefied phenol contains 80% phenol and 20% water. It has antiseptic, local anesthetic and antipruritic action.
- Emollients are substances, which are used for local action on skin and mucus membrane as softening agents. They soften the skin by forming an occlusive oil film on the skin and thus prevent drying of skin.
- Lotions can be also used on mucosal surface, e.g., eye lotions, mouth washes.
- It is important that lotions are dispensed in oval bottles that vertically rubbed down (fluted) in black or amber colored bottles. {This warns the user that the contents are not to be taken orally.}

1. Define Lotion.
2. Explain difference between lotions and liniments.

POWDERS

- A powder is a solid dosage form, which contains one, or more ingredients mixed with each other in a dry and finely divided state.
- A powder must weigh at least 100 mg. If the quantity is less, it is made up to 100 mg by adding a suitable diluent, e.g., lactose, sodium bicarbonate, magnesium oxide, kaolin.
- The powders are usually dispensed in sachets or may be wrapped in paper.

Classification of Powders

- **Simple powders:** Containing a single constituent weighing 100 mg or more.
- **Compound powder:** Containing more than one constituent, e.g., ORS powder.

Advantages

- Powders would be a suitable form of administration for insoluble salts and for substances, which are incompatible in mixture.
- The dose can be weighed out accurately.
- Powders can be keep well for a long period of time.
- They are easy to dispense even in multiple doses.
- They are comparatively inexpensive .

Disadvantages

- Difficult to mask the taste of ingredients.
- Some people find it difficult to swallow the powder.

Examples:

- ORS (oral rehydration salt)
- Seidlitz powder
- Antacid powder

Prescription of ORS (Original WHO formula) for a (child having dehydration due to diarrhea):

Dr ABC
Address
Date:

For Mr XYZ
Age: Sex: Weight:
Address
Rx:

	g/mL
Sodium chloride	3/5
Sodium bicarbonate	2/5
Potassium chloride	1/5
Glucose	20/

Instructions

Mix and make a powder and dispense.

The whole quantity has to be mixed in 4 tumblerful of full of boiled and cooled water. To be taken as 1 tsp every 2 minutes. Reconstituted solution to be used within 24 hours.

Sign:
Reg. No.:

LABEL:

ORS (WHO formula)

Name: ____________________ Age: ______ Sex: ________
Address: ______________________________________
Mix and prepare a lotion
Mix and make a powder and dispense.
The whole quantity has to be mixed in 4 tumblerful of full of boiled and cooled water. To be taken as 1 tsp every 2 minutes. Reconstituted solution to be used within 24 hours.

Date: ____________________ Sign of Pharmacist

TMC LABS

Composition of ORS-citrate

Rx:

	g/mL
Sodium chloride	3/5
Trisodium citrate	2/9
Potassium chloride	1/5
Glucose	20/

Indications

The WHO ORS is based on composition of cholera stools particularly in children. ORS replaces the fluid and electrolyte lost in diarrhea and thus maintain fluid and electrolyte balance.

Used in:

- Mild-to-moderate diarrhea
- Maintenance therapy of severe diarrhea after correction of dehydration with IV fluids.

Non-diarrheal uses:

Post-surgical, post-burn, post-trauma patients for maintenance of hydration and nutrition.

Action of Ingredients

- **Sodium chloride:** In diarrhea, there is excessive loss of sodium from the stools, which is replaced by the sodium in the ORS.
- **Sodium bicarbonate or sodium citrate:** In the original WHO formula, sodium bicarbonate was used which was then replaced by Na citrate. Sodium bicarbonate becomes caked and develops brown color due to formation of furfural compounds by chemical reaction between sodium bicarbonate and glucose. Therefore, it has been replaced by sodium citrate. This makes the preparation more stable as it has longer shelf life and does not undergo this type of reaction. The citrate and bicarbonate used in the ORS powder corrects the acidosis. It may also promote salt and water absorption.
- **Glucose:** In the ileum and colon, in addition to the active Na K ATPase mediated sodium absorption, there is also glucose facilitated sodium absorption; one sodium ion is transported along with each molecule of glucose absorbed. Thus, glucose helps in the absorption of Na and water across the intestinal epithelium. **Glucose used in ORS is not to provide energy to the patient.**

Method of Administration

The above ORS should be reconstituted in 1 liter or 4 tumblers of boiled and cooled water. The solution once prepared should be used within 12–24 hours to avoid bacterial contamination.

Adult patients should be encouraged to drink reconstituted ORS at every half to one-hour interval. In mild diarrhea (i.e., not more than one stool every 2 hours), patient should approximately consume 100 mL/kg/day, till the diarrhea stops. In moderate diarrhea (more than 1 stool every hour), dose is 10 mL/kg 1 hour.

In children, 1 tsp per minute can provide 200–300 mL/hour of the reconstituted solution. If vomiting is present withhold ORS for 10 minutes. Then start again.

Important Points

- ORS is not designed to stop diarrhea but to restore and maintain the hydration, electrolytes and pH balance till the diarrhea stops.
- When ORS is given to a breastfeeding child, the mother should be advised to continue breastfeeding.

Other Types of ORS

- **Super ORS:** Improvement in WHO ORS is done by adding actively transported amino acids (alanine, glycine), which cotransports Na. The efficacy is only marginal and also not much cost-effective.
- **Cereal-based ORS:** Rice and other food sources of starch are hydrolyzed at the brush border into glucose, which is absorbed. It does not cause osmotic diarrhea even when larger quantities is added.
  Rice has 7% protein, which yields amino acids, which may stimulate salt and water absorption.
- **Home-based ORS:**
  - *Table salt:* One teaspoon or 1 pinch
  - *Sugar:* 4 tablespoon or one handful
  - *Water:* 1 cup

IV Rehydration

- This is given in severe dehydration, and in patients of shock.
- The solutions used are—Ringer lactate, normal saline, and diarrhea treatment solution.

LINIMENT

Liniments are liquid preparations containing one or more active ingredients, generally with rubefacient or counterirritant properties, for external application with friction.

Liniments are usually mixtures of dissolved, suspended or emulsified ingredients.

Examples:

- **Suspension:** Compound calamine liniment
- **Emulsion:** Turpentine liniment

Important differences between lotions and liniments:

Lotions	*Liniments*
Applied to skin or mucosa	Applied only to skin
Applied without friction	Applied with friction
Cooling, soothing, protective properties	Rubefacient, counterirritant, analgesic properties
Do not contain camphor	Contain camphor or other irritants

Liniments are intended for rubbing into the skin and their oil or soap components increase ease of application and massage. Alcoholic liniments penetrate skin more readily than those with an oily base.

Mechanism of Action of Liniments

- Liniments have counter-irritant action (due to the volatile oils used in them). They stimulate the area of the skin, and reduce the ascending traffic of pain signals from underlying deeper or visceral structures supplied by the same segment of the spinal cord. This helps to temporarily decrease pain from the deeper structures.
- Thus, liniments are used in various musculoskeletal aches and pains, as well as in conditions, such as sciatica or arthritis. Liniments may contain additional ingredients that confer analgesic, astringent or emollient properties.

Dispensing labeling requisites:

Liniments should be dispensed in fluted bottles clearly labeled 'FOR EXTERNAL USE ONLY' .

Liniments should not be applied to bruised or broken skin.

Example:

TURPENTINE LINIMENT

Prescription of Turpentine Liniment:

Dr ABC
Address
Date:

For Mr XYZ
Age: Sex: Weight:
Address
Rx:

	g/mL
Turpentine oil	32/50
Camphor	2/5
Soft-soap	3/
Water (qs)	50/

Make liniment.
To be applied on the skin with friction thrice daily.

Sign:
Reg. No.:

LABEL:

TURPENTINE LINIMENT

Name: ____________________ Age: ______ Sex: _______
Address: ____
To be applied on the skin with friction thrice daily.
Date: __________________ Sign of Pharmacist

TMC LABS

Applied topically for temporary relief of minor aches and pains of muscles and joints, sprains, bruises, and fibrositis. It is also used as an adjuvant in the treatment of lumbago, stiff neck, backache, and torticollis.

Action of Ingredients

1. **Turpentine oil:** It is obtained from the plant pinus. It has rubefacient and counterirritant actions. Rubefacient is an irritant substance, which causes hyperemia. Counterirritants are those substances, which tend to relieve pain by stimulating sensory nerves.
   These sensory nerves compete with pain impulses from the affected area for neurotransmission to the higher centers in the brain.

They also increase the blood flow in the area applied and promote healing of chronic conditions of the skin.

2. **Camphor:** It is a volatile oil has cooling and counterirritant action. It enhances the action of turpentine oil It gives characteristic odor to the preparation and decreases the chance of the liniment being taken orally.
3. **Soft soap:** It acts as an emulsifying agent and helps in the application of the liniment.

Important Points

- Liniment is an emulsion (Oil; in water).
- **Other agents used as counterirritants:** Camphor, menthol, thymol, oil of wintergreen, capsaicin, eucalyptus, methyl salicylate. NJ liniment is for topical application only on unbroken skin, not on mucous membrane.
- Vesicants are very strong irritant substances, which can cause increase permeability and causes collection of fluid beneath the epidermis.
- Liniments should be dispensed in fluted bottles (indicates NOT for oral use).

Questions:

1. Define liniments.
2. Explain four differences between liniment and lotion.

OINTMENTS

Ointments are semisolid greasy preparations for application to the skin or mucous membrane.

They have protective and emollient effects. The base used in an ointment is usually anhydrous and contains one or more medicaments. The vehicle of an ointment is known as an ointment base. The choice of the base depends upon the clinical indication for the ointment, and the different types of ointment bases are:

1. **Hydrocarbon bases**: These have poor penetrability, superficial action and good stability and do not turn rancid. They are used when a superficial or simple protective action is desired, e.g., hard paraffin, soft paraffin.
2. **Absorption bases**: These are hydrophilic and can absorb considerable amounts of water. They have better penetrability and are easier to spread, e.g., animal bases, such as wool fat, beeswax, hydrous wool fat.
3. **Water-soluble bases:** These are water-soluble and hence easily removed from the skin. They have excellent penetrability, are non-greasy and spread easily, e.g., macrogols 200, 300, 400.
4. **Pastes:** Pastes differ from ointments in containing a large amount of finely powdered solids and hence are often very stiff. Like ointments they are emollient but are less greasy in nature.
   When applied to the skin, they adhere well, forming a thick coat that protects and soothes inflamed and raw surfaces. They are often used to treat oozing and moist lesions, such as burns and open wounds where they absorb serous fluid and secretions.
5. **Creams:** Creams are semisolid emulsions containing medicinal agents for external use. There are two kinds, aqueous and oily creams in which the emulsions are oil in water and water in oil respectively. Creams are less messy to use and the aqueous creams are relatively non-greasy.
6. **Jellies:** Jellies are translucent, non-greasy semisolid preparations used externally. The gelling agent may be gelatin or a carbohydrate, such as starch. They contain a considerable amount of water and are particularly suitable as vehicles for water-soluble medicaments, such as local anesthetics, spermicides and antiseptics. They are used for medication, lubrication and some miscellaneous uses, e.g., electrocardiography.

Properties and Uses of Common Dermatological Preparations

Surface (disease)	*Preparation*	*Effect*	*Examples*
Dry and scaly (dry eczema, psoriasis)	Ointment	Occlusive emollient	Soft white or yellow paraffin, lanolin
Moist or dry (eczema in various stages)	Cream	Cooling, emollient and moisturizing	Oily or aqueous cream
Wet and oozing (weeping eczema, bullous diseases)	Lotion	Drying, soothing cooling	Calamine lotion

Surface (disease)	***Preparation***	***Effect***	***Examples***
Lichenified (eczema)	Paste	Protective, prevents spreading of active ingredient	Zinc compound paste, Tar paste
Flexures, if sore, moist (intertrigo, psoriasis)	Dusting powders	Lessen friction, drying	Talc (used as a vehicle for antifungal drugs)

Examples:
- Salicylic and benzoic acid ointment
- Sulfur ointment
- Atropine ointment

Prescription of Salicylic and Benzoic Acid Ointment:

Dr ABC
Address
Date:

For Mr XYZ
Age: Sex: Weight:
Address

Rx:

	g/mL
Benzoic acid	1/
Salicylic acid	1/
Yellow soft paraffin	50/

Prepare an ointment.
Direction for use: To apply on the affected part 3 times in a day.

Sign:
Reg. No.:

LABEL:

OINTMENT

Name: ____________________ Age: ________ Sex: ________
Address: ____
To be applied on the affected part 3 times in a day.
Date: ______________________ Sign of Pharmacist

TMC LABS

Whitfield's ointment:

Rx:

	g/mL
Benzoic acid	6/
Salicylic acid	3/
Yellow soft paraffin	50/

Indications

It is used as antifungal ointment especially in ringworm infection. Increase in concentration of salicylic acid makes the ointment more effective in hyperkeratotic lesions, such as corns, warts, psoriasis, athlete's foot.

Action of Ingredients

1. **Benzoic acid:** It is fungi static, therefore, eradication of fungus takes prolonged application, and has to applied till the time infected keratin is shed off. It also has antibacterial property in acidic medium.
2. **Salicylic acid:** It has keratolytic, fungicidal and bacteriostatic action. It is used in hyperkeratotic lesions, such as corns and warts.
3. **Yellow soft paraffin:** Paraffin acts as a hydrocarbon base, facilitates the absorption of the drug in the skin.

Important Points

Ointment should not be applied to broken skin or inflamed skin. Its use should be discontinued if excessive dryness and irritation of the skin occurs.

Questions

1. Define ointment.
2. Enumerate various ointment bases.
3. What are the properties, which affect the choice of the ointment base?
4. What are various methods of preparation of ointments?
5. Explain important features of eye ointment.
6. Define paste, creams, jellies, and explain differences from an ointment.
7. Explain how an ointment is dispensed.

7 CHAPTER

Clinical Pharmacology Section

Practical 9: Rational, correct and legible generic prescription writing for a given condition and communicating the same to the patient.

Exercise: Write a prescription for the following conditions.

7.1: CARDIOVASCULAR SYSTEM

1. **Mr Harish, 60 years of age is a known case of congestive cardiac failure (CCF). He presents to the OPD with signs of acute CCF. Prescribe suitable drugs for this patient.**

   Rx:
   - Tab Enalapril 5 mg once daily for 15 days
   - Tab Metoprolol ER (25 mg) half tablet once daily for 15 days

   Non-pharmacological treatment:
   - Salt and water restriction
   - Weight reduction with regular exercise

   Follow up: After 15 days for evaluation and dose adjustment, if required.

   Dispense: 15 tablets of enalapril 5 mg and 8 tablets of metoprolol 25 mg ER

   Doctor sign and stamp
   Registration no.

   Important points
   - The dose can be gradually increased to the maximum tolerated dose. (Metoprolol ER 200 mg/day, enalapril 40 mg/day).
   - Electrolyte monitoring should carry out throughout the therapy
   - Potassium supplements, potassium-sparing diuretics and ACE inhibitors (increase serum K) and diuretics (decrease potassium). use these drugs cautiously.

2. **Prescribe for a patient with heart failure with LVF (>40%) with fluid retention.**

Rx:
- Tab Enalapril 5 mg 1 tablet once daily for 15 days
- Tab Metoprolol ER (25 mg) half tablet once daily for 15 days
- Tab Furosemide 20 mg twice daily for 15 days

Non-pharmacological treatment:
- Salt and water restriction
- Weight reduction with regular exercise

Follow up: After 15 days with serum electrolytes for evaluation and dose adjustment if required.

Dispense: 15 tablets of enalapril 15 mg, 8 tablets of metoprolol ER 25 mg, and 30 tablets of furosemide 20 mg

Doctor sign and stamp
Registration no.

Important points
- The dose can be gradually increased to the maximum tolerated dose. (Metoprolol ER 200 mg/day, enalapril 40 mg/day, furosemide 600 mg/day in the clinically severe edematous state).
- Electrolyte monitoring should be continued throughout the therapy
- Potassium supplements, potassium-sparing diuretics and ACE inhibitors (increase serum K) and diuretics (decrease potassium). Use these drugs cautiously.

3. **Patient M had difficulty breathing at rest, forgetfulness, mild fatigue, feeling chilled requiring blankets, increased urinary frequency, incontinence, and swelling in her bilateral lower extremities that is new onset and worsening. Subsequently, she has not ambulated from bed for several days except to use the restroom due to feeling weak, fatigued, and short of breath. She was diagnosed with heart failure with LVEF <35% Write a prescription for CCF (moderate)**

Moderate CCF:

Rx:
- Tab Enalapril 5 mg 1 tablet once daily
- Tab Metoprolol 50 mg ER once daily
- Tab Furosemide 20 mg twice daily till edema subsides
- Tab Spironolactone 25 mg once daily

Non-pharmacological treatment
- Salt and water restriction
- Weight reduction with regular exercise

Follow up: After 15 days with serum electrolytes for evaluation and dose adjustment if required.

Dispense: 15 tablets of enalapril 5 mg, 15 tablets of metoprolol 50 mg ER, 30 tablets of furosemide 20 mg and 15 tablets of spironolactone 25 mg

Doctor sign and stamp
Registration no.

Important points

- The dose can be gradually increased to the maximum tolerated dose.
- (Metoprolol ER 200 mg/day, Enalapril 40 mg/daily).
- Electrolyte monitoring should be continued throughout the therapy
- Potassium supplements, potassium-sparing diuretics and ACE inhibitors (increase serum K) and diuretics (decrease potassium). Use these drugs cautiously.

4. **A 62-year-old male smoker with type 2 diabetes mellitus and hypertension presents with a 4-month history of exertional chest pain. Physical examination shows a blood pressure of 152/90 mm Hg but is otherwise unremarkable. The ECG is normal, and laboratory tests show a fasting blood glucose value of 110 mg/dL, glycosylated hemoglobin 6.0%, creatinine 1.1 mg/dL, total cholesterol 160, LDL 135 mg/dL, HDL 38, and triglycerides 147 mg/dL. His exercise stress test is positive. Write a prescription for the patient. (Angina Pectoris)**

Rx:

- Tab Isosorbide mononitrate 10 mg 1 tablet twice daily
- Tab Metoprolol ER 25 mg 1 tablet once daily
- Tab Aspirin 75 mg 1 tablet once daily
- Tab Atorvastatin 10 mg 1 tablet once daily for 15 days

Non-pharmacological treatment

- No smoking or alcohol
- Moderate exercise
- Weight reduction

Follow up: After 15 days for evaluation and dose adjustment if required.

Dispense: 30 tablets of isosorbide mononitrate 10 mg, 15 tablets of metoprolol 25 mg ER, aspirin 75 mg and atorvastatin 10 mg each

Doctor sign and stamp
Registration no.

Important points

- Instead of isosorbide mononitrate, isosorbide dinitrate 40 mg once daily can be prescribed.

- Dose of isosorbide dinitrate for prophylaxis can be increased to max 120 mg/day, atorvastatin 80 mg/day,
- Maximum dose of metoprolol ER 25 mg is 200 mg/day, or atenolol can be increased to max 100 mg/day
- Instead of atenolol and isosorbide dinitrate, calcium channel blockers, such as diltiazem ER can be prescribed.

5. **A 57-year-old male presents to OPD with exertional chest pain. Physical examination shows a blood pressure of 152/90 mm Hg but is otherwise unremarkable. Physical examination shows a blood pressure of 152/90 mm Hg but is otherwise unremarkable. The ECG is normal. What will be advised for this patient? (Acute Angina Pectoris)**

Rx:
- Tab Nitroglycerine 0.5 mg 1 tablet kept under the tongue (sublingual) until every 5 minutes, till a maximum of 10 minutes (can add two more tablets at 5-minute intervals)
- Tab Aspirin 325 mg stat and tab Clopidogrel 300 mg stat
- When the acute attack subsides, start prophylaxis with
- Tab Isosorbide dinitrate 10 mg 1 tablet twice daily for 5 days
- Tab Metoprolol ER 25 mg 1 tablet once daily for 15 days
- Tab Aspirin 75 mg once a day lifelong
- Tab Atorvastatin (10 mg) 1 tablet once daily for 15 days

Follow up: After 15 days for evaluation and dose adjustment if required.

Doctor sign and stamp
Registration no.

Important points
- Nitroglycerine may cause postural hypotension so it should be given in lying down or sitting position.
- Instead of tab Nitroglycerine, tab Isosorbide dinitrate 5 mg tablet sublingually can also be used.
- If there is no relief then suspect acute myocardial infarction or unstable angina and transfer the patient to the ICCU.

  Maximum dose of isosorbide dinitrate for prophylaxis: 120 mg/day
  Maximum dose of atorvastatin for prophylaxis: 80 mg/day

6. **Mathura a 35-year-old executive is diagnosed with essential hypertension. The average BP from 3 consecutive readings is 158/100 mm Hg. Prescribe suitable drugs for this patient. (Mild hypertension)**

Rx:

Tab Enalapril 5 mg 1 tablet once daily for 15 days

Non-pharmacological treatment
- Salt and water restriction
- Weight reduction with regular exercise

- To quit smoking if smoker
- Reduce alcohol intake

Follow up: After 15 days for evaluation and dose adjustment, if necessary.
Dispense: 15 tablets of enalapril 5 mg

Doctor sign and stamp
Registration no.

Important points

- Instead of enalapril, ramipril can be prescribed.
- If patients experience dry cough then replace enalapril with olmesartan 20 mg once day for 15 days.
- Instead of ACE inhibitor ARBs, such as telmisartan, olmesartan can be prescribed.
- Uptitration should be gradual.
- Treatment may have to be continued for life long.

7. **Mr Raj a 50-year-old man is diagnosed with essential hypertension. The average BP from 3 consecutive readings is 162/110 mm Hg. Prescribe suitable drugs for this patient. (Moderate hypertension)**

Rx:

- Tab Enalapril 5 mg 1 tablet once daily for 15 days
- Tab Amlodipine 5 mg 1 tablet once daily for 15 days

Non-pharmacological treatment

- Salt and water restriction
- Weight reduction with regular exercise
- To quit smoking is smoker
- Reduce alcohol intake

Follow up: After 15 days for evaluation and dose adjustment, if necessary.
Dispense: 15 tablets of enalapril 5 mg and amlodipine 5 mg each

Doctor sign and stamp
Registration no.

Important points

- Instead of enalapril, ramipril can be prescribed.
- If patients experience dry cough then replace enalapril with olmesartan 20 mg once a day for 15 days.
- Instead of ACE inhibitor ARBs, such as telmisartan, olmesartan can be prescribed.
- Uptitration should be gradual.
- Treatment may have to be continued for life long.

8. Mr Avi a 45-year-old man recently diagnosed as hypertensive was receiving enalapril, he developed severe dry brassy cough after 10 days. Prescribe an alternative antihypertensive for him.

Rx:

Tab Telmisartan 20 mg 1 tablet once daily for 15 days

Non-pharmacological treatment

Salt and water restriction, weight reduction with regular exercise to quit smoking if smoker, reduce alcohol intake.

Follow up after 15 days for evaluation and dose adjustment, if necessary.

Doctor sign and stamp
Registration no.

9. Prescribe for a patient with mild hypertension with no associated diseases.

Rx:

Tab Hydrochlorothiazide 25 mg half tablet once daily for 15 days

Non-pharmacological treatment

- Salt and water restriction
- Weight reduction with regular exercise
- To quit smoking, if smoker
- Reduce alcohol intake

Follow up: After 15 days for evaluation and dose adjustment, if necessary.

Dispense: 15 tablets of hydrochlorothiazide 25 mg

Doctor sign and stamp

Registration no.

Important points

- Instead of hydrochlorothiazide, tab Enalapril, tab Telmisartan or tab Atenolol can be prescribed.
- Uptitration should be gradual.
- Treatment may have to be continued for life long.

10. Prescribe suitable drugs for essential hypertension (130/94 mmg Hg) patient having stable exertional angina

Rx:

Tab Metoprolol ER (extended release) 25 mg 1 tablet once daily.

Non-pharmacological treatment

- Salt and water restriction
- Weight reduction with regular exercise
- To quit smoking, if smoker
- Reduce alcohol intake.

Follow up: After 15 days for evaluation and dosage adjustment.
Dispense: 15 tablets of metoprolol 25 mg

Doctor sign and stamp
Registration no.

Important points
- Maximum dose of metoprolol: 200 mg/day
- Instead of metoprolol, calcium channel blockers (amlodipine) can be given.

11. **Prescribe suitable drugs for essential hypertension patients having post myocardial infarction**

Rx:
- Tab Ramipril 2.5 mg1 tablet once daily
- Tab Metoprolol 25 mg ER 1 tablet once daily
- Tab Spironolactone 25 mg 1 tablet once daily (only if ejection fraction <35%)
- Tab Aspirin 75 mg once day life long

Non-pharmacological treatment
- Salt and water restriction
- Weight reduction with regular exercise

Follow up: After 15 days for evaluation and dosage adjustment.
Dispense: 15 tablets of ramipril 2.5 mg, metoprolol ER 25 mg, spironolactone 25 mg

Doctor sign and stamp
Registration no.

Important points
- Maximum dose of ramipril: 20 mg/day
- Maximum dose of metoprolol: 200 mg/day

12. **Write a prescription for pregnancy-induced hypertension.**

Rx:
Tab Labetalol 100 mg 1 tablet twice a day
Follow up: After 15 days for evaluation and dosage adjustment.
Dispense: 15 tablets of labetalol 100 mg

Doctor sign and stamp
Registration no.

Important points
- Maximum dose of labetalol: 2400 mg/day
- If uncontrolled tab Nifedipine SR (30 mg) one tablet daily
- Maximum dose of nifedipine SR: 200 mg/day
- Alpha methyl dopa is safe in pregnancy but unavailable in the market
- ARB's and ACE inhibitors are contraindicated in pregnancy.

13. A 45-year-old man with a 2-month history of progressive headache presented to the emergency department with nausea, vomiting, visual disturbance, and confusion for 1 day. He denied fever, weakness, numbness, shortness of breath, and flu-like symptoms. He had a significant medical history of hypertension and was on a β-blocker in the past, but a year ago, he stopped taking medication due to an unspecified reason. Physical examination was unremarkable, and at the time of triage, his BP was noted as 210/123 mm Hg. The clinical presentation, elevated BP, and brain MRI findings were suggestive of a hypertensive emergency, more specifically hypertensive encephalopathy. Prescribe suitable drugs for this patient

Hypertensive crisis

Rx:

Nicardipine infusion rate of intravenous of 5 mg/h. The maximum infusion rate is 30 mg/h. Inj Nitroglycerine 5–10 μg/min IV infusion titrate as per BP response

Doctor sign and stamp
Registration no.

Important points

- Till recent past sodium nitroprusside has to be titrated carefully. (Aim must be to reduce DBP to 100–110 mm of Hg gradually over 24 hours.
- Instead of the above treatment inj Nitroglycerine 5–10 μg/min IV infusion or inj Labetalol 20–80 mg IV bolus every 10 minutes to max total dose of 300 mg can be prescribed.
- Instead, sublingual nifedipine, inj Diazoxide or inj Hydralazine can also be prescribed.

14. Lisa is a 49-year-old woman with a history of type 2 diabetes, obesity, hypertension, and migraine headaches. Physical examination reveals a BP of 154/98 mm Hg and a pulse of 78 bpm. Prescribe suitable drugs for this patient. (Mild hypertension with diabetes)

Rx:

Tab Enalapril 5 mg 1 tablet once daily for 15 days

Non-pharmacological treatment

- Salt restriction (up to 5 mg salt per day caloric restriction for weight control)
- Restriction in intake of cholesterol and saturated fats
- Reducing or eliminating alcohol intake
- Relief of stress
- Regular exercise

Follow up: After 15 days for evaluation and dose adjustment, if necessary
Dispense: 15 tablets of ramipril 2.5 mg

Doctor sign and stamp
Registration no.

Important point

Instead of enalapril, telmisartan/olmesartan 20 mg once a day for 15 days is a suitable alternative.

15. **Prescribe suitable drugs for a patient with "Mild hypertension and bronchial asthma".**

Rx:

Tab Amlodipine 5 mg 1 tablet once daily for 15 days.

Non-pharmacological treatment

- Salt restriction (up to 5 mg salt per day caloric restriction for weight control)
- Restriction in intake of cholesterol and saturated fats
- Reducing or eliminating alcohol intake
- Relief of stress
- Regular exercise

Follow up: After 15 days for evaluation and dose adjustment, if necessary
Dispense: 15 tablets of amlodipine 5 mg

Doctor sign and stamp
Registration no.

Important point

Instead of amlodipine, ramipril or olmesartan can be prescribed.

16. **Ram Basyal age 49 years comes to causality with central chest pain since 1day with radiating to the shoulder with episodes of shortness of breath. Investigations showed moderate mitral regurgitation (MR), dilated left ventricle, mild tricuspid regurgitation (TR), ECG: ST segment elevation. Prescribe suitable drugs for this patient. (Acute myocardial infarction)**

Rx:

- Complete bed rest
- Sublingual NTG (0.5 mg) every 3 min till 10 minutes
- Inj Morphine 4 mg iv immediately followed by 2 mg every 5–15 minutes till pain is relieved or till toxicity, such as hypotension or respiratory depression is evident.
- O_2 (100%) 2 liters by nasal catheter. Titrate as per requirement

- Tab Aspirin 325 mg stat (chewed immediately)
- Inj Tenecteplase (0.5 mg/kg) single IV bolus injection. OR
- Inj Alteplase 15 mg iv Bolus injection followed by 50 mg over 30 min then 35 mg over next 1 hour
- Inj Metoprolol 5 mg iv every 5 minutes for a total of 3 doses
- Inj NIG 5 μg/min continuous iv infusion increase by 5 μg/min every 5 minutes up to 20 μg/min. Titrate as per requirement
- Inj (low molecular weight heparin) 30 mg iv bolus plus 1 mg/kg SC once, then every 12 hourly
- Inj low low molecular weight heparin 4000 IU SC (60 mg) bolus dose, then repeat every 2 hours
- Tab Clopidogrel 300 mg loading dose then 75 mg daily
- Tab Atorvastatin 40 mg stat then Atorvastatin 40 daily

Doctor sign and stamp
Registration no.

Important points
- NTG is more preferred in patients with active chest pain, need to watch for hypotension.
- For treatment of complications, e.g., arrhythmias inj Lignocaine 2% 50 mg LV as a bolus followed by a drip rate of 1 mg/min. or DC shock. For Bradycardia: Inj Atropine 0.3–0.5 mg LV.
- Monitor metoprolol dose subsequent dose, however, prescribed with caution in decompensated patients.
- General measures, such as diet, and bowel care should be taken care of.
- Rehabilitation is done with aspirin (75 mg) once a day, -blocker (Atenolol), ACE inhibitors, and modification of risk factors, such as smoking, alcohol, Rx: of hypertension, diabetes and hyperlipidemia should be taken care of.
- Before giving streptokinase, Inj Hydrocortisone 100 mg can be given IV to suppress allergic reactions. Instead of alteplase/tenecteplase streptokinase, urokinase can also be given.

17. A 45-year-old, Mr Bhaskar, an obese person, was asked to test for lipid profile. The report showed elevated total cholesterol and LDL while HDL, VLDL and TGs were normal. After counseling for lifestyle and dietary changes also he was found to be overweight. He also told that his mother died of myocardial infarction before 50 years of age. Prescribe suitable drugs for this patient.

Rx:
- Tab Atorvastatin 10 mg 1 tablet once daily at bed time for 15 days
- Tab Aspirin 75 mg 1 tablet once daily after food for 15 days

Non-pharmacological treatment

- Salt restriction (up to 5 mg salt per day caloric restriction for weight control)
- Restriction in intake of cholesterol and saturated fats.
- Reducing or eliminating alcohol intake
- Relief of stress
- Regular exercise

Follow up: After 15 days for evaluation and dose adjustment, if necessary

Dispense: 15 tablets of atorvastatin 10 mg and aspirin 75 mg each

Doctor sign and stamp
Registration no.

Important point

Maximum dosage of atorvastatin: 80 mg at bedtime.

18. Mr Jacob is a 65-year-old diabetic with hypertension who is treated for acute anterior wall myocardial infarction in your hospital. He is now fit for discharge after 6 days of therapy. What will you prescribe for him at discharge?

Rx:

- Tab Aspirin 75 mg 1 tablet once daily
- Tab Metoprolol ER 25 mg 1 tablet once daily
- Tab Enalapril 5 mg 1 tablet once daily

Non-pharmacological treatment

- Modification of risk factors, such as smoking, alcohol, Rx: of hypertension, diabetes and hyperlipidemia should be taken care of.

Follow up: After 15 days for dose adjustment, if necessary

Dispense: 15 tablets of aspirin 75 mg, metoprolol er 25 mg and enalapril 5 mg each

Doctor sign and stamp
Registration no.

19. A 19-year-old boy is brought to the emergency department after being stung by a bee. He had been well until he was stung on his right forearm, while playing in the yard. He initially complained of localized pain and swelling. Fifteen minutes later, he began to complain of shortness of breath. His parents observed him to be wheezing. His parents brought him immediately to the local emergency department, he is diagnosed as having anaphylactic shock. Write a prescription for this patient.

Rx:

- Inj Adrenaline 0.01 mL/kg (0.5 mL to 1 mL) of 1:1000 solution IM. Repeat every 5 minutes.

- Inj Hydrocortisone 100 mg IV stat repeat every 6 hourly.
- Inj Chlorpheniramine 4 mg slow IV repeat every 8 hourly.

Doctor sign and stamp
Registration no.

20. Mr Rameez a 47-year-old man is diagnosed with essential hypertension. The average BP from 3 consecutive readings is 162/94 mm Hg. Prescribe suitable drugs for this patient.

Rx:

Tab Hydrochlorothiazide 25 mg half tablet once daily for 15 days

Non-pharmacological treatment

- Salt restriction (up to 5 mg salt per day caloric restriction for weight control)
- Restriction in intake of cholesterol and saturated fats
- Reducing or eliminating alcohol intake
- Relief of stress
- Regular exercise

Follow up: After 15 days for evaluation and dosage adjustment

Dispense: 8 tablets of hrdrochlorthiazide 25 mg

Doctor sign and stamp
Registration no.

Important point

Instead of hydrochlorothiazide, amlodipine, enalapril/ramipril, olmesartan/telmisartan can be prescribed. Treatment may have to be continued for life long.

21. Hypercholesterolemia (LDL-CH >190 mg/dL in a patient without coronary artery disease.

Rx:

Tab Atorvastatin 20 mg one tablet at bedtime

Non-pharmacological treatment

- Modification of risk factors, such as smoking, and alcohol
- To review after 6 weeks with lipid profile
- LFTs to be started at the beginning of therapy, to repeat after 3 months

Follow up: After 15 days for dose adjustment, if required

Dispense: 15 tablets of atorvastatin 20 mg

Doctor sign and stamp
Registration no.

Important points

- Rx: of associated comorbidities, such as hypertension, and diabetes should be taken care of.
- The dose of atorvastatin is to be gradually increased to a maximum of 80 mg/day.

22. **Hypertriglyceridemia (TG 200–499 mg/dL in a patient with risk of coronary artery disease.**

Rx:

- Tab Atorvastatin 40 mg 1 tablet at bed time
- Tab Gemfibrozil 600 mg 1 tablet twice daily before meals

Non-pharmacological treatment

- Modification of risk factors, such as smoking, alcohol
- Rx: of hypertension, diabetes should be taken care of
- To review after 6 weeks with lipid profile

Follow up: After 15 days for dose adjustment, if required

Dispense: 15 tablets of atorvastatin 40 mg and 30 tablets of gemfibrosil 600 mg

Doctor sign and stamp
Registration no.

Important points

- The dose of atorvastatin is to be gradually increased to a maximum of 80 mg/day
- The maximum dose of gemfibrozil is 1200 mg/day
- LFTs to be started at the beginning of therapy, to repeat after 3 months

7.2: CENTRAL NERVOUS SYSTEM

1. **A 30-year-old male patient presented to your clinic with complaints of insomnia for 2 days. Detailed history reveals that he has had toothache for the past 2 days. Prescribe suitable drug(s) for this patient.**

Rx:

Tab Zolpidem 5 mg 1 tablet at bedtime (HS) for 3 days

Tab Ibuprofen 400 mg 1 tablet after food for 3 days

Tab Pantoprazole 20 mg 1 tablet in morning for 3 days

Non-pharmacological advice:

Cognitive behavioral therapy (CBT) to be used in combination with medication

Follow up: After 7 days for review

Dispense: 3 tablets of zolpidem 5 mg, ibuprofen 400 mg and pantoprazole 20 mg each

Doctor sign and stamp
Registration no.

Important points

- Alternatively eszopiclone, zaleplon or flurazepam/clonazepam could be prescribed
- The cause of insomnia has to be investigated
- Hypnotics are best used only intermittently
- If a benzodiazepine is used for > 15 days the dose should be tapered slowly

2. **A 20-year-old female Ms Kala, experiences seizures characterized by sudden loss of consciousness and then rigidity of the body for a few minutes. This is followed by jerking of the body musculature that lasts for 3–5 minutes followed by a state of flaccidity. Immediately after the seizure, she recovers consciousness but remains in a confused state. Prescribe suitable drug(s) for this patient. (Generalized tonic clonic seizures i.e., GTCS)**

Rx:

Tab Phenytoin sodium 100 mg 1 tablet thrice daily after food for 15 days

Follow up: After 15 days for evaluation and dose adjustment if necessary.

Dispense: 45 such tablets of phenytoin sodium 100 mg

Doctor sign and stamp
Registration no.

Important points

- The dose of phenytoin has to be increased gradually to a dose that control seizures.
- The maximum dose of phenytoin is 600 mg per day.
- Maximum dose of carbamazepine 1200 mg/day)
- Instead of phenytoin tab Carbamazepine (200 mg BD), sodium valproate (10 mg/kg/day) can be prescribed.
- Newer antiepileptics, such as lamotrigine, topiramate, and levetiracetam can be prescribed.
- Treatment for epilepsy has to be continued for at least 5 years.

3. **Febrile convulsions**

Rx:

- Diazepam (10 mg/5 mL) 2.5 mL rectally as a retention enema,
- If a seizure does not stop, repeat after 10 minutes

Doctor sign and stamp
Registration no.

4. **Leanne 6-year-old girl with parents noticing that she seems to have problems listening and to be daydreaming a lot in class. Mother gives h/o of Leanne having daydreams or 'trances' as she calls them, which sometimes occur when she is in the middle of doing or saying something, and they interrupt her activity. Leanne's birth and early medical history, including her development, have been normal. There was a history of epilepsy on her father's side of the family. Prescribe suitable drug(s) for this patient. (Petit-mal epilepsy)**

Rx:

Syrup Sodium Valproate (200 mg/5 mL) 10 mg/kg/day in two divided doses for 15 days.

Follow up: After 15 days for evaluation and dose adjustment if necessary. LFTs are to be started at the beginning of therapy, to repeat after 3 months.

Doctor sign and stamp
Registration no.

Important points

- The dose of valproate can be increased gradually to reach maintenance dose of 20–40 mg/kg/day.
- Higher doses of sodium valproate should be prescribed with caution for the fear of causing fatal hepatitis in children.
- Alternatively ethosuximide (250 mg/5 mL) 10 mL once daily for 15 days. (initial dose for ethosuximide for children 3–6 years is 250 mg per day and for children >6 years, 500 mg per day. The dose is individualized based on patients' responses. (maximum dose is 20 mg/kg/day).
- Lamotrigine can be used as an alternative.

5. **A 22-year-old woman was referred to an epilepsy center because of intractable seizures. A combination of carbamazepine and valproate reduced the seizure frequency to 2 per month, but maximally tolerated dosages of each drug failed to render her seizure-free. She is married and would like to have children. Prescribe suitable drug(s) for this patient.**

Rx:

Tab Lamotrigine XR 50 mg 1 tablet once daily for 2 weeks

Tab Folic acid 5 mg 1 tablet once a day

Follow up: After 15 days for revaluation and dose adjustment

Dispense: 14 tablets of lamotrigine XR 50 mg and folic acid 5 mg each

Doctor sign and stamp
Registration no.

6. **Prescribe a drug therapy for a patient of trigeminal neuralgia.**

Rx:

Tab Carbamazepine 100 mg 1 tablet twice a day gradually increased by 200 mg every 2 days untill relief of pain.

Follow up after 1 week for evaluation.

Doctor sign and stamp
Registration no.

Important point

Dose of carbamazepine can be increased to 1200 mg/day.

7. **Status epilepticus**

Rx:

- To maintain airway, breathing and circulation (ABC)
- Inj Lorazepam 4 mg (0.1 mg/kg) at the rate of 2 mg/min loading dose to be injected slowly IV, repeated once after 10 min if required. If not controlled, up to a maximum of 0.3 mg/kg can be repeated.
- If seizures continue inj Fosphenytoin 100–150 mg/min as IV infusion
- If seizures continue inj Phenytoin 50 mg/min as IV infusion
- If seizures continue then inj Phenobarbitone 60 mg/min as IV infusion
- If still not controlled inj Midazolam 0.2 mg/kg loading dose followed by 0.75–1 μg/kg/min as maintenance dose.

Doctor sign and stamp
Registration no.

Important point

Instead of lorazepam, inj Diazepam 10 mg IV slowly every 15 minutes up to a maximum of 30 mg till convulsions are controlled. The dose of diazepam can be repeated 4 hourly, to a maximum of 100 mg/day.

8. **A 70-year-old male farmer was referred to a movement disorders outpatient clinic due to a 1-year non-disabling intermittent resting tremor of the left hand, that later progressed to the contralateral hand. On neurological examination, the patient had normal cognition. An intermittent mild resting tremor was observed in the left hand, as well as mild signs of asymmetrical cogwheel rigidity and bradykinesia (left > right). Prescribe suitable drug(s) for this patient. (Parkinsonism)**

Rx:

Fixed dose combination of tab Levodopa + Carbidopa (100 mg + 25 mg) 1/2 tablet thrice daily

Follow up: After 15 days for dose evaluation and dose adjustment, if necessary

Dispense: 23 tablets of the FDC tab Levodopa + Carbidopa (100 mg + 25 mg)

Doctor sign and stamp
Registration no.

Important points

- The dose is gradually increased till optimum improvement is achieved (600–700 mg per day of levodopa). It can be increased to 1000 mg per day in divided doses.
- Other drugs, such as trihexyphenidyl, or pramipexole or amantadine can be started.

9. **Drug-induced Parkinsonism**

Rx:

Tab Benzhexol (trihexyphenidyl) 2 mg ¼ tablet twice daily increased to maximum 1 tablet twice daily.

Follow up: After 15 days

Dispense: (maximum) 15 tablets if benzhexol 2 mg

Doctor sign and stamp
Registration no.

Important point

Instead of tab Benzhexol (Trihexyphenidyl), tab Biperiden or tab Promethazine can be used.

10. **Acute dystonic reaction after inj Metoclopramide.**

Rx:

Inj Promethazine (25 mg) IM stat

Doctor sign and stamp
Registration no.

11. **Write a prescription for a patient with Jet lag.**

Rx:

Tab Melatonin 3 mg 1tablet once daily in the evening for 3 days.

Doctor sign and stamp
Registration no.

Important point

Tab Zolpidem can be used as an alternative

12. **Headache (Adult)**

Rx:

Tab Ibuprofen 400 mg stat as and when required after food.

Doctor sign and stamp
Registration no.

Important points

- Instead of ibuprofen, tab Diclofenac, tab Paracetamol can be given.
- NSAIDs can be given along with PPIs to decrease gastric irritation.

13. **A 40-year-old female with previous history of recurrent headaches, is diagnosed as migraine without aura. Prescribe for both acute attack and prophylaxis.**

Rx:

- Tab Sumatriptan (25 mg) 2 tablets immediately repeat (if required) after 2 hours
- Tab Domperidone 10 mg 1 tab immediately and repeat after if required after 8 hours

Followed by prophylaxis with tab Flunarizine 10 mg once day.

Follow up: After 7 days for review

Dispense: 4 tablets of sumatriptan 25 mg, 2 tablet of domperidone 10 mg and 7 tablets of flunarizine 10 mg.

Doctor sign and stamp
Registration no.

Important point

Alternatively for prophylaxis with tab Propranolol one tablet 40 mg twice daily for 6 weeks. Maximum dose of propranolol is 240 mg/day.

14. **A 40-year-old female with previous history of recurrent headaches, is diagnosed as migraine with acute severe migraine attack. Prescribe for both acute severe attack and prophylaxis.**

Rx:

- For severe attacks
- Sumatriptan injection 6 mg/0.5 mL. 6 mg SC may be repeated after 1 hour. (Max 12 mg/day).
- Inj Metoclopramide 10 mg IM single dose.
- Followed by prophylaxis with tab Flunarizine 10 mg once a day.

Doctor sign and stamp
Registration no.

Important points

- Sumatriptan is available as an intranasal spray.
- Instead of sumatriptan other triptans, such as rizatriptan can be given.
- Concurrent administration of ergotamine with triptans is contraindicated.

15. **A 44-year-old female visited a psychiatric clinic with symptoms of depression. She stated that she had daily weeping spells, anxiety, restlessness, fatigue and low mood. Prescribe for this patient.**

Rx:

- Tab Sertraline 50 mg 1 tablet once daily for 2 weeks
- Tab Lorazepam 2 mg 1 tablet at bedtime

Non-pharmacological advice: Psychotherapy

Follow up: After a week for evaluation and dose adjustment

Dispense: 7 tablets of sertraline 50 mg and lorazepam 2 mg

Doctor sign and stamp
Registration no.

Important points

- Sertraline can be increased by 50 mg every week can be increased to a maximum of 200 mg/day.
- Alternatively, escitalopram can be prescribed (10 mg) 1 tablet once daily for 7 days.
- Instead of lorazepam other benzodiazepines, such as clonazepam (0.25 mg) can be prescribed.

16. **Bipolar depression**

Rx:

Tab Lamotrigine XR 25 mg 1 tablet once daily for 2 weeks

Follow up: After 2 weeks for evaluation and dose adjustment

Dispense: 15 tablets of lamotrigine XR 25 mg

Doctor sign and stamp
Registration no.

Important point

Lamotrigine can be increased to a max dose of 200 mg/day.

17. **Manic disorder (Bipolar disorder)**

Rx:

- Tab Sodium valproate 750 mg. 1 tablet once a day
- Titrate the dose by 250 mg/day every 2 weeks
- LFT to be done after 2 weeks

Follow up: After 14 days

Dispense: 21 tablets of sodium valproate 500 mg

Doctor sign and stamp
Registration no.

Important point

Sodium valproate can be increased to maximum of 2000 mg/day

18. **A relative of patient Aman gives a history of Aman talking to someone who is not there. She adds that he is spending a lot of time in his room by himself and has accused her of tampering with his things. He is diagnosed with schizophrenia. Prescribe suitable drug(s) for this patient.**

Rx:

- Tab Risperidone 1 mg 1 tablet twice daily day for 7 days
- Tab Trihexyphenidyl 1 mg 1 tablet thrice daily for 7 days

Follow up: After 7 days for evaluation and dose adjustment

Dispense: 14 tablets of risperidone 1 mg

Doctor sign and stamp
Registration no.

Important points

- Risperidone can be increased to a maximum dose of 8 mg/day
- Instead of risperidone others, such as olanzapine, and haloperidol can be prescribed.

19. **Patient suffering from panic disorder**

Rx:

- Tab Clonazepam 0.25 mg 1 tablet twice a day for 7 days.
- Tab Sertraline 50 mg 1 tablet once daily for 7 days

Non-pharmacological advice: Psychotherapy

Follow up: After a week for evaluation and dose adjustment.

Dispense: 14 tablets of clonazepam 0.25 mg and 14 tablets of sertraline 50 mg

Doctor sign and stamp
Registration no.

20. **Patient with generalized anxiety disorder.**

Rx:

- Tab Clonazepam 0.25 mg 1 tablet twice a day for 7 days.
- Tab Sertraline 50 mg 1 tablet once daily for 7 days

Advise psychotherapy.

To follow after a week for evaluation and dose adjustment

7.3: ENDOCRINOLOGY

1. **A 40-year-old woman, Mrs Sudha presented with weakness, fatigue, cold intolerance, constipation, dry skin and menorrhagia. Laboratory investigations revealed high levels of TSH and low levels of T3 and T4. Prescribe suitable drugs(s) for this patient. (Hypothyroidism)**

   Rx:
   - Tab Levothyroxine sodium 50 μg 1 tablet once daily, to be taken on empty stomach
   - To follow after one month for evaluation and dose adjustment.

   Follow up: After one month for evaluation and dose adjustment.

   Dispense: 28 tablets of levothyroxine sodium (50 μg)

   Doctor sign and stamp
   Registration no.

   Important point
   - Serum TSH levels should be measured every 6 weeks until it normalizes. If TSH remains above the normal reference the dose of T4 can be increased by 12 to 25 ug/day to a maximum of 200 ug.
   - Once euthyroidism is achieved the maintenance dose is identified, and treatment is continued lifelong with yearly monitoring of TSH.

2. **A 34-year-old pregnant lady Mrs Kala presented to your clinic with the complaints of anxiety, loose stools, loss of weight in spite of increased appetite and heat intolerance. Clinical examination revealed warm and moist skin, tachycardia and tremor. Laboratory investigation revealed low levels of TSH and increased levels of free T3 and T4. Prescribe suitable drugs(s) for this patient. (hyperthyroidism)**

   Rx:
   - Tab Carbimazole 10 mg 1 tablet thrice daily for 6 weeks
   - Tab Propranolol 10 mg 1 tablet thrice daily for 6 weeks

   Follow up: After 6 weeks along with serum T3 and T4 levels

   To report immediately if complaints of sore throat and fever. Hemogram to be done if symptoms of sore throat and fever.

   Dispense: 126 tablets of carbimazole 10 mg and propranolol 10 mg each

   Doctor sign and stamp
   Registration no.

   Important points
   - To continue the same dose of carbimazole till the patient becomes euthyroid (usually within 12 weeks and then taper carbimazole gradually and continue on once-daily maintenance dose for 2 years.

- Treatment should be continued till euthyroidism is achieved, after which the dose of antithyroid drugs is reduced.
- The dose required to maintain the euthyroid state is 5 mg thrice daily.
- Propranolol is added if hyperthyroidism is associated with tremors, sweating, tachycardia can be increased to a maximum of 120 mg/day.

3. **Hyperthyroidism in adult male patient > 40 years old in whom surgery is contraindicated.**

Rx:
- Tab Carbimazole 10 mg one tablet thrice daily for 4 weeks.
- Once euthyroidism is achieved, solution I^{131} (4–10 mCi) orally on an empty stomach.

Follow up: To follow up after 1 month for clinical evaluation, also after 3 months for thyroid function test.
Dispense: 84 tablets of carbimazole 10 mg

Doctor sign and stamp
Registration no.

Important points
- The dose is calculated on basis of previous tracer studies and thyroid size. Higher doses are required for multinodular goiter.
- If euthyroidism is not achieved with carbimazole within 4 weeks then continue the therapy for next 2 more weeks.
- The dose of carbimazole can be increased to maximum of 60 mg.

4. **A 33-year-old woman presented to an outside facility with increasing shortness of breath, orthopnea, paroxysmal nocturnal dyspnea and increasing lower limb edema—findings suggestive of biventricular heart failure. Further questioning revealed a two-to three-month history of unintentional weight loss, heat intolerance, diarrhea, abdominal pain and palpitations. The patient showed signs of tachycardia (118 beats per minute) and tachypnoea (22 breaths per minute). Laboratory testing was significant for severe hyperthyroidism and thyroid storm (thyrotoxic crisis). Write a prescription for this patient.**

Rx:
Tab Propylthiouracil loading dose 600 mg orally/nasogastric tube followed by 250 mg every 4 hours, then gradually reduce.
Saturated solution of potassium iodide (SSKI) (50 mg iodide/drop) 5 drops stat then orally every 6 hours. (to be administered after one hour after first dose of propylthiouracil
- Inj Propranolol IV 2 mg slowly every 6 hourly
- Inj Hydrocortisone 100 mg IV 8 hourly

Doctor sign and stamp
Registration no.

Important points

- Instead of propranolol esmolol can be prescribed
- The administration of iodine should be delayed for at least one hour after thioamide administration.
- Rehydration, anxiolytics, external cooling, antibiotics are other measures taken care off
- Instead of SSKI Lugol's iodine can be given

5. **A 15-year-old male patient presents to the medicine OPD with a history of increased thirst, increased frequency of urination and unexplained loss of weight. His random blood sugar was 280 mg%. He was diagnosed to have type 1 DM. Prescribe suitable drug(s) for this patient.**

Rx:

Inj Human soluble insulin (30%) and isophane insulin (70%). (40 U/ mL). 0.5 U/kg/day subcutaneously 2/3rd before breakfast and 1/3rd before dinner.

Follow up: After a week for dose adjustment depending upon glycemic control.

Doctor sign and stamp
Registration no.

Important point

Average dose in type 1 diabetes is 0.6–0.8 U/kg/day and in type II diabetes dose is usually 0.2–1.6 U/kg/day.

6. **A 39-yea-old marine was brought to the OPD complained of severe weakness, dizziness, and sleepiness during the preceding 4 weeks of boot camp. In a previous episode 3 weeks earlier, he reported generalized tiredness, unquenchable thirst, and the repeated need to urinate. Although he ate all of his rations as well as whatever he could get from his fellow trainees, he had lost 7 kilos. Laboratory, on admission, showed glucose of 400 mg/dL. Prescribe suitable drug(s) for this patient. (Type II diabetes mellitus)**

Rx:

Tab Metformin (500 mg) 1 tablet twice daily after meals for 3 weeks, to be increased by one tablet every 2 weeks till blood sugar are normal

Non-pharmacological methods.

- Caloric restriction, to avoid sugar
- Regular exercise

Follow up: After 15 days for dose adjustment, if required

Dispense: 30 tablets of metformin 500 mg

Doctor sign and stamp
Registration no.

Important point

The dose can be increased by 500 mg weekly up to a maximum dose of 2000 mg once daily or in two divided doses. (once blood sugar controlled, estimate blood sugar every 3 weeks and HbA1c every 3 monthly.

7. **BL is a 58-year-old woman who has been referred to the pharmacist clinician for clinical assessment and diabetes management. Her multiple medical conditions include type 2 diabetes diagnosed in 1995. She is currently on metformin, glimepiride and vildagliptin. But blood sugar is constantly high and she is scheduled for surgery in 10 days. Write a prescription for her. (Diabetes mellitus with impeding surgery)**

Rx:

- FDC of tab Metformin SR 500 mg + glimepiride 1 mg one tablet daily with breakfast
- Tab Vildagliptin 50 mg one tablet twice daily
- Inj Human soluble insulin [(30%) and Isophane insulin (70%)] (40 U/mL) 0.5 U/kg/day subcutaneously 2/3rd before breakfast and 1/3rd dinner. (dose would vary with blood sugar levels)

Follow up: After a week for dose adjustment depending upon glycemic control.

Doctor sign and stamp
Registration no.

8. **Gestational Diabetes**

Rx:

Inj Human soluble insulin (30%) 4 units before each meal

Follow up: After a week for dose adjustment depending upon glycemic control.

Doctor sign and stamp
Registration no.

Important point

Oral antidiabetics, such as metformin is considered safe during pregnancy

9. **Prescribe for a patient with type 2 diabetes mellitus not controlled on metformin monotherapy.**

Rx:

- Tab Metformin 500 mg one tablet twice daily after food
- Tab Glimepiride 1 mg one tablet daily before breakfast

Non-pharmacological methods.

- Caloric restriction, to avoid sugar)
- Exercise

Follow up: After 4 weeks for blood glucose monitoring

Dispense: 56 tablets of metformin 500 mg and 28 tablets of glimepiride 1 mg

Doctor sign and stamp
Registration no.

Important point

Instead of glimepiride glibenclamide, pioglitazone, vildagliptin or acarbose could be started

10. **A 55-year-old woman Mrs Devi came to your clinic with complaints of backache, dull aching in nature for the past two months. Personal history revealed that she attained menopause two years back. A radiological examination of the lumbar spine revealed areas of demineralization. You diagnose her to have postmenopausal osteoporosis. Prescribe suitable drug(s) for her.**

Rx:

- Tab Alendronate 10 mg once a day with a glass of water on an empty stomach in the morning.
- Patient is advised not to lie down, or take food for at least 30 mins.
- Tab Calcium carbonate 500 mg one tablet twice daily for 8 weeks.
- Vitamin D granules, (60,000 IU sachet) one sachet to be given once a week for 8 weeks followed once a month.

Follow up: After 15 days

Dispense: 15 tablets of alendronate 10 mg, 30 tablets of calcium carbonate 500 mg and 2 sachets of vitamin D 60,000 IU/sachet

Doctor sign and stamp
Registration no.

Important points

- Alternatively alendronate can be given weekly at a dose of 70 mg. Tab Risedronate 35 mg/week can be prescribed.
- To monitor vitamin D levels.

11. **A 33-year-old woman with 'brittle' type 1 diabetes treated with continuous subcutaneous insulin infusion (insulin pump). She gives history of gastroparesis (delayed stomach emptying). Some 36 hours prior to emergency hospital admission she complained of abdominal pain and vomiting after attending a party. Her condition deteriorated before transfer to hospital. The ambulance team reported a rapid decline in Glasgow Coma Score (GCS) from 13 to 3 in only 10 minutes, sinus tachycardia, undetectable peripheral pulse, and hypotension (BP 99/52 mm Hg). Clinical examination revealed severe dehydration and respiratory distress (respiration rate 40 breaths/min). Initial**

(fingerstick) blood glucose was above the upper detection limit of the analyzer and blood ketones were >8.0 mmol/L. Prescribe suitable drug(s) for her. (Diabetic Ketoacidosis)

Rx:

- Inj Plain insulin 0.1 U/kg given IV bolus followed by 0.1 units/kg/hour IV infusion in normal saline, then glucose level goes below 150 mg/dL, reduce to 0.05U/kg/hr, stop when the patient is able to take oral feed.
- Normal saline IV at the rate of 1L/hr for 5 hours, then 0.45% NS at 500 mL/hr for the next 6 hrs.
- Inj KCL 20 mEq/hr as IV infusion. (serum K is monitored)
- Inj Cefotaxime 1 g IV BD for 3 days.

Doctor sign and stamp
Registration no.

Important points

- Blood sugar to be monitored every 4–6 hours till patient become euglycemic.
- Sodium bicarbonate to be prescribed if pH falls to 7 or below.

12. **Heena is an 82-year-old woman who presented to her primary care physician with symptoms of anxiety, sweating, chills, irritability or impatience, confusion, rapid heartbeat and feeling lightheaded after injection of insulin this morning after missing her meals. Write a prescription for this patient. (Hypoglycemia)**

Rx:

- 50 mL of 25% dextrose intravenous bolus dose followed by inj Dextrose (5%) given as a rapid infusion.

To monitor blood glucose every 30 minutes until it is maintained at 100 mg%.

Doctor sign and stamp
Registration no.

Important points

- Once blood glucose normalizes oral intake of food can be started along with adjustment of anti-diabetic drugs to prevent future hypoglycemia attacks.
- Inj Glucagon 1 mg IM/IV can be used as alternative.

13. **A 45-year-old woman presents with darkening areas of skin (hyperpigmentation), severe fatigue, unintentional weight loss, gastrointestinal problems, such as nausea, vomiting and abdominal pain. a random cortisol was 2 nmol/L (102–535 nmol/L). Write a prescription for this patient. (Addison's disease).**

Rx:

- Inj Hydrocortisone sodium 100 mg IV bolus then 100 mg every 8 hourly as continuous infusion.
- 2 liters of normal saline as quickly as possible. Once the patient stabilizes continue 0.9 normal saline at slow rate over next 48 hours. (monitor signs for volume overload.)
- Inj Cefotaxime 1 g V BD for 3 days.

Next day

- Tab Prednisolone 5 mg, 3 tablets in the morning and 1 tab in the evening.
- Tab Fludrocortisone (0.1 mg) once day in the morning.

Treatment to continue lifelong.

Follow up: After 15 days for evaluation and dose adjustment, if necessary.

Dispense: 60 tablets of prednisolone 5 mg and 15 tablets of fludrocortisone 0.1 mg

Doctor sign and stamp
Registration no.

14. A 35-year-old woman comes with a request for postponement of menses as she has a ceremony at home. Prescribe suitable drug(s) for her.

Rx:

Tab Norethindrone enanthate [NEE] 5 mg 1 tablet thrice a day for 3 days before the onset of menses for the time required

Doctor sign and stamp
Registration no.

15. A 21-year-old married woman requires contraception to postpone pregnancy. Prescribe a suitable method of contraception for her.

Rx:

- Fixed dose combination of tab Ethinyl estradiol + Levonorgestrel (20 μg + 0.1 mg)
- 1 tablet daily beginning on the 5th day of menstruation for the next 21 days followed by a 7-day free period.
- Next course should be started on the 5th day of next menstrual cycle.

Doctor sign and stamp
Registration no.

Important points

- Instead of oral contraceptive pills depot medroxyprogesterone acetate 150 mg deep intramuscularly depot preparation can be prescribed.
- Before starting OC pills check BP, do a per vaginal examination
- Blood sugar and blood pressure is also measured regularly after starting OC pills.

- Fixed dose combination of tab Ethinyl estradiol + Levonorgestrel (30 μg + 0.15 mg), ethinyl estradiol + desogestrel (20 μg + 0.15 mg) are available. Some contraceptive tablets may contain 21 pills and 7 placebo/iron pills. The course is taken until the last pill is over and the second packet is started without interruption.
- The woman was advised to take the tablet on a regular basis at the same time every day.
- In case of missed pills:
  - » If one tablet is forgotten, it should be taken as soon as the female remembers as per schedule and continue the course as required.
  - » If two pills are forgotten, then two pills are to be taken immediately as soon as she remembers and the next day again continue the course as usual having a backup method to prevent pregnancy.
  - » If three pills are forgotten then discard the current pack and use a backup method for 7 days and start with the new pack.

16. Postcoital contraception

Rx:

- Tab Levonorgestrel 0.75 mg taken within the first 72 hours following unprotected intercourse followed by another tablet within 12 hours.
- This is recommended to be taken within 24 hours.

Doctor sign and stamp
Registration no.

Important point

Alternatively levonorgestrel (0.25 mg) and ethinyl estradiol 50 ug. two tablets within the first 72 hours of unprotected intercourse 2 tablets 12 hours later

17. Ms Reema, a 25-year-old woman, primiparous with one miscarriage, presented to her general practitioner when eight weeks pregnant complaining of nausea and vomiting. Prescribe suitable drug(s) for her.

Rx:

Tab Doxylamine + pyridoxine (10 mg + 10 mg) 2 tablets at bedtime as long as necessary.

Doctor sign and stamp
Registration no.

Important point

Instead of doxylamine any other first generations antihistamines, such as diphenhydramine meclizine dimenhydrinate can be prescribed

18. Immunization schedule in pregnant women.

Rx:

Injection Tetanus toxoid 0.5 mg intramuscularly given at 24 weeks of gestation followed by a second dose after 4 weeks.

Doctor sign and stamp
Registration no.

19. Prevention of anemia in pregnancy

Rx:

- Tablet Ferrous sulphate 200 mg one tablet once daily from the fourth month onwards till lactation is completed. It should not be taken with milk, food coffee. Can be taken along with citrus fruit juices
- Tablet Folic acid 5 mg 1 tablet once-daily till lactation is completed
- To test for hemoglobin every 3 months

Doctor sign and stamp
Registration no.

Important points

- Ferrous sulfate 200 mg contains 60 mg of elemental iron.
- If patient is not tolerating oral therapy parenteral iron therapy can be given
- To advise small frequent meals with avoiding of spicy and fatty foods

20. Write a prescription for a woman requiring to suppress lactation after a stillborn baby.

Rx:

Tab Cabergoline (0.5 mg) 1 tablet once at bedtime

Doctor sign and stamp
Registration no.

21. Write a prescription for a woman having spasmodic dysmenorrhea after insertion of an intrauterine contraceptive device in her uterus

Rx:

- Tab Mefenamic acid + Dicyclomine (250 mg + 10 mg) 1 tablet thrice daily after meals..

Consider removal if symptoms persist.

Doctor sign and stamp
Registration no.

22. Write a prescription for preventing postpartum hemorrhage

Rx:

Inj Methyl ergometrine (0.2 mg/mL) IM after delivery of anterior shoulder of fetus.

Doctor sign and stamp
Registration no.

23. Hypocalcemic tetany

Rx:

- Inj Calcium gluconate (90 mg elemental Ca/10 mL).
- 10 mL to be added to 50 mL of 5% dextrose and injected over 10 minutes followed by a slow IV infusion over 6 hours.

Doctor sign and stamp
Registration no.

24. Julia is a 51-year-old newly postmenopausal woman suffering from intense hot flashes and night sweats, as well as anxiety, insomnia, and stress. Prescribe a suitable hormone replacement therapy for her.

Rx:

Conjugated Estrogen 1.25 mg/day for 25 days each month + norethisterone 2.5 mg/day for last 12 days of each month.

Doctor sign and stamp
Registration no.

7.4: BLOOD AND AUTACOIDS

1. 23-year-old patient Mrs Mahalakshmi, in her 1st trimester was found to be slightly anemic on routine check-up. Her hemoglobin was found to be 8 g/dL, and further blood tests showed a normal serum concentration of vitamin B_{12}. Prescribe suitable drug(s) for this patient. (Severe iron deficiency anemia during pregnancy)

Rx:

Iron carboxymaltose 20 mg/kg body weight single **dose.** 1000 mg iron diluted in 100 mL saline and infused intravenously over 15 minutes
To repeat after a week if required.
Follow up: After one month to estimate Hb levels.

Doctor sign and stamp
Registration no.

2. **A 30-year-old female patients presented with complaints of easy fatigability, and tiredness. Examination revealed pallor and a hemoglobin of 10 g%. Peripheral smear shows microcytic hypochromic anemia. Prescribe suitable drug(s) for this patient.**

Rx:

- Tab Ferrous sulfate 200 mg containing (60 mg elemental iron) 1 tablet thrice daily for 1 month
  - Should not be taken with milk, food, or coffee, may be taken with fruit juice
  - To include iron rich foods in diet

Follow up: After 3 weeks for estimation of hemoglobin.
To continue for 3–6 months after hemoglobin normalizes to replete stores.

Doctor sign and stamp
Registration no.

Important points

- Folic acid and B_{12} may be added to ferrous sulfate to prevent unmasking of their deficiency.
- A total of 200 mg elemental iron daily in 3 divided doses, is a more important consideration in treatment.
- Hemoglobin is to be monitored every month
- if the patient is non-compliant/intolerant to oral therapy, parenteral iron therapy can be given

3. **Write a prescription for pernicious anemia (age 40 years)**

Rx:

- Inj Cyanocobalamin 1000 µg IM once daily for 10 days followed by
- Inj Cyanocobalamin 1000 µg IM weekly for 5 weeks followed by
- Inj Cyanocobalamin 1000 µg IM once a month life long.

Follow up: weekly for the first 6 weeks for monitoring of reticulocyte count and serum vitamin B_{12} levels.

Doctor sign and stamp
Registration no.

7.5: SKIN DISEASES

1. **An 11-year-old girl with a chief complaint of intense body itchiness between the fingers, wrist, palm, armpit, back and chest with nocturnal exacerbation On dermatological examination, found erythematous papules, round shaped with a well-defined border, discrete presentation and distributed bilaterally. A cardinal diagnosis of scabies was made. Prescribe suitable drugs for her.**

Rx:

- Permethrin 5% cream apply all over the body except face and head. Wash after 8–12 hours.
- Tab Ivermectin 200 μg/kg as a single dose; may repeat in 14 days if necessary
- Tab Levocetirizine (5 mg) 1 tablet once daily for 15 days.

All members to be treated simultaneously with permethrin, clothes, underclothes should be washed in boiling not water for at least 10 minutes.

Follow up: After a week for evaluation.

Dispense: 1 tube 5% permethrin cream, 2 tablets of ivermectin (weight-based) 10 tablets of levocetirizine 5 mg

Doctor sign and stamp
Registration no.

Important points

- All members are to be treated simultaneously with permethrin, clothes, and underclothes should be washed in boiling not water for at least 10 minutes.
- Alternatively, emulsion benzyl benzoate (25%) and lotion gamma benzene hexachloride (1%)

2. **Pediculosis capitis.**

Rx:

- Shampoo permethrin 1% cream applied locally lathered in lace and keep for 10 minutes and rinse it off.
- To comb hair with fine-toothed comb to remove dead lice and nits.
- To treat all family members simultaneously

Doctor sign and stamp
Registration no.

3. **A 25-year-old man, Mr PG complained of ringworm lesions on the fingers, web of fingers, forearms and cheek. A diagnosis of tinea corporis was made. Prescribe suitable drugs for him.**

Rx:

Miconazole 2% cream to be applied twice daily for 3 weeks.

Follow up: After 2 weeks for review

Dispense: 1 tube of miconazole 2% cream

Doctor sign and stamp
Registration no.

Important point

For large skin areas, tinea pedis, tinea manuum, onychomycosis, tab Fluconazole 150 mg once a week for 2-4 weeks for varying durations.

4. **Prescribe for a patient with tinea capitis, tinea barbae, tinea pedis, tinea mannus**

   Rx:

   Tab Terbinafine (250 mg) 1 tablet once daily for 14 days

   Follow up: After 2 weeks for review

   Dispense: 14 tablets terbinafine 250 mg

   Doctor sign and stamp
   Registration no.

5. **Mithali is a 15-year-old girl who has several open and closed comedones on her face with a small number of inflammatory lesions. Write a prescription for her. (Mild acne vulgaris)**

   Rx:

   Gel Benzoyl peroxide (2.5%) applied on the lesion once daily till the lesions heal.

   Follow up: After 3 months for clinical evaluation and assessing response to treatment.

   Important points:
   - Alternatively Gel adapalene (0.1%) applied once daily at bedtime can be prescribed.
   - Cream tretinoin (0.025%) applied locally at bedtime and to be washed in the morning.

6. **A 23-year-old male patient comes with complaints of multiple papulopustular acne scattered lesions over the face, neck and back for 6 months. Prescribe suitable drugs for him. (Acne vulgaris with pustules)**

   Rx:
   - Cap Doxycycline (100 mg) once a day for 1 month
   - Gel Clindamycin (1%) applied over the lesion twice daily
   - Gel Adapalene (0.1%) applied on the face once daily at bedtime

   Follow up: After 2 weeks for review

   Dispense: 15 capsules of doxycycline 100 mg, 1 tube of gel clindamycin (1%) and 1 tube of gel adapalene (0.1%)

   Doctor sign and stamp
   Registration no.

7. **A 25-year-old male complains of progressive loss of terminal hair of the scalp after puberty, hair loss is most prominent in the vertex and frontotemporal regions. Write a prescription for him. (Male pattern baldness)**

Rx:

- Minoxidil (5%) lotion 1 mL applied topically on the scalp twice daily for 4 months.
- Tab Biotin 5 mg 1 tablet once daily.

Follow up: After 1 month for review

Dispense: 60 mL bottle of minoxidil 5% lotion, 30 tablets of 5 mg biotin

Doctor sign and stamp
Registration no.

Important points

In addition, finasteride (1 mg) in men can be prescribed.

8. **Sunburns.**

Rx:

- Calamine lotion for topical application thrice daily for 7 days
- Cold compresses to the affected area as often as required

Follow up: After 7 days

Dispense: 1 bottle of calamine lotion (120 mL)

Doctor sign and stamp
Registration no.

9. **Superficial burns (<5% of total body area).**

Rx:

- Cold water compresses locally
- Silver sulphadiazine cream 1% applied locally to affected area thrice daily for 5 days

Follow up: After 7 days

Dispense: 1 tube of 1% Silver sulphadiazine cream

Doctor sign and stamp
Registration no.

Important points

Instead of SSD mupirocin cream 2%, sodium fusidate 2% ointment can be used

10. **Pyoderma**

Rx:

- Cap Cefadroxil 500 mg 1 capsule twice daily for 7 days
- Mupirocin cream 2%, applied twice daily for 7 days

Follow up: After 1 weeks for review

Dispense: 7 capsules of cefadroxil 500 mg, 1 tube of mupirocin cream 2%

Doctor sign and stamp
Registration no.

7.6: RESPIRATORY SYSTEM

1. **Write prescription for 18 year old female presenting with acute attack of bronchial asthma (mild).**

Rx:

- Salbutamol metered dose inhaler via spacer 100 (μgm/puff) 2 puffs repeated every 5 minutes up to 5 puffs.
- Oxygen with flow rate adjusted to achieve SaO2 >90%.

Doctor sign and stamp
Registration no.

Important points

- If no relief then give inj Terbutaline 0.25 mg subcutaneous stat and salbutamol nebulisation every 20 minutes (for 3 doses).
- If still no relief inj Aminophylline 250 mg iv diluted in 25 mL of 5% dextrose over a period of 15–20 minutes + inj Hydrocortisone 100 mg IV stat.

2. **Prescribe for a 12-year-old girl Miss Rani with h/o dyspnea and wheezes for atleast 2 times during the night in a month. On examination, her PEF was >80%. She was diagnosed to have mild persistent asthma. Prescribe suitable drugs for this patient.**

Rx:

- Formoterol (6 μg per puff) + budesonide (100 μg/puff) MDI 2 puffs twice a day through a spacer.
- Patient must be instructed to gargle, following the use of inhaled corticosteroids to prevent topical side effects.

Follow up: After a month for clinical evaluation and assessment of response.

Dispense: Formoterol (6 μg per puff) + budesonide (100 μg/puff) metered dose inhaler

Doctor sign and stamp
Registration no.

Important point

Alternatively any long-acting β_2 agonist (salmeterol) with inhaled corticosteroid—(fluticasone/beclomethasone/flunisolide/ciclesonide) can also be used.

3. **Status asthmaticus (reference Emergency Pharmacotherapy).**

Rx:

- Inj Hydrocortisone hemisuccinate 200 mg IV bolus then 100 mg IV stat followed by 100 mg 8 hourly.)
- Nebulized salbutamol 5 mg/2.5 mL + ipratropium bromide 0.5 mg/2.5 mL in normal saline every
- 20 minutes for 3 doses then intermittent inhalation every 4 hours
- Intermittent humidified O_2 (40%) inhalation at every 4–6 liters/min
- Inj Aminophylline 250 mg diluted in 25 mL of glucose solution injected in 25 minutes. This is followed by a 50 mg IV infusion every 8 hours (avoid in patients with propensity for cardiac arrhythmias)
- Sodium bicarbonate (7.5%) 50 mL IV
- Inj Cefotaxime 500 mg iv 8 hourly

Doctor sign and stamp
Registration no.

4. **Mr Kalim, 50 years of age with mild persistent asthma since 10 years has been on several drug regimens for asthma over the years. He now comes to you and asks for the simplest regimen possible which can be taken orally. What will you prescribe for him?**

Rx:

Tab Montelukast 10 mg 1 tablet once daily

Follow up: After a month for clinical evaluation and assessment of response

Dispense: 30 tablets of montelukast 10 mg

Doctor sign and stamp
Registration no.

5. **A patient comes with sneezing, runny nose and mild fever. A diagnosis of common cold is made. Write a prescription for him.**

Rx:

- Tab Paracetamol 500 mg 1 tablet thrice daily
- Tab Levocetirizine 5 mg one tablet twice daily till relief
- Oxymetazoline hydrochloride nasal spray (5 mg/ mL) 2 drops into each nostril TDS
- Steam inhalation: with tincture benzoin

Follow up: After 7 days

Dispense: 21 tablets of paracetamol 500 mg, 14 tablets of levocetirizine, 10 ml bottle of oxymetazoline 5 mg/mL and 100 mL bottle of tincture benzoin

Doctor sign and stamp
Registration no.

Note: Instead of levocetirizine, azelastine spray or montelukast can be used.

6. **Write a prescription for a patient with dry cough.**

   Rx:

   Dextromethorphan 10 mg/5 mL syrup 1 teaspoon thrice daily for 3 days

   Follow up: After 3 days

   Dispense: 1 bottle of 100 mL Dextromethorphan 10 mg/5 mL syrup

   Doctor sign and stamp
   Registration no.

   Important point

   Syrup Codeine Phosphate (10 mg/5 mL in viscous base) 5 mL thrice daily can be prescribed

7. **Productive cough with lower respiratory tract infection**

   Rx:

   - Expectorant syrup (Ambroxyl- 15 mg + Guaifenesin 50 mg + Menthol 2.5 mg + Terbutaline 1.25 mg)/5 mL. 1 teaspoon thrice daily.
   - Cap Amoxicillin 500 mg 1 tablet thrice daily for 4 days

   Follow up: After 7 days

   Dispense: 12 capsules of Amoxicillin 500 mg and 21 tablets of Tab Bromhexine 8 mg

   Doctor sign and stamp
   Registration no.

8. **A 20-year-old girl Ms Kala presented to your clinic with complaints of nasal congestion, running nose, paroxysms of sneezing associated with nasal itching, eye irritation and sometimes chest tightness also. Detailed history reveals that she is exposed to airborne dusty material in her workplace. She gets repeated attacks whenever she is exposed to dust in her workplace. Physical examination of the nasal cavity reveals a pale, edematous and inflamed nasal mucosa. (sinusitis). Prescribe suitable drug(s) for this patient.**

Rx:
- Cap Amoxicillin 500 mg one capsule thrice a day for 5 days
- Bromhexine elixir (5 mg/5 mL) 10 mL thrice daily
- Steam inhalation

Follow up: After 7 days
Dispense: 15 capsules of amoxicillin 500 mg and 1 bottle of bromhexine elixir (5 mg/5 mL)

Doctor sign and stamp
Registration no.

Important point
Instead of amoxicillin, azithromycin can be prescribed.

7.7: GASTROINTESTINAL SYSTEM

1. **A 32-year-old sales executive presented to your clinic with the complaints of upper abdominal pain. The pain is burning in nature, aggravated by fasting and relieved by taking food. History reveals that he frequently skips his meals. You perform a upper GI endoscopy and it reveals duodenal ulcers. Prescribe suitable drug(s) for this patient.**

Rx:
Kit containing:
- Cap Omeprazole 20 mg 1 capsule twice daily before meals
- Cap Amoxicillin 1000 mg 1 capsule twice daily
- Tab Clarithromycin 500 mg 1 tablet twice daily
- The kit is to be taken for 2 weeks
- To continue with omeprazole 20 mg one capsule daily before breakfast for 4 weeks.

Follow up: After 4 weeks
Dispense: 30 capsules of amoxicillin 1000 mg, 58 tablets of omeprazole 20 mg and 30 tablets of clarithromycin 500 mg

Doctor sign and stamp
Registration no.

Important points
- Alternatively other triple drug regimen can be advised.
- Omeprazole 20 mg one tablet twice daily
- Clarithromycin 500 mg one tablet twice daily, and
- Metronidazole 400 mg one tablet twice daily for 14 days.

2. **A 33-year-old male presents with a one-month history of episodes of mid-epigastric pain, a "burning" sensation in his chest, an associated dry cough, and occasional regurgitation. The pain worsens after eating and when he is lying flat. The patient has increasing postprandial fullness and early satiety. Write a prescription for him. (gastroesophageal reflux disease, i.e., GERD)**

   Rx:

   Tab Omeprazole 20 mg 1 capsule once day 1/2 hour before breakfast for 6 weeks for 6 weeks.

   Non-pharmacological advice:

   Avoiding spicy foods, smoking alcohol. To follow up for dose evaluation.

   Follow up: After 6 weeks

   Dispense: 42 tablets of omeprazole 20 mg

   Doctor sign and stamp
   Registration no.

   Important points
   - To follow diet and exercise program for weight reduction
   - Raise head while sleeping to prevent reflux of gastric contents to restrict fatty foods, alcohol, acidic foods, caffeine containing foods alternatively omeprazole H_2 blockers, such as ranitidine can be given for symptomatic relief
   - Antacids containing magnesium an aluminum hydroxide gel could be given

3. **A patient is going on a sea cruise and suffers from motion sickness. Write a prescription for the same.**

   Short journey

   Rx:

   Tab Promethazine 25 mg one tablet 1/2 hour before journey.

   Doctor sign and stamp
   Registration no.

   Important point

   Instead tab Meclizine, tab Hyoscine can also be prescribed.

   For long journeys

   Rx:

   Scopolamine 1.5 mg as transdermal drug delivery system behind the pinna applied 1/2 hour before the journey.

   Doctor sign and stamp
   Registration no.

   Important point

   Protection last for 3 consecutive days.

4. A 66-year-old patient presents with ovarian cancer and will receive carboplatin and paclitaxel every 3 weeks prior to surgery. She is experiencing nausea due to her intra-abdominal disease and opioid analgesia administered as needed. Prescribe for chemotherapy induced vomiting.

Rx:

- Inj Ondansetron 8 mg iv by slow injection over 15 min ½ hour before chemotherapy infusion, followed by 8 mg iv 4 hours apart. then 8 mg iv twice a day for 5 days
- Tab Aprepitant 125 mg administered one hour prior to chemotherapy treatment on day 1 and 80 mg in morning on day 2 and day 3
- Tab Dexamethasone 8 mg to be administered orally one hour prior to chemotherapy treatment on day 1 and 4 mg in morning on day 2 and 3

Follow up: After 5 days

Dispense: 2 tablets of aprepitant 125 mg and aprepitant 80 mg each, 2 tablets of dexamethasone 8 mg and dexamethasone 4 mg each

Doctor sign and stamp
Registration no.

5. Postoperative nausea and vomiting (PONV)

Rx:

Inj Ondansetron 8 mg IV given before induction, then 4 mg IV 8 hourly

Doctor sign and stamp
Registration no.

6. A patient has to undergo colonoscopy. Prescribe suitable drugs for bowel evacuation for colonoscopy.

Rx:

Tab Bisacodyl 5 mg—2 tablets at bedtime on the night before colonoscopy.

Dispense: 2 tablets of bisacodyl 5 mg

Doctor sign and stamp
Registration no.

7. A 25-year-old woman suffers from piles complicated by constipation. Prescribe symptomatic treatment for constipation.

Rx:

- Liquid Paraffin emulsion 25 mL at bed time.
- Ispaghula Granules 15 mg every night for 3 consecutive days.
- Ointment Lignocaine 2% applied locally twice daily

Non-pharmacological advice:

To take plenty of oral fluids and fiber rich diet to carry out regular exercise.

Follow up: After 3 days

Dispense: 3 sachet of ispaghula granules, liquid paraffin bottle

Doctor sign and stamp
Registration no.

Important points

- Instead of ispaghula powder polyethylene glycol-based powder (PEG) could be taken
- Prucalopride is prescribed preferably only in refractory constipation

8. **Fissure in ano**

Rx:

- Ointment Lignocaine 2% applied locally twice daily for 1 week
- Ointment Nitroglycerine 2% applied locally twice daily for 6 weeks
- Liquid Paraffin emulsion 25 mL at bedtime till fissure heals
- Sitz bath once or twice daily

Follow up: After 6 weeks

Dispense: 1 tube of ointment lignocaine 2% and ointment nitroglycerine 2% each and 1 liter bottle liquid paraffin emulsion

Doctor sign and stamp
Registration no.

Important points

- Instead of ointment nitroglycerine, nifedipine ointment can be applied locally.
- Instead of liquid paraffin, cap Docusate sodium and solution lactulose can be could be prescribed with plenty of water.

7.8: ANTIBIOTICS-CHEMOTHERAPY

1. **Mr Mohan a 16-year-old boy had cough and fever for 2 days. On examination, the pharynx was congested and the throat swab on staining revealed gram-positive cocci. Prescribe suitable drug(s) for him. (Upper respiratory tract infection, i.e., URTI)**

Rx:

- Cap Amoxicillin 500 mg 1 capsule thrice daily for 7 days
- Tab Paracetamol 5 mg 1 tablet thrice daily till fever subsides
- Syrup Ambrolite (30 mg/5 mL) 5 mL thrice daily

Follow up: After 7 days

Dispense: 21 capsules of amoxicillin 500 mg, 21 tablets of paracetamol 500 mg and 100 mL bottle of syrup Ambrolite (30 mg/5 mL)

Doctor sign and stamp
Registration no.

Important point

Instead of Amoxicillin, Erythromycin, tab Azithromycin, tab Cefadroxil can also be prescribed.

2. **Prescribe for a 19-year-old boy with community-acquired pneumonia with no antibiotic exposure in the last 3 months.**

Rx:

Tab Azithromycin 500 mg 1 tablet once a day for 5 days

Follow up: After 5 days

Dispense: 5 tablets of Azithromycin 500 mg

Doctor sign and stamp
Registration no.

Important point

Instead of azithromycin clarithromycin or amoxicillin can also be given.

3. **Community-acquired pneumonia (CAP) patients with comorbidities, diabetes, renal failure or antibiotic exposure in the last 3 months.**

Rx:

- Amoxicillin plus clavulanate (750/125 mg) 1 tablet twice daily for 5 days
- Tab Paracetamol 500 mg thrice daily for 5 days.
- Salt water/$KMnO_4$ gargles
- Syrup Ambrolite (30 mg/5 mL) 5 mL TDS

Follow up: After 5 days

Dispense: 5 tablets of amoxicillin plus clavulanate (750/125 mg), 15 tablets of paracetamol 500 mg and 100 mL bottle of syrup Ambrolite (30 mg/5 mL)

Doctor sign and stamp
Registration no.

Important points

- Instead of amoxicillin plus clavulanate, levofloxacin, gemifloxacin, the new generation fluoroquinolones can be used should be used with caution because they are also used in treatment of tuberculosis can mask symptoms of tuberculosis hence to be used rationally.

- History of antibiotic exposure in the previous 3 months, hence important to take patients history and start with antimicrobial different from the class that patient had received earlier.

4. **Pneumonia in patient admitted to hospital in ICU.**

Rx:
- Inj Ceftriaxone 2 g IV once a day for 10 days
- Inj Levofloxacin 7500 mg IV once a day 10 days

Follow up: After 48 hours after the injection, with culture report.

Doctor sign and stamp
Registration no.

Important point
Instead of ceftriaxone injection, moxifloxacin 400 IV once for 10 days could be prescribed.

5. **Prescribe for a 18-year-old adult male who is suffering from acute tonsillitis. The patient is allergic to penicillin.**

Rx:
- Tab Azithromycin 500 mg 1 tablet once a day for 5 days
- Tab Paracetamol 500 mg 1 tablet thrice daily till fever subsides

Follow up: After 5 days
Dispense: 5 tablets of Azithromycin 500 mg and 15 tablets of paracetamol 500 mg

Doctor sign and stamp
Registration no.

Important point
Instead of erythromycin, Tab Cefadroxil, Tab Amoxicillin can also be prescribed.

6. **Meningococcal meningitis.**

Rx:
Inj Ceftriaxone 2 g IV every 12 hourly for 10 days.

Follow up: After 48 hours after the injection, with culture report.

Doctor sign and stamp
Registration no.

Important points
- If the person is hypersensitive to penicillin, then inj Chloramphenicol 4 g IV in divided doses every four hourly may be administered until the patient is able to take oral medication.
- For prophylaxis cap Rifampicin 600 mg BD daily for 2 days.
- If the organism is not known then inj Ceftriaxone 2 g BD IV for 7 days.

Chemoprophylaxis for closed contact of patient suffering from Meningococcal meningitis
- Followed by prophylaxis
- Cap Rifampicin 600 mg 1 capsule twice daily for 14 days

Important point
Instead of rifampicin, azithromycin ciprofloxacin can also be prescribed.

7. **Gonococcal urethritis**

Rx:
- Inj Ceftriaxone 250 mg IM as a single dose
- Tab Azithromycin 500 mg 2 tablets single dose
- Sex partner to be evaluated and treated simultaneously

Follow up: After 48 hours

Dispense: 2 tablets of Azithromycin 500 mg

Doctor sign and stamp
Registration no.

Important point
Patient infected with gonorrhea is co-infected with chlamydia, should also be given azithromycin.

8. **50-year-old Mr Sameer with a prosthetic heart valve is to undergo tooth extraction and scaling. Prescribe for this patient regarding prophylaxis against subacute bacterial endocarditis.**

Rx:
Cap Amoxicillin 2 g orally 1 hour before procedure.

Doctor sign and stamp
Registration no.

Important point
Note: if patient allergic to penicillin then vancomycin 15 mg/kg single dose 60 min prior to surgery can be given.

9. **26-year-old Mrs Kala presented with complaints of fever and burning sensation while passing urine. On examination, she had right-sided flank tenderness. Laboratory investigation showed WBC count to be 28,000 cells/mL, Urine culture showed gram negative bacilli. A presumptive diagnosis of acute glomerulonephritis/pyelonephritis was made. Prescribe for this patient.**

Rx:
- Injection Ceftriaxone 1 g iv every 24 hours
- After information from antibiotic sensitivity testing is available a most specific antibiotic is to be selected
- Therapy should continue for 10 to 21 days

Doctor sign and stamp
Registration no.

Important points

- Instead, imipenem 500 mg every 6–8 hours or piperacillin tazobactam 4 g combination every 6 hours, inj Ceftazidime 2 g IM 12 hourly can be given for 7 days.
- Follow up of culture should be performed to 2–4 weeks after cessation of therapy to demonstrate cure.
- Urinary tract infections due to *Pseudomonas* have to be treated aggressively. Drugs, such as gentamicin, piperacillin and IIIrd generation cephalosporins can be used against *Pseudomonas* infection.

10. **A 23-year-old woman comes with complaints suggestive of acute cystitis, all characterized by dysuria, increased frequency, and urgency. Write a prescription for her.**

Rx:

- Tab Ciprofloxacin 500 mg twice a day for 7 days
- Liq mist disodium hydrogen citrate 5 mL thrice a day for 3 days

Non-pharmacological advice: Plenty of oral fluids

Follow up: After 7 days

Dispense: 14 tablets of Ciprofloxacin 500 mg, 100 mL bottle of liquid mist disodium hydrogen citrate

Doctor sign and stamp
Registration no.

Important points

- Instead of ciprofloxacin, cotrimoxazole, (1 tablet twice daily for 3 days), fosfomycin 3 g single dose, cap Amoxicillin, Nitrofurantoin can also be prescribed.
- Prescribe for a pregnant women suffering from uncomplicated cystitis.

Rx:

- Tab Amoxycillin 500 mg 1 tablet thrice a day for 7 days
- Tab Fosfomycin 3 g single dose

Important point

Instead of amoxicillin, cephalosporin fosfomycin, nitrofurantoin can also be prescribed.

11. **Prescribe for a 30-year-old pregnant female diagnosed to be suffering from chlamydial urethritis.**

Rx:

Tab Azithromycin 500 mg 2 tablets single dose, simultaneously treat sex partner

Follow up: After 7 days

Dispense: 2 tablets of Azithromycin 500 mg

Doctor sign and stamp
Registration no.

Important points

- Patient infected with gonorrhea is co-infected with chlamydia, and should also be given azithromycin.
- Alternatively doxycycline can be prescribed for both partners.

12. **30-year-old Mr muthu complains of lower abdominal pain, flatulence and occasional diarrhea. A stool culture showed *E. histolytica* and he was diagnosed to have mild intestinal amoebiasis. Prescribe suitable drug(s) for this patient.**

Rx:

- Tab Metronidazole 400 mg 1 tablet thrice daily for 7 days
- Tab Diloxanide furoate 500 mg 1 tablet thrice daily for 10 days

Follow up: After 10 days

Dispense: 21 tablets of Metronidazole 400 mg, 30 tablets of Diloxanide furoate 500 mg

Doctor sign and stamp
Registration no.

Important points

- Instead of metronidazole, tab Secnidazole 1 g single dose or tab Tinidazole 2 g once day for 3 days also be prescribed.
- In pregnant women, paromomycin (500 mg) 1 tablet thrice daily for 7–10 days can be used as alternative.
- Luminal amebicides fail to eradicate the luminal forms in 10–15% of patients, therefore a follow up stool examination is recommended after completion of therapy. A second course of luminal amebecides is required after completion of therapy.

13. **Amebic liver abscess.**

Rx:

- Inj Metronidazole 15 mg/kg intravenously followed by 7.5 mg/kg/6 hour latter to be repeated every 6 hours for 14 days.
- Tab Diloxanide furoate 500 mg thrice daily for 14 days.

Non-pharmacological advice:

To avoid alcohol along with Metronidazole

Follow up: After 7 days

Dispense: 42 tablets of diloxanide furoate 500 mg

Doctor sign and stamp
Registration no.

Important points

- Luminal amebicides fail to eradicate the luminal forms in 10–15% of patients, therefore a follow up stool examination is recommended

after completion of therapy. A second course of luminal amebicides is required after completion of therapy.
- If patient can tolerate oral then tab, metronidazole 800 mg one tablet thrice daily for 14 days.
- Instead of diloxanide furoate 8-hydroxyquinolines, such as quiniodochlor 250 mg thrice daily can be used.
- If patient is pregnant then instead of metronidazole, tab Chloroquine phosphate 250 mg 2 tablet twice daily for two days then one tablet twice daily

14. 38-year-old patient Mr Selvam presented to your clinic with the complaints of periodic attacks of sequential chills, fever and sweating for the past three days. Peripheral blood smear examination reveals *P. vivax* parasites. Prescribe suitable drug(s) for this patient.

Rx:
- Tab Chloroquine phosphate 500 mg 2 tablets stat (1000 mg), then 500 mg 8 hours later, followed by 500 mg once day for 2 more days.
- Tab Metoclopramide 10 mg before each chloroquine tablet
- Tab Primaquine 15 mg once daily for 14 days after laboratory testing for G6PD deficiency is negative.

Non-pharmacological advice: Plenty of oral fluids.

Follow up: After 14 days

Dispense: 5 tablets of Chloroquine phosphate 500 mg, 5 tablets of metoclopramide 10 mg and 14 tablets of primaquine 15 mg

Doctor sign and stamp
Registration no.

Important points
- Chloroquine phosphate tablet 250 mg = 150 mg base.
- In endemic areas tab Primaquine is given only for 5 days. Avoid this drug in patients with G6PD deficiency.
- In pregnant females, they should not receive primaquine but can be given secondary prophylaxis with tab Chloroquine 250 mg once a week till delivery after which primaquine can be given.
- If *P. vivax* is resistant to chloroquine then the following treatment for *P. falciparum* malaria is given. Artesunate combination therapy (ACT) regimen.

15. Acute attack of falciparum malaria. (chloroquine resistant malaria) (uncomplicated).

Rx:
- Fixed dose combination of artemether 80 mg + lumefantrine 480 mg one tablet twice a day for 3 days to be taken with fatty meal
- Tab Primaquine 45 mg single dose after G6PD testing is negative

Follow up: After 3 days

Dispense: 9 tablets of FDC artemether 80 mg + lumefantrine 480 mg and 1 tablet of primaquine 45 mg

Doctor sign and stamp
Registration no.

Important points

Other ACT regimens:

- Tab Artesunate 100 mg BD for 3 days + tab Sulfadoxine 500 mg + pyrimethamine 75 mg (FDC) single dose.
- Alternatively, instead of sulfadoxine + pyrimethamine, tab Mefloquine 750 mg on 2nd day and 500 mg on 3rd day with plenty of water can be given along with artesunate.
- Single-dose primaquine is given to kill gametes and to cut down transmission to mosquitoes.

16. A patient suffering from complicated *P. falciparum* malaria.

Rx:

- Inj Artesunate 2.4 mg/kg IV followed by 2.4 mg 1 kg after 12 and 24 hours then 2.4 mg/kg once daily for 7 days later, switch to 3 days oral ACT regimen.
- Inj Diazepam can be given if there are convulsions.

Follow up: After 7 days

Doctor sign and stamp
Registration no.

Important points

- Associated symptoms with complicated *P. falciparum* malaria also needs to be treated.
- Alternatively, instead of artesunate inj Artemether, or inj Quinine can be given.
- Switch to oral ACT, once patient can take and tolerate oral medications.

17. Prescribe for a traveler who is planning to visit an area endemic for malaria.

Rx:

- Tab Atovaquone/proguanil (250/100 mg) 1 tablet once daily with food starting 1 day before entering the endemic area, continued during the stay and for 7 days after leaving the endemic area.

Doctor sign and stamp
Registration no.

Important points

- Mefloquine is the only drug for pregnant women travelling to areas with drug-resistant malaria.
- Alternatively, mefloquine, doxycycline one tablet daily with food starting one day before entering the endemic area, continued during the stay and up to 4 weeks after leaving the endemic area.
- For prophylaxis of malaria in chloroquine-sensitive area: Tab Chloroquine phosphate base 300 mg once a week, starting 2 weeks before entering the endemic area, continued during the stay and up to 6 weeks after leaving the endemic area.

18. Mr Rajan, 26-year-old presented with complaints of gradual onset of malaise, headache and fever for the past week. Detailed history revealed that fever raised slowly to the maximum. Physical examination showed a temperature of 40°C, pulse rate of 76/min. Laboratory investigations revealed leukopenia and a positive widal test. Prescribe suitable drug(s) for this patient (Typhoid fever).

Rx:

- Tab Ciprofloxacin 500 mg 1 tablet twice daily for 14 days.
- Tab Paracetamol 500 mg 1 tablet as and when required for fever.

Follow up: After 2 days if fever persists

Dispense: 28 tablets of Ciprofloxacin 500 mg, 6 tablets of Paracetamol 500 mg

Doctor sign and stamp
Registration no.

Important points

- Instead of ciprofloxacin, 3rd generation cephalosporins: Inj Ceftriaxone 2 g IV every 12 hourly for 2 days, then 2 g IV daily till 2 days after fever subsides. Generally, 4–5 days of treatment is required. cefoperazone and Cefotaxime also can be used.
- In the past drugs, such as chloramphenicol, co-trimoxazole, amoxicillin and furazolidone were used for the past for treatment of typhoid, but for the fear of resistance now they are not used.
- Prescribe for a patient who is diagnosed as typhoid carrier.

Rx:

- Tab Ciprofloxacin 500 mg 1 tablet twice a day for 4 weeks
- Follow up with stool examination after 4 weeks

19. Prescribe for a patient suffering from bacterial conjunctivitis.

Rx:

Ciprofloxacin (0.03%) eye drops 2 eye drops instilled into the lower conjunctival sac every 6 hourly for 7 days.

Follow up: After 7 days

Dispense: 10 mL bottle of ciprofloxacin (0.03%) eye drops

Doctor sign and stamp
Registration no.

Important point

Other fluroquinolones, such as moxifloxacin and ofloxacin can be prescribed.

20. A 30-year-old female presented to your clinic with complaints of episodic fever for the past two weeks. Detailed history revealed that the fever occurs at irregular intervals and is associated with tender and inflamed lymph nodes. The patient resides in an area endemic to filariasis. Laboratory investigation shows microfilaria in blood. Prescribe suitable drug(s) for this patient. (Filariasis)

Rx:

- Tablet Diethylcarbamazine citrate 100 mg 1 tablet thrice daily for 3 weeks.
- Tab Albendazole 400 mg 1 tablet twice a day for 12 days can be added to Diethylcarbamazine citrate.

Follow up: After 3 weeks

Dispense: 63 tablets of Diethylcarbamazine citrate 100 mg

Doctor sign and stamp
Registration no.

Important points

- Diethylcarbamazine citrate along with albendazole exerts a significant microfilaricidal activity
- Prescribe for tropical pulmonary eosinophilia

Rx:

Tablet Diethylcarbamazine citrate 100 mg 1 tablet thrice a day for 2 weeks.

Doctor sign and stamp
Registration no

21. 35-year-old Mr Ravi (44 kg) presented with the complaints of cough with expectoration for the past one month. Detailed history reveals that he has loss of appetite and weight. He also has evening rise of temperature. Sputum examination reveals acid fast bacilli. Chest radiograph shows apical pulmonary infiltrates. Prescribe suitable drug therapy for this patient. (Tuberculosis)

Rx:

- Fixed dose combination of tab Isoniazid (INH) + tab Rifampicin + tab Pyrazinamide + tab Ethambutol (75/150/400/275) 3 tablets daily in morning on empty stomach for 2 months.
- After 2 months if sputum conversion happens then fixed dose combination of tab Isoniazid (INH) + tab Rifampicin + tab Ethambutol (75/150/275) 3 tablets daily in morning on empty stomach for 4 months.
- Tab Pyridoxine 10 mg 1 tablet once daily for 6 months

Follow up: After every 15 days for assessment and appearance of side effects.

Doctor sign and stamp
Registration no.

Important points

Drug doses for adult TB

	Number of tablets (FDCs)	
	Intensive phase	*Continuationphase*
	HRZE	*HRE*
Weight category	*75/150/400/275*	*75/150/275*
40 kg	2	2
41–55 kg	3	3
56–70 kg	4	4
>70 kg	5	5

22. Neetu, a 10-year-old girl weighing 24 kg comes with the complaints of cough for the past one month. Parents give history of child having loss of appetite and weight. She also has evening rise of temperature. Sputum examination reveals acid fast bacilli. Chest radiograph shows apical pulmonary infiltrates. Prescribe suitable drug therapy for this patient. (Tuberculosis)

Rx:

- Tab Isoniazid (INH) 10 mg/kg once daily for 2 months
- Tab Rifampicin 15 mg/kg once daily for 2 months
- Tab Pyrazinamide 30 mg/kg once daily for 2 months
- Tab Ethambutol 20 mg/kg once daily for 2 months
- This is followed by continuation phase
- Tab Isoniazid (INH) 10 mg/kg once daily for 4 months
- Tab Rifampicin 15 mg/kg once daily for 4 months
- Tab Ethambutol 30 mg/kg once daily for 4 months

Follow up: After 1 month for assessment and appearance of side effects.

Doctor sign and stamp
Registration no.

23. **A 45-year-old male Mr Krishna presented with the complaints of multiple pale patches in the skin. Physical examination revealed the skin lesion to be pale, anesthetic and macular. There was also superficial nerve thickening. Laboratory examination revealed acid fast bacilli in skin lesions. Prescribe suitable drug therapy for this patient. (Leprosy)**

Rx:
- Tab Dapsone 100 mg 1 tablet once a day for 1 year
- Cap Rifampicin 600 mg 1 tablet once a month under supervision for 1 year.
- Tab Clofazimine 50 mg 1 tablet once a day and 300 mg once a month under supervision
- Total duration of therapy is for 12 months.
- Total duration of therapy is for 12 months.

Follow up: Every month for assessment of response
Dispense (for 1 month): 28 tablets of dapsone 100 mg and clofazimine 50 mg each, 1 capsule of rifampicin 600 mg and 1 tablet of clofazimine 100 mg each

Doctor sign and stamp
Registration no.

24. **An adult female patient of 42 years, weight 60 kg is diagnosed to be suffering from paucibacillary leprosy. Prescribe suitable drug therapy for this patient.**

Rx:
- Tab Dapsone 100 mg 1 tablet once a day for 6 months
- Cap Rifampicin 600 mg 1 tablet once a month under supervision for 6 months.

Total duration of therapy is for 6 months.

Follow up: Every month for assessment of response
Dispense (for 1 month): 28 tablets of dapsone 100 mg and 1 capsule of rifampicin 600 mg

Doctor sign and stamp
Registration no.

25. **A patient after initiation of antileprosy regimen comes with acute onset of erythema and swelling of previous lesions with painful neuritis with or without loss of nerve function accompanied by pain and tenderness in the effected nerves. Prescribe suitable for the condition. (Lepra reaction)**

Rx:
Tab Prednisolone 40 mg 1 tablet once daily for 1 week. Patient is to be examined weekly and the dose of corticosteroid is reduced gradually after 2 weeks.

Follow up: Patient is to be examined weekly and the dose of corticosteroid is reduced every 2 weeks.

Dispense: 7 tablets of Prednisolone 40 mg

Doctor sign and stamp
Registration no.

Important point

Maximum dose of prednisolone is 1 mg/kg/day

26. **Prescribe drugs for deworming in a 10 year child.**

Rx:

Tab Albendazole 400 mg single dose

Dispense: 1 tablet of tab Albendazole 400 mg

Doctor sign and stamp
Registration no.

Important point

Instead of albendazole, Tab Mebendazole 100 mg twice a day for 3 days

27. **A 34-year-old female (55 kg) with a past medical history of type 2 diabetes mellitus (BMI 31 kg/m^2) who was brought to the emergency room with a new onset tonic-clonic seizure. MRI demonstrated a well-defined ring enhancing cystic lesion in occipital suggesting granulomatous (Neurocysticercosis). Prescribe suitable drugs for her.**

Rx:

- Tab Albendazole 15 mg/kg daily in two divided doses after fatty meals for 15 days
- Tab Prednisolone 40 mg/day to be started 2 days before and continued till 2 weeks after completing anthelminthic course, thereby gradually taper the dose.
- Tab Lamotrigine XR 50 mg 1 tablet once daily for 2 weeks

Follow up: After 2 weeks for dose adjustment of lamotrigine and prednisolone.

Dispense: 30 tablets of albendazole 400 mg

Doctor sign and stamp
Registration no.

28. **Prescribe for a patient suffering from tapeworm infection.**

Rx:

Tab Praziquantel 10 mg/kg single dose

Doctor sign and stamp
Registration no.:

29. A 30-year-old married lady came to the gynecology OPD with complaints of vaginal discharge and pruritus for the past week. Per speculum examination revealed a creamy, foul-smelling discharge with vascular congestion of the vagina and cervix. No other abnormality was detected on the vaginal examination. A wet smear of the vaginal discharge demonstrated the presence of *Trichomonas vaginalis*. Write down the prescription for this patient. What instructions will you give to this patient?

Rx:

Tab Metronidazole 400 mg 1 tablet thrice daily for 7 days

Clotrimazole 100 mg vaginal tablets once daily for 7 days

Non-pharmacological advise:

- No sexual intercourse during the treatment.
- The male partner should also given the same course.
- Repeat course could be given after 4 weeks.

Follow up: After 7 days

Dispense: 21 tablets of metronidazole 400 mg and 1 vaginal tablet of clotrimazole 100 mg

The male partner should also be given the same course.

A repeat course could be given after 4 weeks.

Doctor sign and stamp
Registration no.

30. A 20-year-old woman complains of itching and irritation, in the vagina. A burning sensation, while urinating with thick, white, odor-free vaginal discharge with a cottage cheese appearance. Write a prescription for her. (Candidial vaginitis)

Rx:

- Tab Fluconazole 150 mg 1 tablet as a single dose.
- Clotrimazole vaginal pessary 100 mg at bedtime every night for 7 days

Follow up: After 7 days

Dispense: 1 tablet of fluconazole 150 mg and 7 vaginal tablet of clotrimazole 100 mg

Doctor sign and stamp
Registration no.

31. A 50-year-old man presented with fever, blisters and pain on the left side of his face for the past 2 days. The pain was very severe, continuous, radiating up to the forehead and ear, and had a tingling sensation. The unilateral distribution of painful, grouped vesicles in a dermatomal pattern suggested herpes zoster. Write a prescription for him.

Rx:
- **Tab Acyclovir 200 mg 1 tablet 5 times a day for 10 days**
- Tab Pregabalin 150 mg in three divided doses for 10 days
- Ointment acyclovir (5%) to be applied every four hourly for 5 days.

Follow up: After 10 days

Dispense: 50 tablets of acyclovir 800 mg, 30 tablets of ibuprofen 400 mg and 1 tube of ointment acyclovir (5%)

Doctor sign and stamp
Registration no.

Important point

Instead of acyclovir, famciclovir and valacyclovir can be prescribed.

7.9: AUTONOMIC NERVOUS SYSTEM

1. **A middle aged Asian woman with depression was brought to emergency attention after drinking of 60 milliliter of organophosphate insecticide in a suicidal attempt. She had vomiting, excessive retching, diarrhea, miosis, hypersalivation and bilateral crepitation on chest during admission. Write a prescription for her. (Organophosphate poisoning)**

   Rx:
   - Gastric lavage with potassium permanganate (1:1000) solution
   - Inj Atropine 2 mg IV repeated every 10 minutes till signs of atropinization.
   - Inj Pralidoxime 1 g IV given over 20 minutes and repeated if required after 1 hour

   Doctor sign and stamp
   Registration no.

   Important points
   - Signs of atropinization are (dilated pupils, dry mouth, dry skin, tachycardia)
   - Pralidoxime can be used to maximum of 12 g
   - Supportive measures include gastric lavage, maintenance of patent airway, blood pressure

2. **An 11-year-old girl, under rifampicin and isoniazid for lymph node tuberculosis, who developed jaundice as side effect of this treatment. She was given *Atropa belladonna* by an herbalist in a therapeutic interest. Since then, the patient presented—dry mouth, confusion, incoherent speech, inability to recognize members of the family, she also presented uncontrollable vomiting, visual disturbances, hearing and visual hallucinations. Write a prescription for her.**

Rx:
- Gastric lavage with tannic acid
- Patient kept in dark quiet room
- Cold sponging applied
- Inj Physostigmine 2 mg slow IV and repeated every 3 hours till symptoms improve

Doctor sign and stamp
Registration no.

3. **Write a prescription for a mydriatic to be used for fundoscopy.**

Rx:
2.5% Phenylephrine one eye drop instilled in each eye

Doctor sign and stamp
Registration no.

4. **Write a prescription for a mydriatic for refractive error.**

Rx:
Tropicamide-instill one or two drops of 1% solution in the eye(s), repeat in five minutes.

Doctor sign and stamp
Registration no.

5. **A 19-year-old boy is brought to the emergency department after being stung by a bee. He had been well until he was stung on his right forearm, while playing in the yard. He initially complained of localized pain and swelling. Fifteen minutes later, he began to complain of shortness of breath. His parents observed him to be wheezing. He also said that he felt very weak and dizzy. His parents brought him immediately to the local emergency department and was diagnosed as having anaphylactic shock. Write a prescription for this patient.**

Rx:
- Inj Adrenaline (0.5 mL to 1 mL) of 1:1000 solution IM repeat every 5 minutes. (to a maximum of 3 doses)
- Inj Hydrocortisone 200 mg IV loading then 100 mg every 6 hours
- Inj Pheniramine 25 mg slow IV repeat every 6 hours
- Humidified oxygen
- 5% glucose saline 500 mL over 4 hours

Doctor sign and stamp
Registration no.

Important points
- Find out the cause and avoid the etiological agent as far as possible.
- Inj Adrenaline can be given iv slowly (1:10,000 solution).

6. **Write a prescription for a patient with cardiogenic shock.**

   Rx:
   - Inj Dobutamine 2 μg/kg/min as IV infusion. To be titrated to the individual requirement.
   - Inj Soda Bicarbonate (7.5%) 100 mL IV.

   Doctor sign and stamp
   Registration no.

   Important points
   - Instead of inj Dobutamine dopamine or inj Amrinone can be given.
   - The dose of dopamine is given in the range of 5–15 μg/kg/min. The drip rate may be increased if the BP response is not adequate.

7. **A 34-year-old woman presents with bilateral severe visual. Her best-corrected visual acuity (BCVA) was counting fingers in both eyes. Intraocular pressures were 49 mm and 51 mm of Hg in right and left eyes respectively, with conjunctival chemosis, corneal edema, shallow anterior chamber and closed angles on gonioscopy. Write a prescription for acute congestive glaucoma.**

   Rx:
   - Inj Mannitol (20%) 1.5 g/kg IV over 60 minutes
   - Inj Acetazolamide 500 mg IV followed by tab Acetazolamide 250 mg 2 tab twice a day for till IOP is normalized.
   - Pilocarpine drops (2%) 1 drop every 10 minutes (total 4 doses)
   - Timolol eye drops (0.5%) one drop 12 hourly.

   Doctor sign and stamp
   Registration no.

   Important point
   - Medical therapy is always followed by surgical treatment, i.e., laser iridotomy.
   - Instead of timolol latanoprost can be instilled.
   - After IOP is normalized definitive treatment is laser iridectomy.

8. **A patient, a 61-year-old female retired school teacher, reports no problems with driving, watching TV, computer or reading. She admits to mild eye burning feeling after reading for long periods of time or in the afternoons. She denies any flashes, floaters, pain, redness or double vision. IOP (tonoapplantation) was: once day: 21 mm Hg. OS: 23 mm Hg. She was diagnosed as chronic simple glaucoma. write a prescription for her.**

   Rx:

   Latanoprost (0.005%) eye drops. One drop instilled in affected eye(s) once daily in the evening

Follow up: After 6 weeks to evaluate Intraocular pressure and fundoscopy

Dispense: 10 mL bottle of latanoprost (0.005%) eye drops

Doctor sign and stamp
Registration no.

Important point

Timolol 0.25% eye drops twice daily can be used as an alternative.

9. **A 56-year-old man has a 2-year history of increasing voiding symptoms—weak stream, intermittent flow, straining to urinate, incomplete emptying, hematuria (>3–4 RBC/high-powered field) on urine microscopy in the absence of infection with prostate volume (on transrectal ultrasonography, i.e., TRUS): 55 mL. The condition was diagnosed as benign hypertrophy prostate. Write a prescription.**

Rx:
- Cap Tamsulosin 0.4 mg 1 capsule once a day for 2 weeks
- Tab Finasteride 5 mg 1 tablet once a day for 2 weeks.

Follow up: After 2 weeks for evaluation.

Dispense: 14 capsules of tamsulosin 0.4 mg and 14 tablets of finasteride 5 mg

Doctor sign and stamp
Registration no.

Important point

Tamsulosin (uricoselective) is preferred over prazosin affects the dynamic component. While—Finasteride reduces the static component of the obstruction.

10. **A 71-year-old male complains of intermittent weakness and muscle fatigue progressively worsening over the past month. He had symptoms of profound leg weakness. He reports having noted "eye strain" and intermittent double vision that seems to be worse when reading at bedtime. The anti-acetylcholine receptor binding antibody was 12.04 nmol/L (normal <0.40 nmol/L), the blocking antibody was 52% (normal <26%), and modulating antibody was 84% (normal <45%), which is consistent with a diagnosis of myasthenia gravis. Write a prescription for him.**

Rx:
- Tab Pyridostigmine 60 mg 1 tablet thrice daily for 15 days
- Tab Prednisolone 20 mg 1 tablet once a day for 15 days

Follow up: After 15 days to discontinue Prednisolone or adjust dose

Dispense: 45 tablets Pyridostigmine 60 mg of and 15 tablets of prednisolone 20 mg

Doctor sign and stamp
Registration no.

11. **Write a prescription for severe postural hypotension.**

Rx:
- Tab Midodrine 5 mg 1 tablet thrice a day
- Tab Midodrine to be taken shortly before, or upon arising in the morning, midday and late afternoon (not later than 6 PM).
- Tab Fludrocortisone 0.1 mg 1 tablet once a day
- Patients should avoid large carbohydrate-rich meals, limit alcohol intake, and ensure adequate hydration. Patients should be encouraged to keep a symptom diary and avoid identified precipitating factors.

Follow up: After 7 days

Dispense: 21 tablets of Midodrine 5 mg and 7 tablets of Fludrocortisone 0.1

Doctor sign and stamp
Registration no.

Important point

Midodrine is to be taken shortly before, or upon arising in the morning, midday and late afternoon (not later than 6 PM). Doses may be given in 3-hour intervals, if required, to control symptoms, but not more frequently.

12. **Write a prescription for essential tremors.**

Rx:

Tab Propranolol 10 mg 1 tablet once daily: Gradually titrated every 7 days to 20 mg/twice daily

Follow up: After 7 days

Dispense: 7 tablets of Propranolol 10 mg

Doctor sign and stamp
Registration no.

Important point

Maximum dose of propranolol is 320 mg/day.

13. **Write a prescription for epistaxis.**

Rx:
- Gentle pressure applied over the nostril with thumb and index finger.
- Adrenaline pack (1:1000) in the bleeding nostril.

Doctor sign and stamp
Registration no.

Important points
- Instead of adrenaline, oxymetazoline can be used.
- Tranexamic acid and ethamsylate can be used as an add-on drug.

14. A 26-year-old female presented in the emergency room complaining of a two-week history of right flank pain. Her past medical history was unremarkable but included an episode of pyelonephritis two years ago. The kidney-ureter-bladder X-ray revealed ureteric stones. write a prescription for her.

Rx:

- Inj Diclofenac sodium (75 mg/3 mL) 3 mL IM STAT
- Inj Drotaverin IM 20 mg thrice daily

Doctor sign and stamp
Registration no.

15. A 20-year-old girl Ms Kala experiences vomiting whenever she travels to a hilly area. Prescribe suitable drug(s) for this patient who is to embark on a picnic trip by bus to a hilly area. (Motion sickness).

Rx:

Tab Promethazine 25 mg, the first dose taken one hour before the start of the journey then 4 times a day till vomiting subsides.

Doctor sign and stamp
Registration no.

16. A 68-year-old woman with a 2-year history of repetitiveness, memory loss, and executive function loss. MRI revealed mild generalized cortical atrophy. Neurocognitive assessment at the first clinic visit revealed a Mini-Mental State Examination (MMSE) score of 14/30; poor verbal fluency (patient was able to produce only 5 animal names and 1 F-word in 1 min) as well as poor visuospatial and executive skills. Patient was diagnosed as Alzheimer's disease. Write a prescription for her.

Rx:

Tab Donepezil 5 mg 1 tablet administered per day in the evening before sleep

Follow up: After 4 weeks

Dispense: 28 tablets of Donepezil 5 mg

Doctor sign and stamp
Registration no.

Important point

Other cerebroselectives, such as rivastigmine, galantamine can be used.

7.10: MISCELLANEOUS

1. **A 52-year-old woman Mrs Mamta presented with pain, redness and warmth over her first toe. A laboratory examination of fluid taken from an inflamed joint revealed crystals of uric acid and she was diagnosed to have acute gout. Prescribe for this patient.**

   Rx:

   Tab Diclofenac 50 mg 1 tablet thrice a day for 2 days after meals, gradually tapered as pain subsides: After the pain subsides tab Allopurinol 100 mg one tablet once a day.

   Non-pharmacological advice:

   Dietary modification with a low purine diet may be given.

   Follow up: After 1 week

   Dispense: 20 tablets of diclofenac 50 mg (2 strips) and 7 tablets of allopurinol 100 mg

   Doctor sign and stamp
   Registration no.

   Important points

   - Other NSAIDs can be prescribed, such as naproxen, ibuprofen and diclofenac
   - As an alternative to indomethacin can be prescribed. Tab Colchicine 12 mg every 4 hourly till the pain subsides or till GI symptoms occur.

2. **Prescribe for a patient of rheumatoid arthritis.**

   Rx:

   - Tab Methotrexate 2.5 mg, 3 tablets once a week
   - Tab Folic acid 5 mg once weekly

   Follow up: After 1 month for clinical evaluation

   Dispense: 12 tablets of Methotrexate 2.5 mg and 4 tablets of folic acid 5 mg

   Doctor sign and stamp
   Registration no.

   Important point

   Before starting methotrexate CBC, LFT, serum creatinine.

3. **Mr Ranga, 40 years of age presents to the emergency having sustained a snake-bite this morning at 3 AM. He presents to the casualty now (7 AM) with pain and swelling at the site of the bite. The patient has a clotting time of 23 minutes. How will you manage a case of viper envenomation?**

Rx:

- ASV (anti-snake venom) 10 vials stat as infusion over 30 minutes followed by dose of 10 vials after 1 hour, if no improvement within first 1 hour.
- Additional infusions containing 5 10 vials (50–100 mL) should be repeated hourly until progressive swelling in the bitten part ceases and systemic signs and symptoms disappear.

Doctor sign and stamp
Registration no.

7.11: EMERGENCY PHARMACOTHERAPY

1. **A 28-year-old type 1 diabetic Mr Ramu presented to the emergency department with the complaints of marked fatigue, nausea and vomiting and mental confusion. Detailed history reveals that he is a diabetic for the past ten years and he is irregular in taking insulin injections. Physical examination shows dehydration, rapid deep breathing and a fruity breath odor. Laboratory investigations show blood glucose—480 mg/dL, urine ketones—strongly positive. Prescribe suitable drug(s) for this patient. (Diabetic ketoacidosis).**

   Rx:

   - Inj Plain Insulin 0.1 U/kg given IV bolus followed by 0.1 units/kg/hour IV infusion in 2 liters of normal saline.
   - Normal Saline IV at the rate of 1L/hr. Once vitals stabilized, change to normal saline.
   - Inj KCL 20 mEq/hr as IV infusion. (serum K is monitored)
   - Inj Cefotaxime 1 g IV BD for 3 days.

   Doctor sign and stamp
   Registration no.

   Important points

   - Blood sugar to be monitored every 4–6 hours till the patient become euglycemic.
   - Sodium bicarbonate to be prescribed if pH falls to 7 or below.

2. **A 36-year-old known epileptic patient M Kannan, was brought to the emergency department for repeated seizures without recovery or regaining consciousness for the past 20 minutes. Detailed history reveals that he is very irregular in taking antiepileptic medications. Prescribe suitable drugs for him. (Status epilepticus)**

Rx:

- To maintain airway, breathing and circulation (ABC)
- Inj Lorazepam 4 mg (0.1 mg/kg) at the rate of 2 mg/min loading dose to be injected slowly IV, repeated once after 10 min if required. If not controlled, up to a maximum of 0.3 mg/kg can be repeated.
- If seizures continue inj Fosphenytoin 100–150 mg/min as IV infusion
- If seizures continue inj Phenytoin 50 mg/min as IV infusion
- If seizures continue then Inj Phenobarbitone 60 mg/min as IV infusion
- If still not controlled inj Midazolam 0.2 mg/kg loading dose followed by 00.75–1 μg/kg/min as maintenance dose.

Doctor sign and stamp
Registration no.

Important points

- After convulsions stop change over to tab Phenytoin 100 mg thrice daily for 15 days.
- Dose of diazepam can be repeated 4 hourly, to a maximum of 100 mg/day.
- Instead of inj Phenytoin, inj Phenobarbitone can be administered.

3. **A 40-year-old known asthmatic Mr Kumar presented to the emergency department with difficulty in breathing. Physical examination revealed pallor and slight cyanosis. He was diagnosed with status asthmaticus. Prescribe suitable drug(s) for the treatment of this condition.**

Rx:

- Inj Hydrocortisone Hemisuccinate 100 mg iv stat followed by 100 mg 8 hourly)
- Nebulized Salbutamol + Ipratropium bromide intermittent inhalation every 4 hours
- Inj Terbutaline 0.25 mg SC
- Intermittent humidified O_2 (40%) inhalation at every 4–6 liters/min
- Inj Aminophylline 250 mg diluted in 25 mL of glucose solution injected in 25 minutes. This is followed by a 100 mg IV infusion every 8 hours
- Sodium bicarbonate (7.5%) 50 mL IV
- Inj Cefotaxime 500 mg iv 8 hourly

Doctor sign and stamp
Registration no.

4. **A middle aged Asian woman with depression was brought to emergency attention after drinking of 60 mL of organophosphate insecticide in a suicidal attempt. She had vomiting, excessive retching,**

diarrhoea, miosis, hypersalivation and bilateral crepitation on chest during admission. Write a prescription for her.

Rx:

- Gastric lavage with potassium permanganate (1:1000) solution
- Inj Atropine 2 mg IV repeated every 10 minutes till signs of atropinization.
- Inj Pralidoxime 1 g IV given over 20 minutes and repeated if required after 1 hour

Doctor sign and stamp
Registration no.

Important points

- Signs of atropinization are (dilated pupils, dry mouth, dry skin, tachycardia).
- Pralidoxime can be used to maximum of 12 g
- Supportive measures include gastric lavage, maintenance of patent airway, blood pressure.

5. **Mr Dwaraka is a 55-year-old patient who presents to the casualty with acute chest pain for the past 3 hours not responding to nitrates. He is a non-smoker, non-diabetic. The patient has hypertension for the last three years and is on treatment with Tab Atenolol 50 mg once day. ECG shows ST elevation in lead II, III and aVF. What treatment will you give him now?**

Rx:

- Complete bed rest
- Sublingual NTG (0.5 mg) every 3 min till 10 minutes
- Inj Morphine 10 mg + inj Metoclopramide 10 mg IV, then 2 mg every 10 min till pain stops.
- O_2 (100%) 2 liters for 4 hours by nasal catheter.
- Tab Aspirin 300 mg stat (chewed) and tab Clopidogrel 400 mg stat
- Inj Tenecteplase (0.5 mg/kg) single
- IV Bolus injection inj Alteplase 15 mg iv bolus injection followed by 50 mg over 30 min then 35 mg over next 1 hour.
- Inj Atenolol 10 mg iv followed by 100 mg orally.
- Inj NIG 5 μg/min continuous iv infusion increase by 5 μg/min every 5 minutes up to 20 μg/min.
- Inj Enoxaparin (low molecular weight heparin) 30 mg iv bolus plus 1 mg/kg SC once, then every 12 hours.
- Tab Atorvastatin 80 mg stat

Doctor sign and stamp
Registration no.

Important points

- For treatment of complications, e.g., arrhythmias inj Lignocaine 2% 50 mg LV as bolus followed by a drip rate of 1 mg/min. or DC shock. For bradycardia—inj Atropine 0.3–0.5 mg LV.
- General measures, such as diet, and bowel care should be taken care of.
- Rehabilitation is done with aspirin (75 mg) once day, beta-blocker (atenolol), ACE inhibitors, and modification of risk factors , such as smoking, alcohol, Rx of hypertension, diabetes and hyperlipidemia should be taken care of.
- Before giving streptokinase, inj Hydrocortisone 100 mg can be given IV to suppress allergic reactions. Instead of streptokinase, inj Urokinase or alteplase can also be given.

8 CHAPTER

Critical Appraisal of Prescriptions

AUTONOMIC NERVOUS SYSTEM

1. **Comment on the following prescription for a patient who has consumed 200 mL of parathion. Do not criticize the format of the prescription.**

   Rx:

   Inj Atropine 0.5 mL IM twice daily
   Inj Neostigmine 50 mg thrice daily
   Inj Pralidoxime 50 mg thrice daily

   Dr ABC
   Reg. No:

   Criticism:
   - Atropine is the drug of choice in Parathion (irreversible anticholinesterase) poisoning. But the dose given here is incorrect.
   - Neostigmine is contraindicated in parathion poisoning as it an anticholinesterase, would increase the ACh levels and aggravate cholinergic effects.
   - Pralidoxime is a cholinesterase reactivator; it combines with the phosphorylated cholinesterase to form oxime-phosphonate, which diffuses away easily, which leaves the reactivated enzyme. Treatment should be started as early as possible, before the enzyme becomes aged. The dose given here is incorrect.

2. **Comment on the following prescription for a patient with anaphylactic shock:**

   Rx:

   Inj Adrenaline (5 mg) IV stat
   Cap Ampicillin (500 mg). 1 cap three times daily.
   Tab Prednisolone (50 mg). 1 tab three times daily.

   Dr ABC
   Reg. No:

Criticism:
- Adrenaline is the correct drug but dose and route wrong.
- Ampicillin itself can cause allergy, C/I in anaphylactic shock.
- A parenteral steroid, such as hydrocortisone/dexamethasone is to be used, prednisolone can be used latter, after 1–2 days of parenteral steroids.

3. **Comment on the following prescription for a patient with open-angle glaucoma:**

Rx:
Homatropine eye drops 1% twice daily
Mannitol 20% 2 g/kg iv stat
Timolol 0.25% eye drops twice daily

Dr ABC
Reg. No:

Criticism:
- Homatropine is anticholinergic drug, because of its mydriatic and cycloplegic action can lead to rise in IOP hence contraindicated in narrow angle and open-angle glaucoma.
- Mannitol is osmotic diuretic, indicated as first-line treatment in acute congestive glaucoma. It has no role in open-angle glaucoma.
- Timolol is a appropriate drug and the dose is also correct. Latanoprost can be used as an alternative.

CARDIOVASCULAR SYSTEM

1. **Comment on the following prescription for a patient having moderate congestive cardiac failure (CCF) in a patient having paroxysmal atrial tachycardia.**

Rx:
Tab Hydrochlorothiazide 12.5 mg once daily
Tab Atenolol 50 mg thrice daily.
Inj Furosemide (10 mg per nmL) 2 mL daily/1 m
Tab Verapamil 20 mg 8 hourly.

Dr ABC
Reg. No:

Criticism:
- Hydrochlorothiazide (medium efficacy diuretic-relieves edema) can be given in moderate CCF but 12.5 mg is an antihypertensive dose. The dose required for CCF is higher (25–50 mg per day.) if the edema is more than high efficacy furosemide can be used
- Atenolol is 2nd add on drug in a patient of CCF with paroxysmal atrial tachycardia, but the dose mentioned here is not correct. It has to be started with low doses.

- Syrup KCl or potassium sparing diuretic (spironolactone) should be given in conjunction with concurrent use of above diuretics (as they cause hypokalemia).
- Enalapril (arteriovenous vasodilator), is first line in CCF.
- Verapamil is not indicated in CCF. It can precipitate failure as it decreases cardiac output.

2. **Comment on the following prescription for a patient discharged from the hospital following treatment for acute myocardial infarction with history of coronary artery disease. He was on irregular treatment for hypertension for 2 years prior to this event. He is a non-smoker, does not have diabetes, obesity or dyslipidemia. He is prescribed the following drugs at discharge:**

Rx:
Tab Metoprolol 200 mg thrice daily
Tab Alprazolam 5 mg at night
Tab Nitroglycerine 10 mg whenever required

Dr ABC
Reg. No:

Criticism:
- Tab Metoprolol (cardioselective β-blocker) can be prescribed for post-MI patient but the dose is very high. They may act by preventing reinfarction and sudden ventricular fibrillation at the next attack.
- Alprazolam 5 mg can be prescribed for few days post-MI. It reduces anxiety and insomnia because of associated stress.
- Nitroglycerine is used for acute chest pain. Instead, Tab Isosorbide dinitrate 10 mg can be continued for prophylaxis.
- Aspirin 75 mg or clopidogrel (antiplatelet drugs) should be prescribed post-MI.

3. **Comment on the following prescription for a 55-year-old male patient having BP of 140/100 mg of Hg and detected as having type II diabetes mellitus. Do not criticize the format of the prescription.**

Rx:
Tab Propranolol 40 mg twice daily
Tab Glibenclamide 50 mg twice daily
Tab Hydrochlorothiazide 50 mg twice daily

Dr ABC
Reg. No:

Criticism:
- Propranolol (non-selective beta-blocker), is contraindicated in diabetics. It prolongs hypoglycemia by inhibiting the compensatory mechanisms (i.e., warning signs of hypoglycemia, such as palpitation, tremor, and anxiety). They block beta 2 receptors in the liver inhibiting the glycogenolysis. [UNAWARENESS HYPOGLYCEMIA]

- Hydrochlorothiazide (50 mg) given over a long period of time can cause hyperglycemia (by inhibiting insulin release) hence contraindicated in a patient of hypertension with diabetes.
- Glibenclamide can be given for Type II DM, but the dose given here is incorrect. It is started in the dose of 5 mg once or twice daily. Non-pharmacological measures are not included.

4. **Comment on the following prescription for a male patient having an acute attack of angina pectoris. He also suffers from bronchial asthma. Do not criticize the format of the prescription.**

Rx:

Tab Glyceryl trinitrate 5 mg oral once daily

Tab Propranolol 20 mg stat

Tab Aspirin 600 mg stat, with one tablet to be continued life long

Dr ABC

Reg. No:

Criticism:

- Glyceryl trinitrate (GTN) is a drug of choice for acute attack of angina, but route of administration is not oral. It is given sublingually to avoid first pass metabolism in the liver, to have faster onset of action. Other nitrates, such as isosorbide dinitrate can also be given sublingually in an acute attack.
- Aspirin (600 mg) not required in this anginal pain. Aspirin at a dose of 75–150 mg, has antiplatelet action which can be prescribed post-MI.
- Propranolol a non-selective beta blocker used only in prophylaxis of classical angina. It has no role in acute attack, can be prescribed to a patient after the acute subsides. It blocks β_2 receptors causing bronchospasm precipitating an attack of bronchial asthma. Instead isosorbide dinitrate, or the calcium channel blockers can be used in this patient.

5. **Comment on the following prescription for a 50-year-old ischemic heart disease patient who is already on tab Aspirin 165 mg once daily and tab Isosorbide dinitrate 10 mg thrice daily is diagnosed to have hypertension in a routine medical check-up. He was prescribed**

Rx:

Tab Nifedipine 10 mg thrice daily

Tab Hydralazine 25 mg twice daily

Dr ABC

Reg. No:

Criticism:

- Nifedipine is a calcium channel blocker, which can be prescribed but plain nifedipine is not preferred because of shorter duration and because of the adverse effect of reflex tachycardia. Instead, nifedipine SR/Retard preparations or amlodipine can be prescribed.

- Nifedipine and hydralazine (arteriolar vasodilator) both cause reflex tachycardia hence is not to be prescribed individually or even concomitantly.
- Tab Aspirin dose 165 mg is used for antiplatelet action. But lower dose 75 mg is preferred.

6. **Mr Harris, aged 60 years with past history of MI and diabetes is on treatment with metformin 850 mg tds and glibenclamide 5 mg bd for his blood sugars. He presents to the casualty with signs of severe congestive heart failure and high blood sugars (blood glucose 340 mg/dL). The patient is given the following drugs:**

   Rx:

   Inj Morphine 5 mg iv stat
   Inj Furosemide 40 mg iv q8h
   Inj Mannitol 100 mL iv q8h
   Tab Metformin 850 mg tds
   Tab Pioglitazone 30 mg od

   Dr ABC
   Reg. No:

   Comment on the choice of each of the above drugs for this patient.

   Criticism:
   - Morphine can be given for acute CCF with pulmonary edema for the following:
     » Reduces preload on heart by causing vasodilatation and peripheral pooling of blood
     » Shift blood from pulmonary to systemic circulation relieving pulmonary congestion and edema
     » Calms the patient, reduces the anxiety and sympathetic stimulation thus reducing cardiac work
   - Furosemide also reduce pulmonary edema associated with CCF (same first two mechanisms as above).
   - Mannitol is contraindicated in pulmonary edema associated with CCF.
   - Since blood sugar is on the higher side i.v. regular/soluble insulin is to be given. All oral antidiabetics (Pioglitazone and metformin) need to be stopped and patient switched over to insulin. Pioglitazone causes fluid retention can aggravate CCF.

7. **Mr Ranjith, 67-year-old man, a known case of diabetes with hypertension for the last 10 years was on the following drugs:**

   Rx:

   Tab Glimepiride 1 mg od
   Tab Metformin 500 mg tds
   Tab Hydrochlorothiazide 25 mg bd
   Tab Aspirin 150 mg od

   Dr ABC
   Reg. No:

The patient is brought to the casualty by his relatives with complaints of malaise, lethargy, loss of appetite, pruritus. Examination reveals hypertension with a blood pressure of 150/90 mm Hg, cardiomegaly, rales and pleural effusion. Laboratory investigations revealed blood urea—70 mg%, serum creatinine—3.2 mg/dL, Na^+- 127 mEq/dL, K^+ - 5.9 mEq/L. Random blood glucose—158 mg/dL. A diagnosis of chronic renal failure is made.

Comment on the above prescription. What important complication (drug related) is the patient at risk now?

Criticism:

- Long-term of aspirin (NSAIDs) is known to cause analgesic nephropathy (by inhibiting renal PGs).
- Hydrochlorothiazide decreases GFR can aggravate renal failure.
- Metformin is excreted unchanged by kidney and is contraindicated in renal insufficiency because risk of adverse effects, such as lactic acidosis may increase.
- Glimepiride is relatively safe in chronic renal failure.

CENTRAL NERVOUS SYSTEM

1. **Comment the following prescription for a patient who complains of tremors of fingers, rigidity of facial muscles and mental depression diagnosed as Parkinson's. Do not criticize the format of the prescription.**

Rx:

Tab Levodopa 100 mg once daily

Tab Pyridoxine 10 mg twice daily

Dr ABC

Reg. No:

Criticism:

- Levodopa is the correct drug for treatment of this patient but it is never given alone because 98% of it gets peripherally decarboxylated by dopa decarboxylase (DDC) enzyme to dopamine which cannot cross the bood brain barrier. It is always available as fixed dose combination with Carbidopa/Benserazide.
- They are Peripheral DDC inhibitors. They prevent the peripheral decarboxylation of levodopa so that more is made available to cross the blood brain barrier to reach the brain. The dose given is incorrect. It is started with the combination of (Levodopa + Carbidopa) (100 mg + 25 mg) thrice daily to max of levodopa of 2 g.
- Pyridoxine is vitamin B_6, which is a cofactor for enzyme dopa decarboxylase, given along with levodopa it would increase the peripheral decarboxylation, thereby decreasing the therapeutic effect of levodopa.

Note: Antidopaminergics (Phenothiazines, haloperidol, metoclopramide but not domperidone) also reverse the therapeutic effect of levodopa.

2. **Criticize the following prescription for a patient to be given lignocaine 2% plus adrenaline 1:10000 for a contused lacerated wound at the tip of the toe.**

Rx:

Inj Lignocaine 2 % plus adrenaline 1:80000

Dr ABC

Reg. No:

Criticism:

- Adrenaline is combined with lignocaine because:
- Adrenaline because of its vasoconstricting action would increase the duration of the action of the lignocaine.
- La remains in the localized area thereby decreasing the systemic toxicity (Heart and CNS).
- The combination of adrenaline with local anesthesia in the dilution of (1:50,000 or 1:200,000).
- However for surgery done at END ARTERIES, i.e., tip of fingers, toes, pinna and penis this combination would be contraindicated as there is no collateral circulation and the area can go in necrosis and turn gangrenous.
- Therefore, at these places only lignocaine ALONE and should not be combined with adrenaline.

3. **Mr Banerjee, is a patient 58 years of age who has undergone a subtotal gastrectomy for carcinoma stomach. He is a known case of ischemic heart disease on regular treatment for two years. In the postoperative period, he has been given the following medication on day 1:**

Rx:

Inj Morphine 5 mg SC q6h

Inj Pentazocine 30 mg IM q6h

Inj Ketorolac 30 mg IM q6h

Inj Lorazepam 4 mg IV q12h

Dr ABC

Reg. No:

Comment on the above prescription assuming that the doses are appropriate.

Criticism:

- Inj Morphine (opioid) or Ketorolac (NSAID) both will control postoperative pain effectively. But since this is postoperative cancer pain morphine would be a better choice.
- Pentazocine is an opioid can control pain but is contraindicated in ischemic heart disease because it stimulates sympathetic system.
- Lorazepam is a benzodiazepine has no role in postoperative period.

4. **Mrs Meena, fifty years of age who underwent hysterectomy was prescribed the following for insomnia due to postoperative pain:**

   Rx:

   Inj Pethidine 2 mg s.c. sos
   Inj Diazepam 10 mg hs after first dose

   Dr ABC
   Reg. No:

   - Half an hour after the injections, she became very agitated and restless. Comment on the situation above, correct and rewrite the above prescription, if necessary.
   - Diazepam probably has caused this paradoxical stimulation.
   - She can be prescribed inj Tramadol 50 mg thrice a day and diclofenac suppository PR twice daily.

5. **Comment on the following prescription for Rishi a 8-year-old boy who has been diagnosed with absence seizures. He is started on:**

   Rx:

   Tab Carbamazepine 100 mg TDS
   Tab Valproate sodium 200 mg TDS

   Dr ABC
   Reg. No:

   Criticism:

   - Carbamazepine is not indicated in absence seizures.
   - Valproate is given in the dose of 20–30 mg/kg body weight. So initial dosage could be started at 400 mg per day, with spaced intervals.

6. **Mr Kumar, a 50-year-old patient, on tab Haloperidol 10 mg tds developed rigidity and bradykinesia. He was diagnosed to have haloperidol induced Parkinsonism. He was started on tab Levodopa (100 mg) + carbidopa (25 mg) tds. There was no improvement in the symptoms of Parkinsonism. Comment.**

   Criticism:

   Haloperidol is a typical antipsychotic acts by blocking the D_2 receptors in the mesocortical and the mesolimbic tract. Haloperidol induced Parkinsonism is an extrapyramidal manifestation which is because of reduced dopamine action in nigrostriatal tract.

   Levodopa (100 mg) + carbidopa FDC will increase the dopamine in the all the tracts. So, it will indirectly neutralize both the effects (anti-psychotic and Parkinson's effect) of haloperidol.

RESPIRATORY SYSTEM

1. **Comment on the following prescription for a male patient having acute attack of bronchial asthma. Do not criticize the format of the prescription.**

   Rx:

   Tab Salbutamol 2 mg twice daily
   Tab Prednisolone 1 mg once daily
   Tab Aspirin 100 mg twice daily

   Dr ABC
   Reg. No:

   Criticism:

   - Salbutamol is a drug of choice in acute attack of asthma but the route of administration is not correct. Salbutamol is given as a metered dose inhaler.
   - Corticosteroids are not indicated in an acute attack of asthma, unless it is a severe attack or in status asthmatics. If given, it is given by intravenous route of administration and later on shifted to oral followed by inhalation route. Prednisolone is not given in acute attack, because it is not available in inhalation form or in parenteral—dosage form. Commonly prescribed parenteral corticosteroids are dexamethasone and hydrocortisone.
   - Aspirin inhibits the cyclooxygenase enzyme-giving rise to preferential production of leukotrienes, which would further aggravate the bronchial asthma attack.

2. **Comment on the following prescription for a patient with headache having acute attack of bronchial asthma. Do not criticize the format of the prescription.**

   Rx:

   Cap Cromolyn sodium (10 mg) three times a day
   Tab Ephedrine (100 mg)
   Tab Prednisolone (1 mg) QID
   Tab Aspirin (100 mg) tabs

   Dr ABC
   Reg. No:

   Criticism:

   - Cromolyn sodium has no role in acute attack of asthma.
     » Ephedrine is non-selective bronchodilator, so salbutamol/formetrol a selective β-2 agonist is preferred.
     » Prednisolone an oral steroid can be given in acute attack but a parenteral steroid, such as hydrocortisone, dexamethasone is preferred.
     » Aspirin an NSAID is C/I in asthma, as it inhibits the cycloxygenase enzyme giving to preferential production of leukotrienes. So paracetamol can be given for headache.

GASTROINTESTINAL SYSTEM

1. **Criticize the following prescription for a patient having rheumatoid arthritis suffering from recurrent peptic ulcers. Do not criticize the format of prescription. Do not prescribe for arthritis.**

   Rx:

   Tab Aspirin 350 mg thrice daily
   Tab Ranitidine 100 mg twice daily
   Tab Sodium bicarbonate 50 mg twice daily

   Dr ABC
   Reg. No:

   Criticism:

   - Aspirin is a NSAID. It inhibits the prostaglandins in the stomach, which are cytoprotective in action. It remains unionized and diffuses in the gastric juice but on entering the mucosal cell, it ionizes causing ion trapping, which irritates gastric mucosa. Aspirin particles coming in contact with gastric mucosa, also promotes back diffusion of the acid causing focal necrosis producing acute ulcers. Hence NSAIDs, especially non-selective COX inhibitors are contraindicated in patient of peptic ulcer. Aspirin no longer used for RA, DMARDs like methotrexate is a drug of choice.
   - Ranitidine/Omeprazole (PPI) are preferred drugs for treatment of peptic ulcer. Omeprazole 20 mg OD is more effective than H_2 blockers in the treatment of peptic ulcer.
   - Sodium bicarbonate is a systemic antacid but has various disadvantages. It gets absorbed systemically to produce alkalosis. Sodium bicarbonate also produces acid rebound (short lasting). It increases the Na load, may worsen edema and CHF and hence not suitable for use in peptic ulcer. Its use is restricted to casual treatment of gastroesophageal reflux.
   - Since the patient has recurrent peptic ulcer, he should be prescribed anti-*Helicobacter pylori* regimen.

2. **Comment on the following prescription for Mr Babu (35 years old) had epigastric pain. After examination and investigation, he was diagnosed to have peptic ulcer and was prescribed the following:**

   Rx:

   Cap Omeprazole 200 mg OD after food
   Tab Aluminum hydroxide 250 mg + Magnesium trisilicate 500 mg TID after food
   Tab Sucralfate 1 g TID after food
   Tab Ibuprofen 400 mg TID before food
   All drugs were prescribed for a period of 4 weeks.

   Dr ABC
   Reg. No:

Criticism:

- Sucralfate is an ulcer protective agent. However, it should not be prescribed with antacids as it interferes with its action. Sucralfate needs acid pH to produce a gel like consistency. Antacids neutralize the pH decreasing the action of sucralfate.
- Ibuprofen an NSAID is C/I in peptic ulcer patient. (NSAIDs inhibit cytoprotective PGs in the stomach).
- Aluminum hydroxide + Magnesium trisilicate is an antacid combination commonly prescribed for epigastric burning pain, GERD. This gives temporary relief and not preferred for long-term use as they are required in large frequent doses, afford little nocturnal protection and have poor patient acceptability.
- Omeprazole is a appropriate drug for this patient, preferred over sucralfate. But subsequently after 4 weeks relapses can occur.

3. **Criticize the following prescription for 55 years old hypertensive, diabetic patient who underwent coronary angioplasty and was prescribed the following drugs:**

Rx:

Tab Enalapril 5 mg once daily
Tab Aspirin 150 mg once daily
Tab Clopidogrel 150 mg od
Tab Metformin 500 mg bd

Dr ABC
Reg. No:

The patient complained of severe epigastric pain and the general practitioner has added cap Omeprazole 40 mg bd to his prescription. Comment on the prescription.

Criticism:

- Epigastric pain is due to gastric irritation probably caused by aspirin, clopidogrel and metformin. Hence, a PPI was prescribed.
- Omeprazole in a microsomal enzyme inhibitor which will inhibit activation of clopidogrel, a prodrug. This will inhibit the antiplatelet action of clopidogrel. Aspirin can be modified to low dose. Hence, substitute omeprazole with pantoprazole/Rabeprazole (which do not inhibit microsomal enzymes).
- Tab Metformin can be taken as SR formulation to reduce gastric irritation.

4. **A 2-year-old child with non-specific diarrhea, moderate dehydration and vomiting was prescribe the following:**

Rx:

Tab Loperamide tds
ORS powder

Inj Vit B complex
Syrup Erythromycin 200 mg tds

Dr ABC
Reg. No:

Comment on the above prescription.

Criticism:

- Loperamide (antimotility drug) is contraindicated in children as it can cause paralytic ileus in a diarrhea patient. Racecadotril can be used as safer antimotility agent. Probiotics can be prescribed.
- Erythromycin can stimulate motilin receptors to aggravate diarrhea. Safer anti microbial may be preferred.
- For a child with moderate dehydration, IV fluids could be added in addition to oral rehydration. Vomiting can be treated with ondansetron orally or parenterally.
- There is no role of Vit B complex in diarrhea.

ENDOCRINE SYSTEM

1. **Comment on the following prescription for a 28-year-old type 1 diabetic Mr Kishan who presented to the emergency department with complaints of marked fatigue, nausea and vomiting and mental confusion. Detailed history reveals that he has been a diabetic for the past ten years and he is irregular in taking insulin injections. Physical examination shows dehydration, rapid deep breathing and a fruity breath odor. Laboratory investigations show blood glucose—580 mg/dL, urine ketones—strongly positive.**

The patient is started on the following therapy:

Rx:

Inj Regular Insulin 5 units sc stat
Tab Metformin 500 mg tds
Inj Dexamethasone 8 mg iv stat
Inj Ceftriaxone 2 mg iv bd
5% Dextrose 2 pints. iv infusion over 4 hours

Dr ABC
Reg. No:

Criticism:

- Inj plain insulin given initially as bolus dose needs to be continued with a IV infusion. Lot of IV fluids (normal saline) need to be infused along with insulin.
- There is no role of metformin (oral antidiabetics) in diabetic ketoacidosis.

- Dexamethasone is not given in diabetic ketoacidosis (DKA), in fact it can cause glycogenolysis and can cause hyperglycemia.
- Ceftriaxone can be given to counter any associated infection.
- Dextrose is not given initially, normal saline is used with insulin followed by dextrose only after correction of blood sugars.

2. **Criticize, the following prescription for a patient pregnant female suffering with thyrotoxicosis. Do not criticize the format of prescription.**

Rx:

Tab Carbimazole 20 mg once daily

Radioactive I^{131} 3 curie once in the OPD

Dr ABC

Reg. No:

Criticism:

- Radioactive I^{131} is contraindicated in pregnancy as it destroys fetal thyroid and can cause cretinism.
- Carbimazole crosses placental barrier and will decrease synthesis and can cause cretinism in the fetus.
- Methimazole and propylthiouracil do not cross placental barrier and therefore safe in pregnancy.

3. **A 23-year-old lady married for three months was prescribed tab Ergometrine 500 μg for the management of migraine prophylaxis. Comment.**

Criticism:

- Ergometrine is not used for migraine prophylaxis. It is used for prevention of post-partum hemorrhage. Ergotamine can be used for acute attack of migraine, NEVER for prophylaxis. It causes vasoconstriction and can cause gangrene of tips of fingers and toes.
- Beta blockers or flunarizine can also be used.

4. **A 32-year-old female was on low-dose combined oral contraceptive pills. She developed a lower respiratory tract infection and was prescribed cap Ampicillin 500 mg tds for 7 days.**

One month later, she again presented to your clinic with complaints of missed periods. She was found to be pregnant. Comment.

Criticism:

- Ampicillin inhibits the intestinal flora. Estrogen undergoes deconjugation by colonic flora. This fails to occur because of ampicillin and interrupting the enterohepatic circulation of OC pills. This can cause failure of OC pills.
- Patient can take an alternate antibiotic tab Azithromycin 500 mg 1 OD for three days.

CHEMOTHERAPY

1. **Comment on the following prescription for a patient (weight 40 kg) suffering from pulmonary tuberculosis. Do not criticize the format of the prescription.**

   Rx:

   Tab Isoniazid 600 mg twice a day for 1 month
   Tab Rifampicin 300 mg once a day for 1 month
   Tab Pyrazinamide 1.5 g once a day for 1 month
   Inj Streptomycin 750 mg twice a day for 1 month

   Dr ABC
   Reg. No:

   Criticism:
   - Tab INH is given but dose is incorrect. Pyridoxine in the dose of 10 mg per day should also be given along with isoniazid to prevent peripheral neuropathy.
   - Rifampicin is given in the dose of 450 mg once daily before breakfast for 6 months.
   - Tab Pyrazinamide 1500 mg once a day for 2 months for first two months.
   - Inj Streptomycin is usually not recommended for treatment of pulmonary tuberculosis, due to need of daily injections, and lower margin of safety (ototoxicity and nephrotoxicity). It is used in drug resistant TB.
   - Another required drug, ethambutol is given as 800 mg once a day.

   After the initial intensive phase of HRZE for 2 months will be followed by 4 months of HRE. [2HRZE + 4 HRE]

2. **Comment on the following prescription for 20-year-old patient suffering from urinary tract infection due to *Pseudomonas*.**

   Rx:

   Cap Amoxicillin 500 mg twice daily
   Inj Gentamicin 40 mg subcutaneous thrice daily
   Tab Aspirin 300 mg SOS

   Dr ABC
   Reg. No:

   Criticism:
   - Amoxicillin is not effective against *Pseudomonas*. Drugs effective against pseudomonas are gentamicin, piperacillin, carbenicillin, fluoroquinolones and 3rd generation cephalosporins. Inj Gentamicin mentioned in the prescription is correct drug but it is given IM or IV. for 10–14 days.
   - Instead of acetyl salicylic acid (aspirin), the urine should be alkalinized by giving disodium hydrogen citrate (CITAL).
   - Antispasmodics, such as dicyclomine or drotaverine could be added to the prescription.

3. Comment on the following prescription for 27-year-old pregnant female having urinary tract infection.

Rx:

Tab Co-trimoxazole (400 + 80 mg) twice daily
Inj Gentamicin 40 mg subcutaneous thrice daily
Tab Vitamin C 500 mg once a day
Tab Aspirin 300 mg SOS

Dr ABC
Reg. No:

Criticism:

- Tab Co-trimoxazole and norfloxacin are effective for lower urinary tract infection due to *E. coli*, but it is to be avoided in pregnant women. UTI in pregnancy should be treated by amoxicillin or by cephalosporins. (cephalexin/cephaloridine)
- Tab Vitamin C should not be given in UTI, as they would further acidify the urine, which would increase the growth of the bacteria. Usually, the urine is made alkaline, because it would inhibit the growth of *E. coli*. Most antimicrobials act better in alkaline urine.
- Instead of aspirin (NSAID with analgesic action), antispasmodics, such as dicyclomine or drotaverine will relieve pain better.

4. Comment on the following prescription for 20-year old patient having high-grade fever due to cerebral malaria.

Rx:

Tab Quinine 600 mg twice daily
Tab Doxycycline 10 mg once daily for 5 days
Tab Primaquine 7.5 mg once daily

Dr ABC
Reg. No:

Criticism:

- Quinine is effective in treatment of cerebral malaria, but safer alternatives, such as parenteral artemisinin's are faster acting, more effective, better tolerated and more conveniently administered. Artemisinin's should be given for adequate period of time to prevent recrudescence. This is followed by oral (ACT) artemisinin combination therapy.
- Doxycycline can be used with quinine but their combination with artemisinin is not documented.
- Primaquine a single dose of 45 mg is given in *P. falciparum* malaria to kill the gametes and cut the transmission to mosquito. Here radical cure is not required.

5. **Comment the following prescription for 28-year-old woman weighing 45 kg started on therapy for pulmonary tuberculosis develops hepatotoxicity after 10 days of treatment.**

   Rx:
   Tab Isoniazid 300 mg OD
   Tab Rifampicin 400 mg BD
   Tab Pyrazinamide 1 g IM twice daily
   Tab Streptomycin 75 mg once daily

   Dr ABC
   Reg. No:

   Criticism:
   Isoniazid(H), rifampicin(R) and pyrazinamide (Z) all can be causative, and hepatotoxicity occurs more frequently, when the combination is used. All of them therefore should be stopped. Then streptomycin + ethambutol (E) + ciprofloxacin can be started. When the reaction clears, the causative drugs should be started one by one to identify the culprit. Generally R is resumed first followed 7 days later by H. If hepatitis is recurs the last added drug is stopped permanently, and the regimen is reconstructed. In case if both R and H are tolerated then do not restart Z but prolongs therapy with R, H, and E to 9 months.

6. **Comment on the following prescription 18-year-old women, with history of hypersensitivity to penicillin is diagnosed to have acute tonsillitis and put on the following treatment:**

   Rx:
   Cap Amoxicillin 500 mg BD
   Tab Ibuprofen 400 mg OD

   Dr ABC
   Reg. No:

   Criticism:
   - The patient is allergic to penicillin, and since amoxicillin is a semi-synthetic penicillin, there is some degree of partial cross sensitivity. Hence, amoxicillin cannot be used for this patient. Other antibiotics, which are effective for tonsillitis, are cephalosporins, and macrolides (azithromycin). But 10% of patients allergic to penicillin also show cross sensitivity to cephalosporins, especially patients with history of immediate type of hypersensitivity to penicillin. Therefore, it is preferable not to give cephalosporin's.
     Therefore, macrolides, such as erythromycin, azithromycin are safer alternatives in this condition.
   - Tab Ibuprofen can be given for analgesic and antipyretic action but the dose given is incorrect, preferably given after food.
   - Potassium permanganate gargles or warm saline gargles can also be given to the patient.

7. **A 45-year-old Mrs Archana underwent elective vaginal hysterectomy and she was given normal therapeutic dose of cefazolin through iv during induction of anesthesia and the drug was continued till she was discharged from the hospital. Comment.**

   Criticism:

   Cefazolin 1g iv single injection is preferred for elective vaginal hysterectomy. This is a clean wound with minimum chances of surgical site infection. The drug should not be continued till she was discharged from the hospital.

8. **Sundar, 40-year-old male was having fever and cough with expectoration for 5 days. He went to a local general practitioner who diagnosed it to be a case of severe lower respiratory tract infection. He was prescribed**

   Rx:

   Tab Paracetamol 500 mg tds for 5 days
   Cap Ampicillin 500 mg qid for 10 days

   Dr ABC
   Reg. No:

   He came back to the general practitioner after 5 days with complaints of diarrhea. He was subsequently prescribed tab Loperamide 2 mg BD for 3 days in addition to above prescribed drugs. Comment.

   Criticism:

   - Ampicillin is an extended semisynthetic penicillin which gets incompletely absorbed when administered by oral route.
   - The unabsorbed drug irritates the lower intestine as well as causes, marked alternation of bacterial flora, which is resulted in diarrhea. *Lactobacillus* (probiotic preparations) should be prescribed simultaneously with ampicillin.
   - In this particular patient, stop ampicillin, instead azithromycin can be prescribed. Loperamide can be discontinued. Paracetamol can be given whenever there is fever.

9. **Comment on the following prescription for 20-year-old patient having high-grade fever due to *P. vivax* malaria. Do not criticize the format of the prescription.**

   Rx:

   Tab Chloroquine 250 mg once a day
   Tab Paracetamol 500 mg once a day

   Dr ABC
   Reg. No:

   Criticism:

   Tab Chloroquine is drug of choice in this patient, but the dose given is incorrect. It is given in the loading dose of 1000 mg chloroquine phosphate stat, followed by 500 mg after 8 hours. Then, chloroquine phosphate 500 mg once daily for next 2 days.

- Tab Paracetamol can be given whenever there is fever.
- An antiemetic, such as domperidone/metoclopramide should be given half an hour before giving: chloroquine as it causes nausea and vomiting.
- Tab Primaquine is required for radical cure after giving chloroquine for eradicating exoerythrocytic phase (Hypnozoites) of *P. vivax* in the liver.

10. Criticize the following prescription for 20-year-old patient having acute invasive intestinal amoebiasis. Do not criticize the format of prescription.

Rx:

Tab Diloxanide furoate 500 mg once a day

Tab Paracetamol 250 mg thrice a day for 2 days

Dr ABC

Reg. No:

Criticism:

Diloxanide furoate is a luminal amoebicide. Metronidazole should be prescribed. It is a intestinal and extraintestinal amoebocide. Metronidazole should be subsequently followed by diloxanide to kill trophozoites in intestine giving a complete cure. An antispasmodic, such as dicyclomine and drotaverine should also be prescribed.

11. Comment on the following prescription for a 20-year-old patient having pulmonary tuberculosis.

Rx:

Inj Streptomycin 1 g daily

Tab Isoniazid (10 mg) 1 tab 8 hourly

Tab Rifampicin (500 mg) 1 cap at bed time

Tab Pyridoxine (100 mg) 1 tab daily

Tab Vitamin C 500 mg OD

Dr ABC

Reg. No:

Criticism:

Streptomycin an aminoglycoside is preferred only in TB resistant to first-line drugs. It has adverse effects, such as nephrotoxicity, ototoxicity. Other limitations being to be given by IM route, streptomycin dependence. Other aminoglycosides, such as amikacin and kanamycin can be used in MDR TB.

INH (isoniazid), rifampicin are correct but doses are wrong. Ethambutol, pyrazinamide, are anti-TB drugs which needs to be added. Pyridoxine is required to prevent neuropathy due to INH, but dose is wrong.

Vitamin C is not required.

12. Criticize the following prescription for 20-year-old patient having enteric fever.

Rx:

Cap Chloramphenicol (100 mg) 1 cap 4 times a day for 4 days
Tab Aspirin (100 mg)1 tab twice a day for 2-3 days

Dr ABC
Reg. No:

Criticism:

Chloramphenicol is not preferred in enteric fever because of the following reasons.

It is bacteriostatic, relapses can occur. It does not prevent and cure carrier state.

- Ciprofloxacin, being bactericidal, brings about quick defervescence, lower incidence of complications and relapse. Ciprofloxacin also prevent carrier state. Thus, ciprofloxacin and third generation cephalosporins are preferred for enteric fever.
- Aspirin given in typhoid can increase chances of ulcers, hence contraindicated. Paracetamol as an antipyretic is more preferred.

MISCELLANEOUS

1. Mrs Anita, a 24-year-old female presented with symptoms of fatigue and body ache. Her hemoglobin was 8.5 g% and peripheral smear showed megaloblasts. She was treated with:

Rx:

Folic acid 5 mg OD for 2 months

Dr ABC
Reg. No:

She returned back with worsening of lower limb cramps and his peripheral smear showed normal RBC's. Comment.

Criticism:

Folic acid 5 mg should never be given alone to patients, with symptoms of vitamin B_{12} deficiency, because hematological response can occur, but neurological deficit may worsen because of diversion of B_{12} in the body to hematopoiesis. This cause unmasking of vitamin B_{12} deficiency.

2. A 42-year-old woman presents to the casualty with acute dyspnea. She gives history of traveling in a bus for 10 hours continuously from her native village 3 days ago. On arrival in the casualty, she is tachypneic. Her pulse rate is 114 beats/min and respiratory rate is 30/min, SpO_2 is 92% on room air. Her weight is 90 kg. Helical CT shows a pulmonary embolus. She is given:

Tab Warfarin 5 mg once a day to maintain an INR of 2–3. Comment on the prescription.

Criticism:

Low molecular weight heparin should have been added to warfarin in this emergency situation, as it has faster onset of action. Warfarin has a slow onset of action (1–3 days). After few days, heparin should be discontinued with warfarin maintained at a dose of 5 mg once a day.

9 CHAPTER

Drug Promotional Literature

1. **What is drug promotional literature?**
   a. Drug promotional literature (DPL) is a tool for advertising new drugs entering the market to doctors.
   b. According to the World Health Organization (WHO), medicinal drug promotion is "all informational and persuasive activities by manufacturers and distributors, the effect of which is to induce the prescription, supply, purchase, and/or use of medicinal drugs."
   c. DPLs are prepared by pharmaceutical companies to provide vital details about the new drug to convince doctors to prescribe it to patients.
   d. More often than not, DPL becomes the only source of information about novel drugs to physicians.
2. **Name the guidelines to be followed while preparing DPL.**
   a. WHO has prepared ethical guidelines for DPL to promote the rational use of medicines. It comprises 11 criteria to judge the completeness of any piece of promotional literature.
   b. In 2012, the Organization of Pharmaceutical Producers of India (OPPI) also released its own criteria that DPL should follow.
3. **What are the WHO criteria?**

   The following are the WHO criteria to be followed by pharmaceutical industries for the completeness of DPL:
   1. The names of the active ingredients using either international nonproprietary names or the approved generic names of the drug
   2. The brand name
   3. Content of active ingredient per dosage form or regimen
   4. Name of other ingredients known to cause problems (adjuvant)
   5. Approved therapeutic uses
   6. Dosage form or regimen
   7. Side effects and major adverse drug reactions
   8. Precautions, contraindications, and warnings
   9. Major interactions
   10. Name and address of the manufacturer or distributor
   11. Reference to scientific literature as appropriate

4. **What are the OPPI criteria?**

   The following are the OPPI criteria to be followed by pharmaceutical industries for the completeness of DPL:

   1. The name of the product (brand name)
   2. The active ingredients
   3. The name and address of the pharmaceutical company or its marketing agent
   4. The date of production of the advertisement
   5. Approved indications
   6. Dosage
   7. Method of use
   8. A concise statement of contraindications, precautions, and side effects

Exercise 1: Comment on the following DPL:

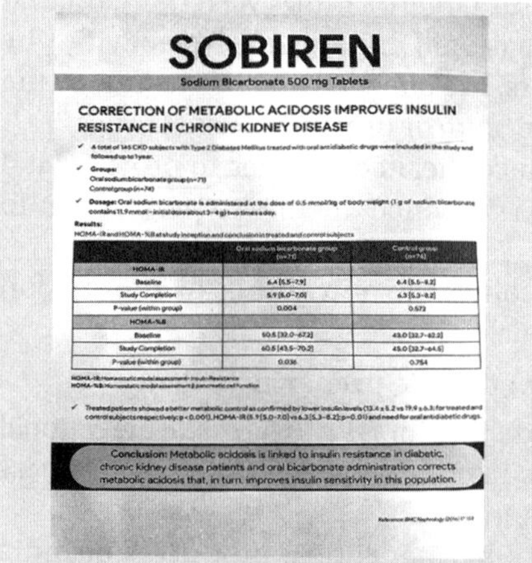

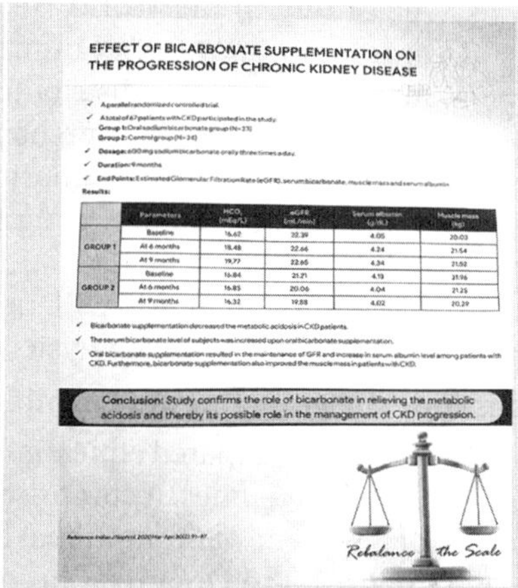

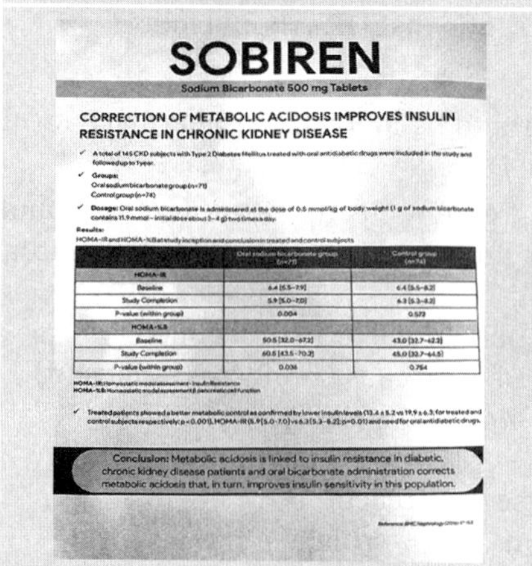

WHO criteria

- The names of the active ingredients using either international nonproprietary names or the approved generlc names of the drug
- The brand name
- Content of active ingredient per dosage form or regimen
- Name of other ingredients known to cause problems (adjuvant)
- Approved therapeutic uses
- Dosage form or regimen
- Side effects and major adverse drug reaction
- Precautions, contraindications, and warnings
- Major interactions
- Name and address of the manufacturer or distributor
- Reference to scientific literature as appropriate

OPPI criteria

- The name of the product (brand name)
- The active ingredients
- The name and address of the pharmaceutical company or its marketing agent
- The date of production of the advertisement
- Approved indications
- Dosage
- Method of use
- A concise statement of contraindications, precautions, and side effects

Exercise 2: Comment on the following DPL:

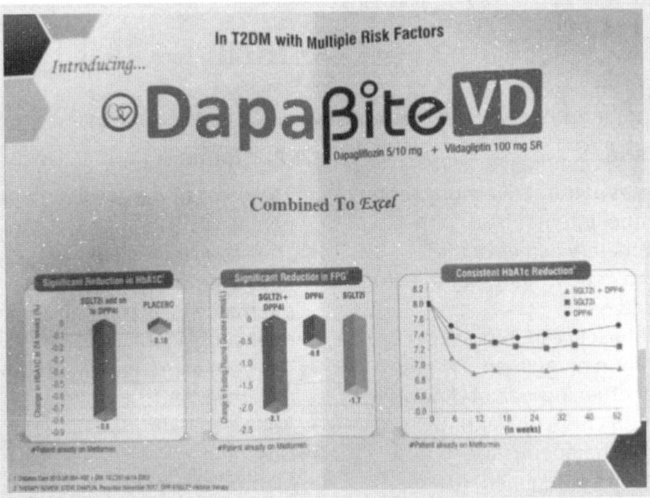

WHO criteria

- The names of the active ingredients using either international nonproprietary names or the approved generic names of the drug
- The brand name
- Content of active ingredient per dosage form or regimen

OPPI criteria

- The name of the product (brand name)
- The active ingredients
- The name and address of the pharmaceutical company or its marketing agent

- Name of other ingredients known to cause problems (adjuvant)
- Approved therapeutic uses
- Dosage form or regimen
- Side effects and major adverse drug reaction
- Precautions, contraindications, and warnings
- Major interactions
- Name and address of the manufacturer or distributor
- Reference to scientific literature as appropriate

- The date of production of the advertisement
- Approved indications
- Dosage
- Method of use
- A concise statement of contraindications, precautions, and side effects

Exercise 3: Comment on the following DPL:

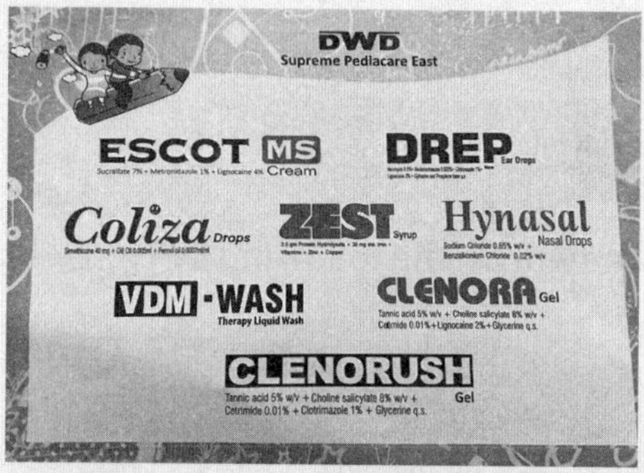

WHO criteria

- The names of the active ingredients using either international nonproprietary names or the approved generic names of the drug
- The brand name
- Content of active ingredient per dosage form or regimen
- Name of other ingredients known to cause problems (adjuvant)
- Approved therapeutic uses
- Dosage form or regimen
- Side effects and major adverse drug reaction
- Precautions, contraindications, and warnings
- Major interactions
- Name and address of the manufacturer or distributor—name only
- Reference to scientific literature as appropriate

OPPI criteria

- The name of the product (brand name)
- The active ingredients
- The name and address of the pharmaceutical company or its marketing agent
- The date of production of the advertisement
- Approved indications
- Dosage
- Method of use
- A concise statement of contraindications, precautions, and side effects

10 CHAPTER

Adverse Drug Reactions

1. Define adverse events (AE) and adverse drug reactions (ADRs).

- Adverse event—an AE is a noxious, undesired, unintended event that happens when a patient is under medical treatment. **An AE may/may not be associated with the drug.**
- Adverse drug reactions—noxious, undesired, unintended reactions to a drug that occurs at doses normally used for treatment, prevention or diagnosis of a disease are called adverse drug reactions (ADRs).

2. What is a serious adverse event (SAE)?

Any AE, adverse reaction or unexpected adverse reaction that at any dose results in:

- Death or immediately threatens life (NOT an event which hypothetically might have caused death if it were more severe)
- Hospitalization or longer than anticipated stay in the hospital
- Persistent or significant disability or incapacity
- Congenital anomaly or birth defect.

3. Classify the types of ADR with examples.

Type	*Description*	*Examples*
A. Augmented	• Predictable • Based on pharmacological action • Dose-related	
	Side effect: Undesired effect at therapeutic effect	Dryness of mouth with atropine
	Secondary effect: Due to action secondary to pharmacological action	Superinfection due to injudicious use of broad-spectrum antibiotics
	Toxicity: Overdose	Paracetamol, diazepam

Contd...

Contd...

Type	*Description*	*Examples*
B. Bizarre	• Unpredictable • Qualitative • Due to immune reaction, genetic abnormality or idiosyncrasy **Allergy** **Idiosyncrasy**	 Penicillin, aspirin Paradoxical excitement seen with barbiturates
C. Chronic	**On prolonged usage (Time-dependent)** • Drug dependence • Organ damage • Cumulative • Immunosuppression	 • Opioid dependence • Hepatotoxicity due to pyrazinamide • Retinal toxicity with chloroquine • Opportunistic infection with corticosteroids
D. Delayed	Mutagenicity, carcinogenicity teratogenicity	Radioactive iodine, sodium valproate, Isotretinoin, thalidomide
E. End of use	Withdrawal	**Sudden stoppage of:** • Beta blockers-MI • Corticosteroids—acute adrenal insufficiency • Phenytoin/Valproate—seizures
F. Failure	Failure of therapy	• Oral contraceptive pills • Antimicrobial resistance

4. What are the differences between type A and type B ADR?

Type A ADR	*Type B ADR*
Mechanism-based adverse reaction	Not based on the drug's known actions but on immunological/genetic factors
Quantitative	Qualitative
Dose-related	Non-dose related
Predictable	Unpredictable
More common	Rare
Less serious	More serious, requiring drug withdrawal
For example, dryness of mouth with atropine	For example, anaphylaxis due to penicillin

5. What are the grades of ADR?

- **Mild**—not requiring intervention
- **Moderate**—requires stopping the drug, specific treatment or prolonged hospitalization
- **Severe**—requires hospitalization, ICU admission, disability (*see* SAE)
- **Fatal**—resulting in death

6. What is causality assessment?

- Causality assessment is the finding of any relationship between a drug and a drug reaction.
- It is an evaluation of the likelihood that a particular treatment is the cause of an observed adverse event.
- Naranjo's algorithm and The World Health Organization-Uppsala Monitoring Centre causality assessment scale are examples of methods for causality assessment. The WHO scale is more commonly used.

World Health Organization-Uppsala Monitoring Centre causality assessment scale

Causality term	Assessment criteria
Certain	• Event or laboratory test abnormality, with plausible time relationship to drug intake • Cannot be explained by disease or other drugs • Response to withdrawal • Plausible (pharmacologically, pathologically) • Event definitive pharmacologically or phenomenologically (i.e., an objective and specific medical disorder or a recognized pharmacological phenomenon) • Rechallenge satisfactory, if necessary
Probable or likely	• Event or laboratory test abnormality, with reasonable time relationship to drug intake • Unlikely to be attributed to disease or other drugs • Response to withdrawal clinically reasonable • Rechallenge not required
Possible	• Event or laboratory test abnormality, with reasonable time relationship to drug intake • Could also be explained by disease or other drugs • Information on drug withdrawal may be lacking or unclear
Unlikely	• Event or laboratory test abnormality, with a time to drug intake that makes a relationship improbable (but not impossible) • Disease or other drugs provide plausible explanations
Conditional or unclassified	• Event or laboratory test abnormality • More data for proper assessment needed, or additional data under examination
Unassessable/ unclassifiable	• Report suggesting an adverse reaction Cannot be judged because information is insufficient or contradictory • Data cannot be supplemented or verified

COMMON ADVERSE DRUG REACTIONS

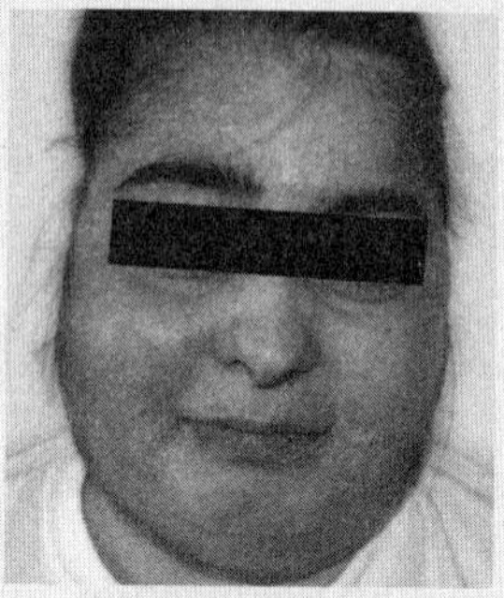

Moon Face

MOON FACE
Cause: Prolonged usage of Glucocorticoids

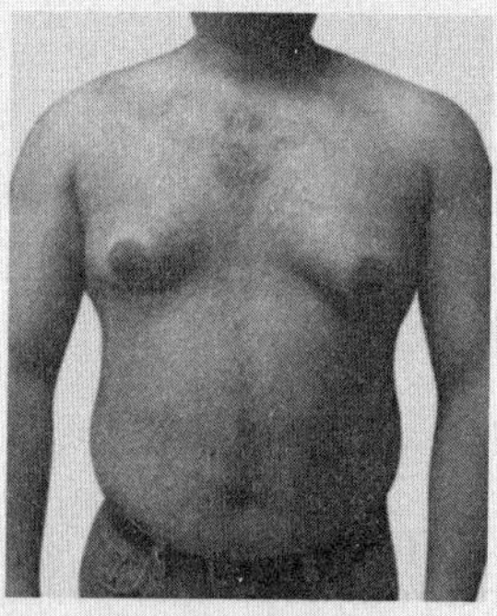

Gynecomastia

B. GYNECOMASTIA
Cause: Spironolactone, ketoconazole, digitalis, cimetidine, inh, chlorpromazine

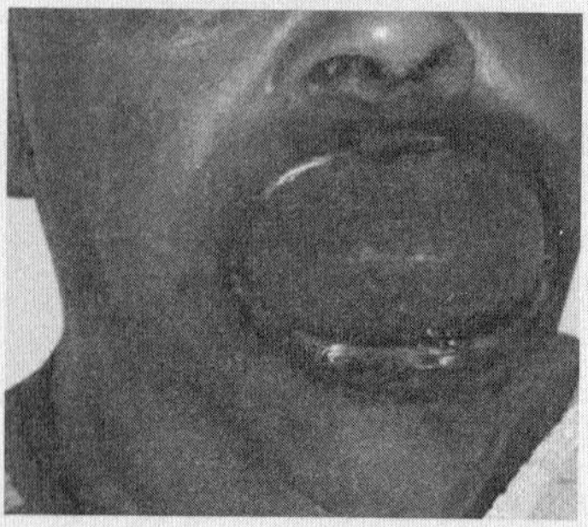

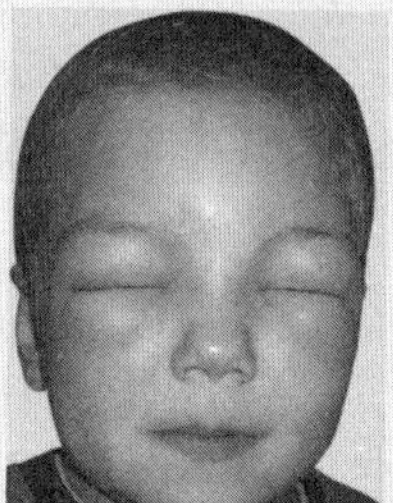

Angioedema

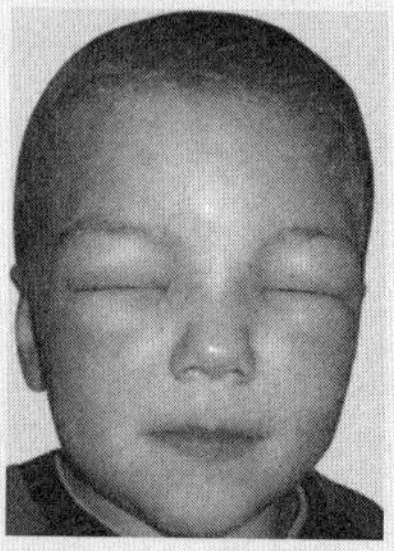

C. ANGIOEDEMA
Cause: Ace Inhibitors, e.g., captopril, penicillin, cephalosporin, salicylates

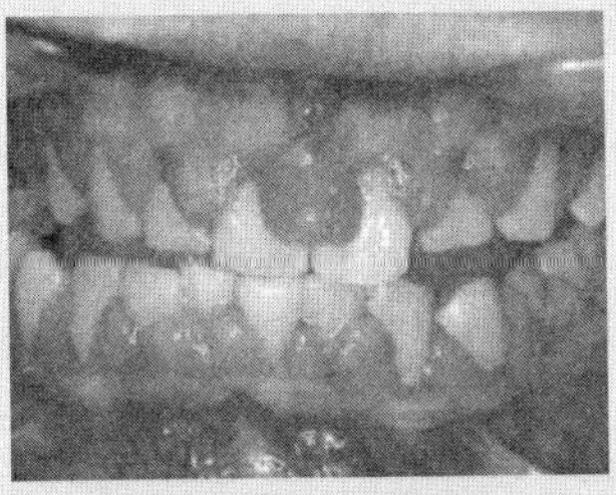

Gum hyperplasia

D. GUM HYPERPLASIA
Cause: Phenytoin, nifedipine, OCP

Note: Never stop the drug or decrease the dose—ADR is seen at therapeutic doses
Rx maintain oral hygiene,
Gingivectomy
In case of excessive hyperplasia, switch to an alternate antiepileptic drug

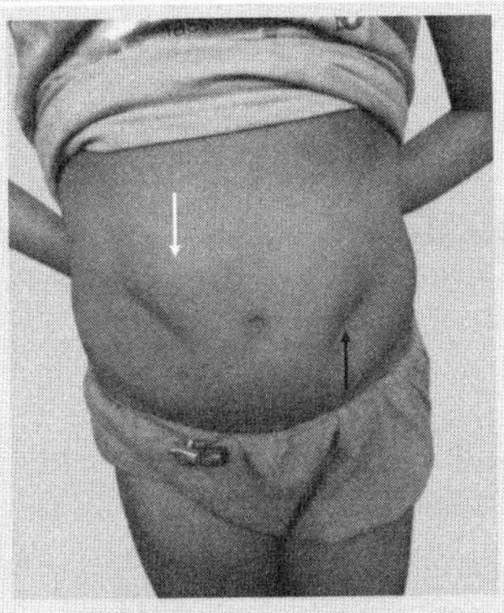

Lipodystrophy

E. LIPODYSTROPHY
Causes: Insulin, antiretroviral drugs—stavudine, protease inhibitors

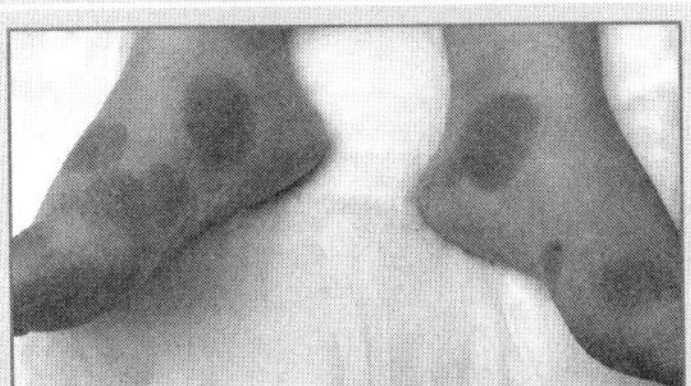

Fixed drug eruptions

F. FIXED DRUG ERUPTIONS
Causes: Sulphonamides, quinine, barbiturates

Note: Rx: Stop the causative drug; treat with topical corticosteroids and oral antihistamines

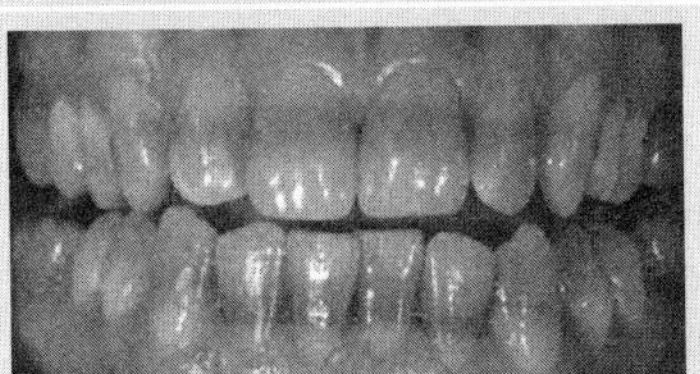

Teeth discolouration

G. DISCOLORATION OF TEETH
Causes: Tetracyclines

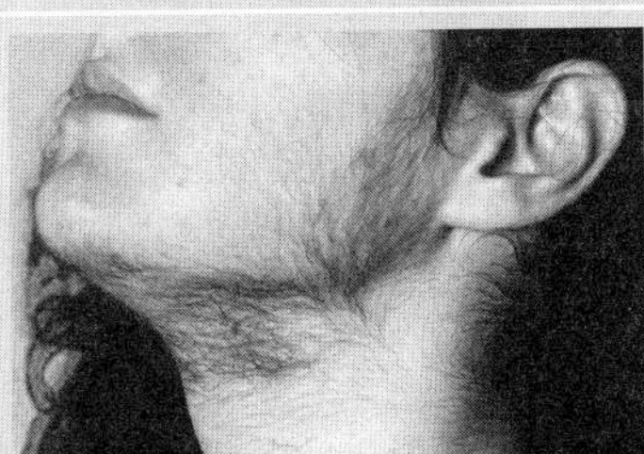

Hirsuitism

H. HIRSUITISM
Causes: Minoxidil, phenytoin, also, spironolactone, testosterone in females, cyclosporine

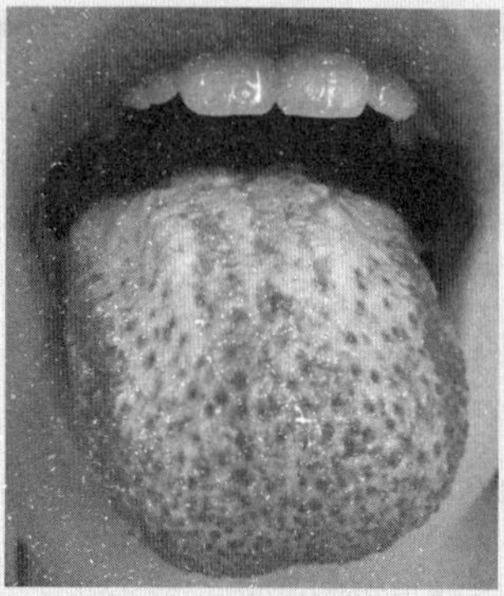

Oral candidiasis

I. ORAL CANDIDIASIS

Cause: Inhaled corticosteroids, budesonide, fluticasone, beclomethasone

Note: Rx: Topical clotrimazole, gargle after each inhalation of glucocorticosteroids use spacer

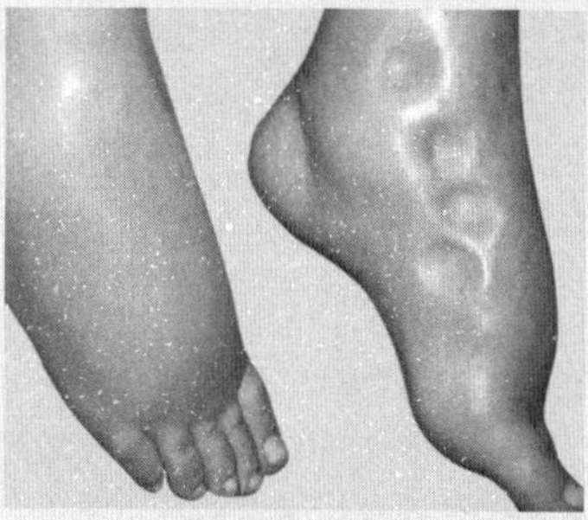

Pitting edema

J. PITTING EDEMA

Cause: Calcium channel blockers, e.g., amlodipine

Note: Rx: Leg elevation, discontinue amlodipine and switch to an alternate antihypertensive agent

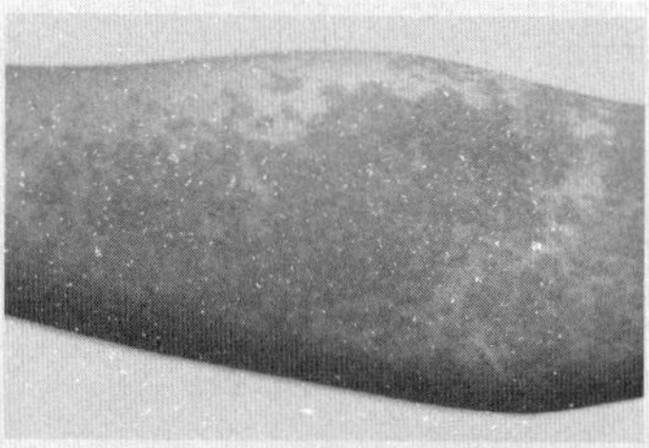

Maculopapular rash

K. MACULOPAPULAR RASH

Cause: Amoxicillin, ampicillin, sulfonamides, anti-epileptic drugs, allopurinol, NSAIDs

Note: Stop causative drug, antihistamine

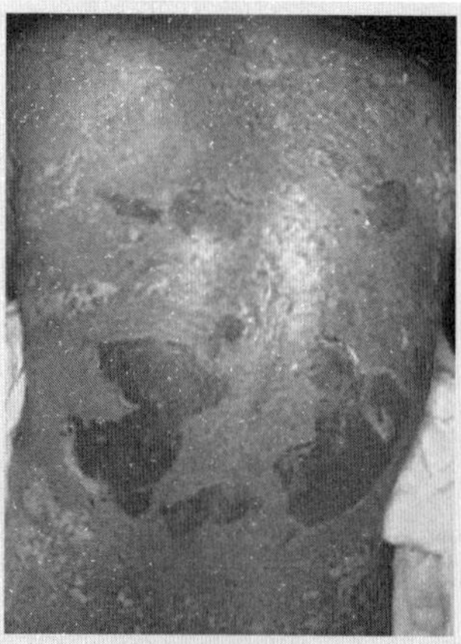

SJS/TEN

L. STEVEN JOHNSON SYNDROME/ TOXIC EPIDERMAL NECROLYSIS

Cause: Allopurinol, aminopenicillins, barbiturates, carbamazepine, cephalosporin, codeine

Note: Rx: Stop causative drug, hospitalization is required—fluid replacement and wound dressing

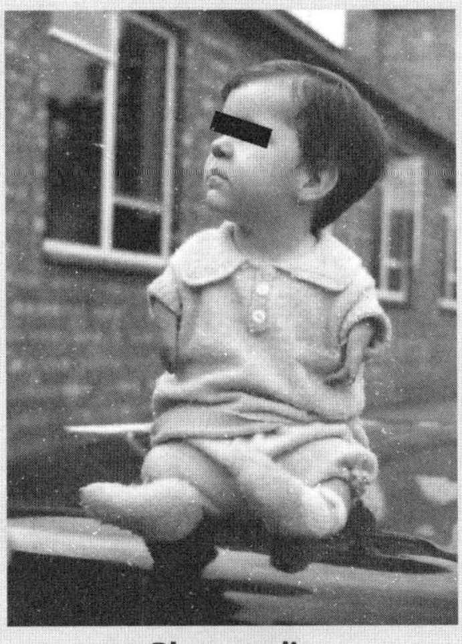

Phocomelia

M. TERATOGENIC EFFECTS

i. **Phocomelia**: 1st known teratogenic malformation (late 1950s)

Cause: Thalidomide
- Was widely used for morning sickness and was withdrawn from the market after teratogenic effects were reported
- Currently reserved for treatment of Multiple myeloma and erythema nodosum leprosum (ENL type II lepra reaction)

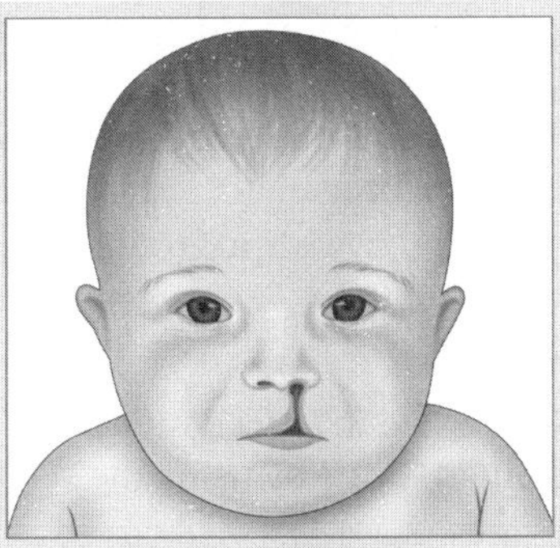

Cleft lip/palate

ii. **Cleft Lip/Cleft Palate**

Cause: Seen when an epileptic female takes **Phenytoin** during pregnancy

Note: If the drug cannot be replaced, add a folic acid supplement and perform frequent USG for detection of any malformation

Preferable switch on to safer antiepileptic drugs—lamotrigine, levetiracetam

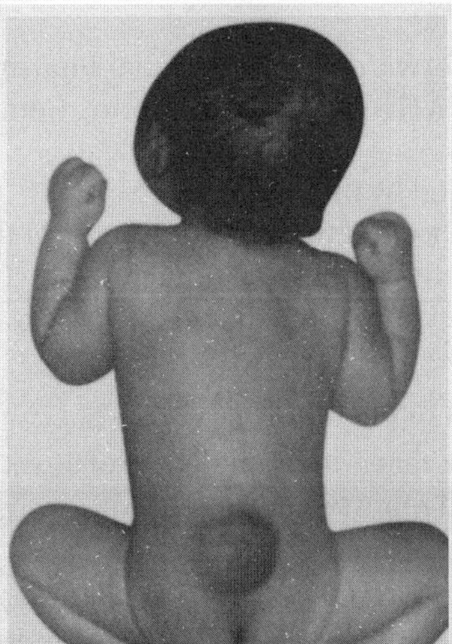

Neural tube defects

iii. **Neural Tube Defects—Spina Bifida**

Cause: Anticonvulsants—sodium valproate

Note: Preferable switch on to safer anti-epileptic drugs—lamotrigine, levetiracetam

Valproate is contraindicated in pregnancy

ADR REPORTING FORM

A. What to report?

- All adverse events should be reported.
- Non-serious, known or unknown, frequent or rare adverse drug reactions due to medicines, vaccines or herbal products.
- Serious adverse drug reactions.

Note: Serious/adverse events following immunization can also be reported in the serious AEFI case notification.

Form available on the website http://www.ipc.gov.in

B. Who can report?

All healthcare professionals (Clinicians, dentists, pharmacists, nurses, etc.) can report adverse drug reactions.

C. Where to report?

Duly filled in Suspected Adverse Drug Reaction Reporting Form can be sent to the nearest Adverse Drug Reaction Monitoring Centre (AMC) or directly to the National Coordination Centre (NCC) for PvPI.

Call on Helpline (Toll Free) 1800 180 3024 to report ADRs or directly mail this filled form to pvpi.ipc@gov.in

A list of nationwide AMCs is available at: http://www.ipc.gov.in, http://www.ipc.gov.in/PvPI/pv_home.html

D. What happens to the submitted information?

- Information provided in this form is handled in strict confidence.
- The causality assessment is carried out at AMCs by using the WHO-UMC scale.
- The analyzed forms are forwarded to the NCC-PvPI through the ADR database.
- Finally, the data is analyzed and forwarded to the Global Pharmacovigilance Database managed by WHO Uppsala Monitoring Centre in Sweden.
- The reports are periodically reviewed by the NCC-PvPI.
- The information generated on the basis of these reports helps in the continuous assessment of the benefit-risk ratio of medicines.
- The Signal Review Panel of PvPI reviews the data and suggests any interventions that may be required.

E. Mandatory fields for suspected ADR Reporting Form (*)

Patient initials, age at onset of reaction, reaction term(s), date of onset of reaction, suspected medication(s) and reporter information.

For Adverse Drug Reaction Reporting Tools

E-mail: pvpi.ipc@gov.in

PvPI Helpline (Toll-Free): 1800 180 3024 (9:00 AM to 5:30 PM, Monday-Friday)

ADR Mobile App: "ADRPvPI"

Exercise 1

19-year-old Mr SAM, was diagnosed with pulmonary tuberculosis on 09/10/2021 and started on ATT (weight-based regimen for 60 kg):

Tab isoniazid 300 mg OD for 6 months
Tab rifampicin 600 mg OD for 6 months
Tab pyrazinamide 1500 mg OD for 2 months

SUSPECTED ADVERSE DRUG REACTION REPORTING FORM

For **VOLUNTARY** reporting of ADRs by Healthcare Professionals

INDIAN PHARMACOPOEIA COMMISSION (National Coordination Centre-Pharmacovigilance Programme of India)

Ministry of Health & Family Welfare, Government of India, Sector-23, Raj Nagar, Ghaziabad-201002

PvPI Helpline (Toll Free) :1800-180-3024 (9:00 AM to 5:30 PM, Monday-Friday)

Initial Case ☐ ✓ Follow-up Case ☐

FOR AMC / NCC USE ONLY

Reg. No. / IPD No. / OPD No. / CR No. :

AMC Report No. :

Worldwide Unique No. :

A. PATIENT INFORMATION *

1. Patient Initials: SAM
2. Age or date of birth: 19 years
3. Gender: M ✓ F ☐ Other ☐
4. Weight (in Kg.) 60 Kg

B. SUSPECTED ADVERSE REACTION *

5. Event / Reaction start date (dd/mm/yyyy): 27/11/2021
6. Event / Reaction stop date (dd/mm/yyyy): —
7. Describe Event/Reaction management with details , if any

19 year old male was diagnosed with Pulmonary TB and started on AKT on 09/10/2021
He presented to the OPD on 1/12/2021 with h/o
- ↓ appetite and abdominal pain ∵ 7days
- yellowing of sclera ∵ 5 days
- 3 episodes of vomiting ∵ 1 day
- No Significant medical, surgical or family history
- General exam → Pallor and icterus present
- Systemic exam → No abnormality detected
- deranged LFT (dated 30/11/2021) HBV, HCV, HIV negative
- provisional diagnosis: Drug-induced Hepatitis due to AKT
- suspected drug was stopped on 1/12/2021; patient is recovering

12. Relevant investigations with dates :

HBV, HCV, HIV – negative
LFT: SGOT – 400 IU/L (↑)
SGPT – 550 IU/L (↑)
ALP – 200 IU/L (↑)
} Dated 30/11/2021

13. Relevant medical / medication history (e.g. allergies, pregnancy, addiction, hepatic, renal dysfunction etc.)

Diagnosed with Tuberculosis – AKT started 9/10/21
No other comorbidities
No relevant medication history

14. Seriousness of the reaction : No ✓ if Yes ☐ (*please tick anyone*)
☐ Death (dd/mm/yyyy) ☐ Congenital-anomaly
☐ Life threatening ☐ Disability
☐ Hospitalization-Initial/Prolonged ☐ Other Medically important

15. Outcome:
☐ Recovered ✓ Recovering ☐ Not Recovered
☐ Fatal ☐ Recovered with sequelae ☐ Unknown

C. SUSPECTED MEDICATION(S) *

S. No.	8. Name (Brand/ Generic)	Manufacturer (if known)	Batch No. / Lot No.	Expiry Date (if known)	Dose (mg)	Route	Frequency	Therapy Dates		Indication	Causality Assessment
								Date Started	Date Stopped		
i	Pyrazinamide	—	—	—	1500	oral	OD	9/10/21	1/12/21	PULMONARY TUBERCULOSIS	Probable
ii	Isoniazide	—	—	—	300	oral	OD	9/10/21	1/12/21		Probable
iii	Rifampicin	—	—	—	600	oral	OD	9/10/21	1/12/21		Probable
iv#											

9. Action taken after reaction (*please tick*)

S. No. as per C	Drug withdrawn	Dose increased	Dose reduced	Dose not changed	Not applicable	Unknown
i	✓					
ii	✓					
iii	✓					
iv						

10. Reaction reappeared after reintroduction of suspected medication (*please tick*) NO

Yes	No	Effect unknown	Dose (if re-introduced)

11. Concomitant medical product including self-medication and herbal remedies with therapy dates (Exclude those used to treat reaction)

S. No.	Name (Brand / Generic)	Dose	Route	Frequency (OD, BD, etc.)	Therapy Dates		Indication
					Date Started	Date Stopped	
i	Ethambutol	1000mg	oral	OD	9/10/21	—	PULMONARY TUBERCULOSIS
ii	Pyridoxine	10mg	oral	OD	9/10/21	—	Prevention of peripheral neuropathy (due to INH)
iii#							

Additional Information :

D. REPORTER DETAILS *

16. Name & Address : Dr ABC , DYPH Hospital

Pin : 400706 Email : abc@gmail.com

Contact No- : 98XXXXX4XX

Occupation : Physician Signature : ABC

17. **Date of this report (dd/mm/yyyy) :** 11/12/2021

Signature and Name of Receiving Personnel :

Confidentiality : The patient's identity is held in strict confidence and protected to the fullest extent. Submission of a report does not constitute an admission that medical personnel or manufacturer or the product caused or contributed to the reaction. Submission of an ADR report does not have any legal implication on the reporter.

Exercise 1: ADR reporting form.

Tab ethambutol 1000 mg OD for 6 months
Tab pyridoxine 10 mg OD for 6 months

On 01/12/2021, he presented with complaints of yellowing of the whites of his eyes for 5 days, 3 episodes of vomiting since 1 day and loss of appetite. On general examination, pallor and icterus were noted and systemic exam showed no abnormality. He has no significant family, medical or surgical history.

Liver Function Test dated 30/11/2021 showed:

SGOT—400 IU/L
SGPT—550 IU/L
ALP—200 IU/L

Tests for hepatitis B, C and HIV were negative.

A provisional diagnosis of drug-induced hepatitis was made. Tab pyrazinamide, tab isoniazid and tab rifampicin were discontinued on 01/12/2021. The patient is currently recovering.

Report the adverse reaction with all the relevant details.

Exercise 2

A 65-year-old Mr MLK, was started on tab largactil (chlorpromazine) 100 mg, 4 tablets at bedtime, following a psychotic episode on 30/05/2023. Four weeks after taking the medicine (since 01/06/2023), the patient began experiencing pain while tilting his head to the left side and limited range of motion of head and neck. On 06/06/2023, the patient presented to the OPD and was diagnosed with antipsychotic-induced torticollis.

The patient has no other relevant surgical, medical or family history and is not currently taking any other medication. A Liver Function Test done on 06/06/2023 showed no abnormality.

The torticollis was treated with tab benztropine 1 mg BD and the patient is currently recovering.

Drug details

Tab largactil (Chlorpromazine)

Dose 100 mg 4 tabs at bedtime

Manufacturer: Wembley Labs

Batch no: LGL0941

Expiry date: 07/2024

SUSPECTED ADVERSE DRUG REACTION REPORTING FORM

For **VOLUNTARY** reporting of ADRs by Healthcare Professionals

INDIAN PHARMACOPOEIA COMMISSION (National Coordination Centre-Pharmacovigilance Programme of India)

Ministry of Health & Family Welfare, Government of India, Sector-23, Raj Nagar, Ghaziabad-201002

PvPI Helpline (Toll Free) :1800-180-3024 (9:00 AM to 5:30 PM, Monday-Friday)

Initial Case ☐ ✓ Follow-up Case ☐

FOR AMC / NCC USE ONLY

Reg. No. / IPD No. / OPD No. / CR No. :

AMC Report No. :

Worldwide Unique No. :

A. PATIENT INFORMATION *

1. Patient Initials: MLK
2. Age or date of birth: 65years
3. Gender: M ✓ F ☐ Other ☐
4. Weight (in Kg.) 72kg

B. SUSPECTED ADVERSE REACTION *

5. Event / Reaction start date (dd/mm/yyyy): 1/06/2023
6. Event / Reaction stop date (dd/mm/yyyy): –
7. Describe Event/Reaction management with details, if any

65 year old Male recieved Tab Chlorpromazine (Tab Largachil 100mg 4 times at bedtime) 4 weeks ago, following a psychotic episode.

Since the past 5 days, he is experiencing pain while tilting his head to the left side and limited range of motion of his head and neck

He was diagnosed with antipsychotic-induced torticollis.

Tab Chlorpromazine was stopped on 06/06/2023.

He was prescribed Tab Benztropine 1mg BD and is recovering

12. Relevant investigations with dates :

LFT: no abnormality detected (06/06/2023)

13. Relevant medical / medication history (e.g. allergies, pregnancy, addiction, hepatic, renal dysfunction etc.)

No relevant history

14. Seriousness of the reaction : No ✓ if Yes ☐ (*please tick anyone*)

☐ Death (dd/mm/yyyy) ☐ Congenital-anomaly
☐ Life threatening ☐ Disability
☐ Hospitalization-Initial/Prolonged ☐ Other Medically important

15. Outcome:

☐ Recovered ✓ Recovering ☐ Not Recovered
☐ Fatal ☐ Recovered with sequelae ☐ Unknown

C. SUSPECTED MEDICATION(S) *

S. No.	8. Name (Brand/ Generic)	Manufacturer (if known)	Batch No. / Lot No.	Expiry Date (if known)	Dose	Route	Frequency	Therapy Dates: Date Started	Therapy Dates: Date Stopped	Indication	Causality Assessment
i	Tab largactil	Wembley	LGL0941	07/2024	100mg	PO	4tablets	30/04/23	06/06/23	psychosis	Probable
ii	(Chlorpromazine)	labs					at bedtime				
iii											
iv#											

9. Action taken after reaction (*please tick*)

10. Reaction reappeared after reintroduction of suspected medication (*please tick*) NA

S. No. as per C	Drug withdrawn	Dose increased	Dose reduced	Dose not changed	Not applicable	Unknown	Yes	No	Effect unknown	Dose (if re-introduced)
i	✓									
ii										
iii										
iv										

11. Concomitant medical product including self-medication and herbal remedies with therapy dates (Exclude those used to treat reaction) NA

S. No.	Name (Brand / Generic)	Dose	Route	Frequency (OD, BD, etc.)	Therapy Dates: Date Started	Therapy Dates: Date Stopped	Indication
i							
ii							
iii#							

Additional Information :

D. REPORTER DETAILS *

16. Name & Address : Dr ABC, DYPH, Nerul, Navi-Mumbai

Pin : 400706 Email : abc@gmail.com

Contact No- : 99XXXXXX

Occupation : Doctor Signature : ABC

17. **Date of this report (dd/mm/yyyy) :**

Signature and Name of Receiving Personnel :

Confidentiality : The patient's identity is held in strict confidence and protected to the fullest extent. Submission of a report does not constitute an admission that medical personnel or manufacturer or the product caused or contributed to the reaction. Submission of an ADR report does not have any legal implication on the reporter.

\# Use separate page for more information

* Mandatory Fields for suspected ADR Reporting Form

Exercise 2: ADR reporting form.

11 CHAPTER

P-Drug

The drugs you are going to prescribe regularly and with which you will become familiar are called P(ersonal)-drugs. The P-drug concept includes the name of a drug, dosage form, dosage schedule and duration of treatment for a specified condition.

A P-drug is selected depending on the safety, tolerability, efficacy and price (STEP) of a drug. While selecting a drug, to be included in the P-drug list, not only is the name of the drug considered in selecting a drug, but its dosage form, schedule and duration of treatment for a particular indication is also considered.

Format for preparing and explaining P-drug:

1. Define the diagnosis.			
2. Specify the therapeutic objective:			
3. Make an inventory of effective groups:			
4. Choose a group according to the criteria			
Efficacy	Safety	Suitability	Cost
Group 1			
Group 2			
Group 3			
Group 4			
4. Choose a P-drug			
Efficacy	Safety	Suitability	Cost
Drug 1			
Drug 2			
Drug 3			
Drug 4			
5. Conclusion: a Active substance, dosage form: b. Standard dosage schedule: c. Standard duration:			
6. Explanation for selection of P-drug:			

1. A 50-year-old male patient complains of bloody, mucoid stools and abdominal pain. There is no history of alcohol abuse. You have diagnosed it as a case of acute amoebic dysentery. Choose an appropriate drug and mention its dosage schedule and duration of treatment.

a. **Diagnosis:** Acute amoebic dysentery

b. **Therapeutic objective:**
   - » Eradicate disease
   - » Prevent further transmission
   - » Symptomatic treatment

c. **Effective drug groups**:
   - » *Nitroimidazoles:* metronidazole, tinidazole
   - » *Alkaloids:* Emetine
   - » *Amide:* Diloxanide furoate
   - » *8-Hydroxyquinolines:* Iodochlor
   - » *Antibiotics:* Tetracycline's

	Safety	***Tolerability***	***Efficacy***	***Price***	***Choice***
Nitro-imidazole	+++	+++	+++	+	Best
Alkaloids: dehydroemetine	+	+	++	+	Not preferred
Amide: Diloxanide furoate	+++	+++	+	+	Cannot bring cure however required for radical cure (luminal amebicides)
8-Hydroxy-quinolines: Iodochlor	+	+	+	+	(luminal amebicides)
Antibiotics: tetracycline's	++	++	+	+	Not preferred

d. **Choose a P-drug** according to according to above steps

	Safety	***Tolerability***	***Efficacy***	***Price***
Metronidazole	+++	++	+++	+
Tinidazole	+++	+++	+++	++
Secnidazole	+++	+++	+++	++
Ornidazole	+++	+++	+++	++
Satranidazole	+++	+++	+++	++

Conclusion:

- » Metronidazole is the cheapest active agent. Oral tablet 400 mg. This should be followed by a luminal amebicide to prevent a carrier state (diloxanide furoate is the rational choice for this).

- » Metronidazole has more adverse effects (anti-abuse reaction) as compared to others. Since the patient is not alcoholic it can be used, otherwise Tinidazole and others can be used.
- » *Dosage schedule:* Metronidazole 400 mg three times a day.
- » Duration of treatment for acute intestinal amoebiasis is usually 5-7 days with 400 mg metronidazole.

2. **Mr Sonavane, a 35-year-old man presented with fever, abdominal pain and generalised weakness for the past 2 days. He gave a history of loose motions 2-3 times a day. Following clinical examination and laboratory investigations (Widal's test), he was diagnosed to be suffering from typhoid.**
   - What will be your therapeutic objective?
   - Which of the following drugs would you select for this patient from the following P-drug list, which you have made for a case of typhoid? Give reasons for selection of the drugs

     a. Chloramphenicol b. Ciprofloxacin
     c. Cefoperazone d. Ampicillin
     e. Cotrimoxazole

   a. **Diagnosis:** Acute typhoid.

   b. **Therapeutic objective**
      - » Eradicate disease.
      - » Symptomatic treatment.

   c. **Effective drug groups** (provided in question)
      - » Chloramphenicol
      - » Ciprofloxacin
      - » Cefoperazone
      - » Ampicillin
      - » Cotrimoxazole
      - » Azithromycin

   d. **Choosing a P drug** according to above steps

	Safety	*Tolerability*	*Efficacy*	*Price*
Chloramphenicol	++	++	+	+
Ciprofloxacin	+++	+++	+++	+
Cefoperazone/ ceftriaxone	+++	+++	+++	++
Cotrimoxazole	+	+	+	+
Ampicillin	++	++	+	+
Azithromycin	+++	+++	+++	++

- » Cefoperazone/ceftriaxone and Ciprofloxacin are fastest acting bactericidal drugs, lesser resistance problems, prevents/No relapses and carrier state.
- » Azithromycin is a second-line alternative in multidrug-resistant typhoid.
- » Chloramphenicol and Cotrimoxazole are not effective with high resistance.

Conclusion:

» Tab ciprofloxacin
» *Dosage schedule:* 500 mg twice daily for 14 days
» Tab Paracetamol 500 mg as and when required for fever
» To follow up after 2 days if fever persists

3. **Khushi Kumari a 3-year-old girl suffering from acute watery diarrhoea with mild dehydration**
   a. **Diagnosis**: Acute watery diarrhoea with mild dehydration.
   b. **Therapeutic objective:** To prevent further dehydration and to rehydrate, the goal is not to cure the infection
   c. **Effective drug groups:**
      » ORS
      » Rice water, homemade sugar/salt solution, fruit juice
   d. **Choosing** an effective group based on efficacy, safety, suitability and cost.

	Safety	*Tolerability*	*Efficacy*	*Price*	*Choice*
ORS	+++	+++	+++	+ (least)	Best
Probiotics	+++	+++	++	+	As adjuvant therapy
Zinc supplements	+++	+++	+	+	As adjuvant therapy
Antibiotics	+	+	+	+	Not required
Antimotility drugs	++	++	+	+	C/I

Conclusion:

» ORS is preferred as a life-saving and helps in rehydration, replacement of ongoing losses
» Maintenance of electrolyte balance
» *ORS:* The active substance, dosage form ORS in powdered dosage form, dissolved in 1 L of water, 250 mL to be sipped every hour
» Dosage will depend upon the amount of dehydration.

4. **A woman of 36 has had an intermittent fever for 6 days, with rigors, headache and anorexia. A thick film of her blood shows many red cells invaded with *P. falciparum*.**
   a. **Diagnosis:** *P. falciparum* malaria
   b. **Specify the therapeutic objective:** Complete cure with no recrudescence
   c. **Choose a group** according to criteria

	Safety	*tolerability*	*Efficacy*	*Price*	*Choice*
Quinoline-methanol Mefloquine	++	++	++	++	Not used alone
Cinchona alkaloid: Quinine	+	+	++	+	Toxic drug

Contd...

Contd...

	Safety	*tolerability*	*Efficacy*	*Price*	*Choice*
Sulfonamides sulfadoxine, and sulfone sulfamethopyrazine	++	++	+	+	Never used alone
Antibiotics tetracycline, doxycycline, clindamycin	++	+	+	++	Never used alone
Artemesins: artesunate, artemether, arteether, arterolane	+++	+++	+++	++	Faster parasite clearance no recrudescence when used in combination
Amino alcohols halofantrine, lumefantrine	+++	+++	+++	++	• Rapid clinical and parasitological cure • High cure rates and low recrudescence rate

d. **Choose a P-drug**

	Safety	*Tolerability*	*Efficacy*	*Price*	*choice*
Mefloquine	++	++	++	++	Not used alone
Quinine	+	+	++	+	Toxic drug
Sulfadoxine, sulfame-thopyrazine	++	++	+	+	Never used alone
Doxycycline	++	+	+	++	Never used alone
Artesunate, artemether	+++	+++	+++	++	Faster parasite clearance no recrudescence when used in combination
Lumefantrine	+++	+++	+++	++	Rapid clinical and parasitological cure. High cure rates and low recrudescence rate

Conclusion:

- » In *P. falciparum* malaria two drugs need to be used in combination.
- » *The active substance, dosage form:* Standard dosage schedule, duration:
  - Fixed dose combination of artemether 80 mg + lumefantrine 480 mg
  - One tablet, twice a day for 3 days to be taken with fatty meal

- » Artemether used alone is quick acting, reduces the parasite load rapidly and kills >95% plasmodia (*P. falciparum*), leaving a small number of malarial parasites to cause recrudescence. Lumefantrine being long acting will eliminate the remaining plasmodia.
- » Gametocyte population is reduced decreasing transmission rate.
- » This combination is used as a part of ACT (Artemisinin combination therapy) therapy in treatment of *P. falciparum* malaria. Combination is administered along with fatty food which enhances mainly lumefantrine absorption to ensure adequate blood levels.
- » Caution is administered when given along with drugs, such as metoprolol undergoing metabolism with CYP2D6.
- » Combination should not be given to the patient receiving QTc prolonging drugs (Artemether prolongs QTc). Should be avoided in 1st trimester of pregnancy.
- » *Advantages of this combination:*
  - Rapid clinical and parasitological cure
  - High cure rate (>95%) low recrudescence rate
  - Decrease parasite resistance
  - Good tolerability profile

5. Write a P-drug for a pregnant female with lower urinary tract infection.

a. **Diagnosis:** Lower urinary tract infection

b. **Therapeutic objectives:**
- » Eradicate disease
- » Prevent relapses
- » Symptomatic treatment

c. **Effective drug groups:**
- » TMP-SMX
- » Fluoroquinolones
- » Norfloxacin
- » Levofloxacin
- » Nitrofurantoin
- » Beta lactams
- » Cefixime
- » Fosfomycin

d. **Choose a group** according to criteria

	Safety	*Tolerability*	*Efficacy*	*Price*	*choice*
TMP-SMX	++	++	+++	++	Good alternative excluded as not safe in pregnancy
Fluoroquinolones norfloxacin	+++	+++	+++	+	Good alternative excluded as not safe in pregnancy
Levofloxacin	+++	+++	+++	+	Good alternative excluded as not safe in pregnancy

Contd...

Contd...

	Safety	Tolerability	Efficacy	Price	choice
Nitrofurantoin					
Beta-lactams cefixime	+++	+++	+++	+	Good alternative
Fosfomycin	+++	+++	+++	+	Preferred choice also safe in pregnancy

e. **Choose a P-drug:**
   - » Fosfomycin
   - » Fosfomycin is used only for the treatment of uncomplicated urinary tract infections. It is administered as a one-time 3-gram oral dose. Overall, it is well tolerated. Side effects that may occur include diarrhea (9%), nausea, vomiting, and esophageal discomfort.
   - » It is also safe in pregnancy.
   - » Fosfomycin is an FDA-approved drug for pregnant women (category B)
   - » Wide spectrum of antimicrobial activity against common uropathogens.
   - » Administered in a single oral dose.

6. Discuss P-drug for a 20-year-old patient with grand-mal epilepsy.

a. **Diagnosis:** Grand-mal epilepsy (generalized tonic-clonic seizures)

b. **Specify the therapeutic objective:**
   - » Symptomatic treatment (no seizures)
   - » Improvement in quality of life

c. **Effective groups:**
   - » Barbiturate phenobarbitone
   - » Hydantoin phenytoin fosphenytoin
   - » Iminostilbene carbamazepine, oxcarbazepine
   - » Aliphatic carboxylic valproic acid (sodium valproate) divalproex
   - » Benzodiazepines clonazepam, diazepam, lorazepam, clobazam
   - » Phenyltriazine lamotrigine

d. **Choose a group/P-drug** according to the criteria:

	Safety	Tolerability	Efficacy	Price	choice
Barbiturate	+	+	++	+	Not preferred because of dulling behavioral effects
Hydantoin phenytoin	++	+++	+++	+	Lots of adverse effects. But first-line alternative for GTC
Iminostilbene carbamazepine	+++	+++	+++	++	First-line alternative for GTC

Contd...

Contd...

	Safety	*Tolerability*	*Efficacy*	*Price*	*choice*
Aliphatic carboxylic valproic acid	+++	+++	+++	+	Broad spectrum, well tolerated first line in GTC
Benzodiazepines clonazepam	++	+++	+	+	Sedation and Tolerance develops to antiepileptic action, hence not preferred
Phenyltriazine lamotrigine	++	+++	+++	++	Broad spectrum, well tolerated first line in GTC

Conclusion:

» Older drugs, such as phenytoin, carbamazepine, and valproic acid are generally used as a first-line therapy since they are as effective as recently marketed drugs and significantly less expensive. Of the newer drugs lamotrigine, and levetiracetam are also now considered first line. (though a little more expensive)

- Active substance, dosage form: Tab sodium valproate
- Standard dosage schedule: Tab sodium valproate 20 mg/day in two divided doses
- Standard duration: 15 days. To follow up after 15 days for evaluation
- Explanation for selection of P-drug: Broad spectrum, well tolerated, cost-effective first line in GTC

7. A 39-year-old marine was brought to the OPD and complained of severe weakness, dizziness, and sleepiness during the preceding 4 weeks of boot camp. In a previous episode 3 weeks earlier, he reported generalized tiredness, unquenchable thirst, and the repeated need to urinate. Although he ate all of his rations as well as whatever he could get from his fellow trainees, he had lost 7 kilos. Laboratory, on admission, showed glucose of 267 mg/dL. Prescribe suitable drug(s) for this patient. (Type II diabetes mellitus). Discuss P-drug for a 45-year-old man with newly diagnosed type 2 diabetes mellitus.

a. **Diagnosis:** Naïve type II diabetes mellitus.

b. **Specific therapeutic objective:**

» Controlling blood sugar levels to prevent long-term complications

» To prevent hypoglycemia due to overdosage of drug or missing meals.

» Education as treatment may be life long

c. **Effective groups:**

» *Biguanides:* Metformin

» *Sulfonylureas:* Glimepiride

» *Thiazolidinedione, eg.:* Pioglitazone

- *DPPIV inhibitors:* Gliptins
- *Alpha glycosidase inhibitors:* Voglibose
- *SGLT-2 inhibitors:* Dapagliflozin

d. **Choose a group/drug** according to the criteria:

	Safety	*Tolerability*	*Efficacy*	*Price*	*choice*
Biguanides: metformin	+++	++	++	+	No hypoglycemia, cheap decreases insulin resistance
Sulfonylureas: glimepiride	++	++	+++	+	Hypoglycemia
Thiazolidinedione, e.g., pioglitazone	++	++	++	++	Mainly used as an adjuvant, No hypoglycemia
DPPIV inhibitors: Gliptins	+++	+++	++	++	Mainly used as an adjuvant, No hypoglycemia
Alpha glycosidase inhibitors: Voglibose	++	+++	++	+	Mainly used as an adjuvant, No hypoglycemia
SGLT-2 inhibitors: Dapagliflozin	++	+++	++	++	Mainly used as an adjuvant, No hypoglycemia

Conclusion:

- *Biguanides:* Metformin
- *Active substance, dosage form:* Metformin 500 mg tablet
- *Standard dosage schedule:* Metformin 500 mg one tablet twice a day after food for 3 weeks. To follow after that for evaluation and dose adjustment
- *Standard duration:* 3 weeks. Then latter can be increased by 1 tablet till euglycemia is achieved.
- *Explanation for selection of P-drug:* Metformin is the first choice—dvantages—no hypoglycemia, in obesity it also reduces appetite to reduce weight, prevents macrovascular and microvascular complications, efficacy is similar to other oral drugs, decreases insulin resistance.

7. **A 33-year-old woman presented to an outside facility with unintentional weight loss. Further questioning revealed a two- to three-month history of, heat intolerance, diarrhea, abdominal pain and palpitations. Examination showed enlargement of thyroid gland, bulged eyes, tremors. The patient showed signs of tachycardia (118 beats per minute) and tachypnea (22 breaths per minute). Laboratory testing was significant for hyperthyroidism (Graves' disease).**

   a. **Define the diagnosis:** Hyperthyroidism due to Graves' disease

b. **Therapeutic objective:**
   » Relief of symptoms
   » To keep thyroid levels under normal
   » Maintain euthyroid status
   » To find out the cause and treat it
c. **Effective groups:**
   » *Thioamides:* Propylthiouracil, methimazole, carbimazole
   » Iodine, iodides of Na and K, organic iodide, logos iodine
   » Radioactive iodine (Iodine-131, -125, and -123).
d. **Choose a group** according to criteria

	Safety	*Tolerability*	*Efficacy*	*Price*	*choice*
Thioamides: Propylthiouracil, methimazole, carbimazole	+++	+++	+++	+	• Definite therapeutic effect is maintained for long-term • Can bring remission in Graves' disease after 1–2 years of treatment
Iodine, iodides of Na and K, organic iodide, logos iodine	++	++	+	+	Quick onset for short-lived action (10 days) after which thyroid escape will occur
Radioactive iodine (131I, 125I, 123I)	++	++	+	+++	• Delayed onset, permanent destruction of thyroid cells, can cause hypothyroidism in 5–10% of cases of Graves' disease • Radioactive not preferred in young adults

Thioamides: Propylthiouracil, methimazole, carbimazole

e. **Choose a P-drug**

	Safety	*Tolerability*	*Efficacy*	*Price*	
Carbimazole	+++	+++	+++	+	Longest duration of action than PTZ
Propylthiouracil (PTZ)	++	+++	+++	+	Shorter duration of action, risk of hepatitis (reserved for early pregnancy, and thyroid storm)

Contd...

Contd...

	Safety	*Tolerability*	*Efficacy*	*Price*	
Methimazole	+++	+++	+++	+	Active from of carbimazole (lesser available)

Conclusion:

- » *Thioamides:* Carbimazole
- » *Active substance, dosage form:* Tablet carbimazole (5–15 mg) one tablet thrice daily
- » *Standard dosage schedule:* Tablet carbimazole one tablet thrice daily
- » To follow after that for evaluation and dose adjustment. Simultaneous administration of propranolol is recommended to reduce tremors and tachycardia.
- » *Standard duration:* 6 weeks. To follow after that for evaluation and dose adjustment
- » Carbimazole gives a definite therapeutic effect and its effect is maintained for long term. Can bring remission in Graves' disease after 1–2 years of treatment. Longer duration of action than PTZ.

8. **A 25-year-old woman comes to the casualty with a history of acute breathlessness since the last 15 minutes. The patient gives a history of three similar attacks in the past which was relieved by taking drugs by inhalation. On examination, pulse rate was 120/min and respiratory rate was 27/min. Auscultation of the chest revealed bilateral expiratory rhonchi with prolonged expiration.**

   a. **Diagnosis**: Acute attack of bronchial asthma
   b. **Therapeutic objective:** To relieve the attack by using an effective bronchodilator with fast onset of action
   c. **Effective groups:**
      - » Bronchodilators
      - » *Beta 2 sympathomimetics:* Short-acting—salbutamol. Terbutaline
      - » *Long acting:* Salmeterol
      - » *Methylxanthines:* Theophylline, aminophylline
      - » *Anticholinergic:* Ipratropium bromide, tiotropium bromide
   d. **Choosing an effective group** based on efficacy, safety, suitability and cost. Choose a P-drug according to the below-given steps:

	Safety	*Tolerability*	*Efficacy*	*Price*
Salbutamol	+++	+++	+++	++
Salmeterol	+++	+++	++	++
Aminophylline	+	+	++	+
Ipratropium bromide	++	++	+	++

Selective beta 2 agonists are short acting; have rapid onset of action and are used by inhalation route. Salmeterol is long-acting and has a delayed onset of action. Aminophylline has to be given orally;

therefore, delayed onset of action, or slow IV, which is inconvenient. Ipratropium is used by inhalation route but onset of action is delayed hence not used.

e. **Choose a P-drug**
   » *Salbutamol:* Highest selectivity, fast onset of action, used by inhalation
   » *Dosage schedule:* 100 μg/MDI

9. A 45-year-old man diagnosed from mild hypertension with BP 148/94 mm Hg. There was left ventricular enlargement in this patient. Choose a P-drug for this patient.

a. **Diagnosis:** Mild hypertension
b. **Therapeutic objective:** To maintain BP <140/90 mm Hg
c. **Effective drug groups:**
   » *ACE inhibitors:* Captopril, enalapril
   » *Angiotensin receptor blocker:* Losartan
   » *Diuretics:* Hydrochlorothiazide, furosemide
   » *Beta blockers:* Atenolol
   » *Calcium channel blockers:* Amlodipine
d. **Choosing an effective group** based on efficacy, safety, suitability and cost.
e. **Choose a P-drug** according to the below given steps:

	Safety	*Tolerability*	*Efficacy*	*Price*
Enalapril	++	++	+++	+
Hydrochlorothiazide	+	+	++	++
Atenolol	+	+	+	+
Amlodipine	+	+	+	++

Conclusion:

– Tab enalapril, 5 mg, 1 tablet OD.

10. A 50-year-old male patient was brought to the casualty with complaints of chest pain. History revealed the patient had few attacks of classical angina previously.

a. **Diagnosis**: Chronic angina pectoris
b. **Therapeutic objective:**
   » To prevent/reduce the frequency/severity of the attack
   » To prevent myocardial infarction and other cardiovascular event
c. **Effective drug groups:**
   » *Organic nitrates:* Glyceryl trinitrate, isosorbide dinitrate
   » *Beta blockers:* Atenolol, metoprolol
   » *Calcium channel blockers:* Amlodipine, verapamil
d. **Choosing an effective group** based on efficacy, safety, suitability and cost.
e. **Choose a P-drug** according to according to above steps

	Safety	Tolerability	Efficacy	Price
Glyceryl nitrate	++	+++	+++	++
Atenolol	++	++	++	+
Amlodipine	++	++	++	+

Conclusion:

Cardioselective beta blocker: Atenolol

11. **A 31-year-old female patient came to the OPD with a complaint of a frontal headache from the past two days. No history of nausea, vomiting or diarrhea was reported. Patient complain of worsening headaches when exposed to sunlight. Choose a P-drug for this patient.**
    a. **Diagnosis**: Mild migraine
    b. **Therapeutic objectives:** To relieve headache
    c. **Effective drug groups:**
       » Simple analgesics/NSAIDs
       » Antiemetics
    d. **Choosing an effective group** based on efficacy, safety, suitability and cost.
    e. **Choose a P-drug** according to the below given steps:

	Safety	Tolerability	Efficacy	Price
Paracetamol	++	+++	+	+
Ibuprofen	+	+	+	+
Naproxen	+	++	+	+
Diclofenac	+	+	+	+

Conclusion:

12. **A 52-year-old male patient comes to the OPD complaining of sore throat and cough. Further history revealed the patient is a chronic smoker and examination showed throat inflammation. The doctor advises the patient to stop smoking and writes a prescription. Choose a P-drug for this patient.**
    a. **Diagnosis:** Irritation of mucous membrane
    b. **Therapeutic objectives:** Suppression of dry cough
    c. **Effective drug groups:**
       » Smoking cessation
       » Cough suppressants (opioids, antihistamines)
    d. **Choosing an effective group** based on efficacy, safety, suitability and cost.
    e. **Choose a P-drug** according to the below-given steps

	Safety	Tolerability	Efficacy	Price
Codeine	++	+	+++	+
Dextromethorphan	+++	+	+++	++
Chlorpheniramine	+	+	+	+++

- *Conclusion:* chosen drug—dextromethorphan syrup, 5 mL, QID X 1 week

13. A 40-year-old patient comes to the doctor with complaints of running nose, sneezing and nasal stuffiness for two days. Choose a P-drug for this case.

a. **Diagnosis**: Common cold

b. **Therapeutic objectives:** To reduce the symptoms of common cold

c. **Effective drug groups:**
   - First-generation antihistamines
   - *Highly sedative:* Diphenhydramine, dimenhydrinate, promethazine
   - *Moderately sedative:* Cinnarizine
   - *Mildly sedative:* Chlorpheniramine
   - *2nd generation antihistamines:* Fexofenadine, loratadine, cetirizine, levocetirizine, mizolastine, ebastine

d. **Choosing an effective group** based on efficacy, safety, suitability and cost.

e. **Choose a P-drug** according to the below given steps

	Safety	Tolerability	Efficacy	Price
Promethazine	++	++	+++	+
Chlorpheniramine	++	++	+++	+
Cetirizine	+++	++	+++	++
Levocetirizine	+++	+++	+++	++

Conclusion:

- Levocetirizine 5 mg in the evening for 1 week

12 CHAPTER

Essential Medicines for a Healthcare Facility

DEFINITION

Essential medicines are those that satisfy the priority healthcare needs of a population. They are selected with due regard to disease prevalence and public health relevance, evidence of efficacy and safety and comparative cost-effectiveness. They are intended to be available in functioning health systems at all times, in appropriate dosage forms, of assured quality and at prices individuals and health systems can afford.

1. **Enlist criteria for selection of essential drugs.**

   WHO has laid down criteria to guide selection of an essential medicine:

   a. Adequate data on its efficacy and safety should be available from clinical studies.
   b. It should be available in a form in which quality, including bioavailability, and stability on storage can be assured.
   c. Its choice should depend upon pattern of prevalent diseases; availability of facilities and trained personnel; financial resources; genetic, demographic and environmental factors.
   d. In case of two or more similar medicines, choice should be made on the basis of their relative efficacy, safety, quality, price and availability. Cost-benefit ratio should be a major consideration.
   e. Choice may also be influenced by comparative pharmacokinetic properties and local facilities for manufacture and storage.
   f. Most essential medicines should be single compounds. Fixed ratio combination products should be included only when dosage of each ingredient meets the requirements of a defined population group, and when the combination has a proven advantage in therapeutic effect, safety, adherence or in decreasing the emergence of drug resistance.
   g. Selection of essential medicines should be a continuous process which should take into account the changing priorities for public health action, epidemiological conditions as well as availability of better medicines/formulations and progress in pharmacological knowledge.

h. Recently, it has been emphasized to select essential medicines based on rationally developed treatment guidelines.

2. **List medicines not included in the NLEM (National List of Essential Medicines) for primary health care.**
   - Antihepatitis B and C drugs
   - Thrombolytic, antiarrhythmic drugs medicines used in shock.
   - Anticancer drugs, hormone antagonist for cancer chemotherapy, immunosuppressants
   - Blood and blood components
   - Drugs sued for dementia
   - Radiocontrast dye media, dialysis solutions
   - Medicines for neonatal care
   - Skeletal muscle relaxants
   - Antibiotics, such as piperacillin + tazobactam, meropenem, ceftriaxone, ceftazidime
   - Newer anti TB, such as bedaquiline, delamanid
   - Anti fungals, such as amphotericin B, anti-HIV drugs

3. **Prepare an essential drug list for an emergency care center.**
   - *Analgesics:* Inj diclofenac, inj hyoscine
   - *Antiemetic:* Inj metoclopramide inj ondansetron
   - *PPIs :* Inj pantoprazole, inj omeprazole
   - *Antiallergics:* Inj chlorpheniramine
   - *Steroids:* Inj hydrocortisone, inj dexamethasone
   - *Bronchodilators:* Inj terbutaline
   - *Sedatives:* Inj diazepam
   - *Anti epileptics:* Inj phenytoin
   - *Diuretics:* Inj furosemide
   - *Local anesthetics:* Inj lignocaine
   - *Cardiac drugs:* NTG, isosorbide nitrate
   - *Inotropes:* Dopamine
   - *Anticholinergic:* Inj atropine
   - Dextrose
   - Inj heparin

4. **Prepare a list of medicines used in the management of HIV for a tertiary care center**

Nucleoside reverse transcriptase inhibitors		
Abacavir + lamivudine	S,T	Tablet 60 mg, 600 + 30 mg
Lamivudine	S,T	Tablet 100 mg, 150 mg
Tenofovir + lamivudine	S,T	Tablet 300 mg + 300 mg
Tenofovir + lamivudine + dolutegravir	P,S,T	Tablet 300 mg + 300 mg + 50 mg
Tenofovir + lamivudine + efavirenz	S,T	Tablet 300 mg + 300 mg + 600 mg
Zidovudine + lamivudine	S,T	Tablet 60, 300 mg + 30, 150 mg

Non-nucleoside reverse transcriptase inhibitors		
Efavirenz	S,T	Tablet 200, 600 mg
Nevirapine	P,S,T	Tablet 200 mg
Integrase inhibitors		
Dolutegravir	S,T	Tablet 50 mg
Raltegravir	S,T	Tablet 400 mg
Protease inhibitors		
Atazanavir + ritonavir	S,T	Tablet 300 mg + tablet 100 mg
Darunavir + ritonavir	S,T	Tablet 600 mg + tablet 100 mg
Lopinavir + ritonavir	S,T	Tablet 100, 200 mg + 25, 50 mg Oral liquid 80 mg + 20 mg/mL

P–Primary health care, S–secondary care center, T–tertiary care center

5. **Prepare an essential drugs list of antibiotics for a tertiary care center.**
6. **Prepare an essential drugs list of antibiotics for a primary care center.**
7. **Prepare a list of cardiovascular medicines for a tertiary care center.**
8. **Prepare a list of essential medicines for a pediatrics clinic.**
9. **Prepare a list of antiplatelet and antithrombotic Medicines for a for a secondary care center.**
10. **Prepare a list of essential medicines for an obstetrics and gynecology ward at a tertiary care center.**
11. **Prepare an essential drugs list of drugs used in endocrine disorders for a tertiary care center.**

Look into the detailed list below and accordingly prepare the above

Sr. No.	*Medicine*	*Level of healthcare*	*Dosage form(s) and strength(s)*
1.	**Non-opioid analgesics, antipyretics and non-steroidal anti-inflammatory drugs**		
	Acetylsalicylic acid	P,S,T	Tablet 300 mg to 500 mg Effervescent/Dispersible/ Enteric-coated tablet 300 mg to 500 mg
	Diclofenac	P,S,T	Tablet 50 mg, injection 25 mg/mL
	Ibuprofen	P,S,T	Tablet 200 mg, 400 mg, oral liquid 100 mg/5 mL (p)
	Mefenamic acid	P,S,T	Tablet 250 mg, oral liquid 100 mg/5 mL (p)
	Paracetamol	P,S,T	Tablet 500 mg, 650 mg. Oral liquid 120 mg/5 mL (p),125 mg/5 mL (p) 250 mg/5 mL (p) injection 150 mg/mL suppository 80 mg, 170 mg
2.	**Opioid analgesics**		
	Fentanyl	S,T	Injection 50 µg/mL

Sr. No.	Medicine	Level of healthcare	Dosage form(s) and strength(s)
	Morphine	P,S,T	Tablet 10 mg, injection 10 mg/mL, 15 mg/mL
	Tramadol	S,T	Capsule 50 mg, 100 mg, injection 50 mg/mL
	Medicines used to treat Gout		
	Allopurinol	P,S,T	Tablet 100 mg, 300 mg
	Colchicine	P,S,T	Tablet 0.5 mg
3.	**Disease modifying agents used in rheumatoid disorders**		
	Azathioprine	S,T	Tablet 25 mg, 50 mg
	Hydroxychloroquine	P,S,T	Tablet 200 mg, 400 mg
	Methotrexate	P,S,T	Tablet 2.5 mg, 5 mg, 10 mg
	Sulfasalazine	S,T	Tablet 500 mg
4.	**Antiallergics and medicines used in anaphylaxis**		
	Adrenaline	P,S,T	Injection 1 mg/mL
	Cetirizine	P,S,T	Tablet 10 mg, oral liquid 5 mg/5 mL (p)
	Dexamethasone	P,S,T	Tablet 0.5 mg, 2 mg,4 mg, oral liquid 0.5 mg/5 mL (p) injection 4 mg/mL
	Hydrocortisone	P,S,T	Tablet 5 mg,10 mg, powder for injection 200 mg,100 mg
	Pheniramine	P,S,T	Injection 22.75 mg/mL
	Prednisolone	P,S,T	Tablet 5 mg,10 mg, 20 mg, Oral liquid 5 mg/5 mL,15 mg/5 mL (p)
5.	**Antidotes and other substances used in management of poisonings/ envenomation**		
	Activated charcoal	P,S,T	Powder (as licensed)
	Atropine	P,S,T	Injection 0.6 mg/mL
	Calcium gluconate	P,S,T	Injection 100 mg/mL
	D- Penicillamine	P,S,T	Capsule 150 mg (p) capsule 250 mg
	Desferrioxamine	S,T	Powder for injection 500 mg
	Methylene blue	S,T	Injection 10 mg/mL
	N-acetylcysteine	P,S,T	Sachet 200 mg, injection 200 mg/mL
	Naloxone	P,S,T	Injection 0.4 mg/mL
	Neostigmine	P,S,T	Injection 0.5 mg/mL
	Pralidoxime chloride (2-PAM)	P,S,T	Injection 25 mg/mL
	Snake venom antiserum	P,S,T	Soluble/liquid polyvalent—as licensed Lyophilized polyvalent—as licensed

Sr. No.	Medicine	Level of healthcare	Dosage form(s) and strength(s)
	Sodium nitrite	S,T	Injection 30 mg/mL
	Sodium thiosulfate	S,T	Injection 250 mg/mL
6.	**Medicines used in neurological disorders**		
	Carbamazepine	P,S,T	Tablet 100 mg, 200 mg, 400 mg, Modified release—tablet 200 mg, 400 mg, oral liquid 100 mg/5 mL (p)
	Clobazam	S,T	Tablet 5 mg,10 mg
	Diazepam	P,S,T	Oral liquid 2 mg/5 mL (p), injection 5 mg/mL, suppository 5 mg
	Levetiracetam	S,T	Tablet 250 mg, 500 mg, 750 mg Modified release tablet 750 mg, oral liquid 100 mg/mL (p) injection 100 mg/mL
	Lorazepam	P,S,T	Tablet 1 mg, 2 mg, injection 2 mg/mL Injection 4 mg/mL
	Magnesium sulfate	S,T	Injection 500 mg/mL
	Midazolam	P,S,T	Tablet 7.5 mg,15 mg, nasal spray 0.5 mg/actuation nasal spray 1.25 mg/actuation, injection 1 mg/mL, injection 5 mg/mL
	Phenobarbitone	P,S,T	Tablet 30 mg, 60 mg, oral liquid 20 mg/5 mL (p)
	Phenytoin	P,S,T	Tablet 50 mg,100 mg, 300 mg Modified release tablet 300 mg, oral liquid 125 mg/5 mL (p), injection 25, 50 mg/mL
	Sodium valproate	P,S,T	Tablet 200 mg, 300 mg, 500 mg, oral liquid 200 mg/5 mL (p)
	Antimigraine medicines		
	Acetylsalicylic acid	P,S,T	Tablet 300 mg to 500 mg Effervescent/Dispersible/Enteric-coated tablet 300 mg to 500 mg
	Ibuprofen	P,S,T	Tablet 200 mg, 400 mg, oral liquid 100 mg/5 mL (p)
	Paracetamol	P,S,T	Tablet 500 mg, 650 mg, oral liquid 120 mg/5 mL (p),125 mg/5 mL (p) 250 mg/5 mL (p)
	Sumatriptan	P,S,T	Tablet 25 mg, 50 mg
	Amitriptyline	P,S,T	Tablet 10 mg, 25 mg, 75 mg
	Flunarizine	P,S,T	Tablet 5 mg, 10 mg
	Propranolol	P,S,T	Tablet 10 mg, 20 mg, 40 mg

Sr. No.	Medicine	Level of healthcare	Dosage form(s) and strength(s)
7.	**Antiparkinsonism medicines**		
	Levodopa + Carbidopa	P,S,T	Tablet 100, 100, 250 mq + 10, 25, 25 mg
	Trihexyphenidyl	P,S,T	Tablet 2 mg
8.	**Medicines used in dementia**		
	Donepezil	S,T	Tablet 5 mg, 10 mg
9.	**Anti-infective medicines: Anthelminthics**		
	Albendazole	P,S,T	Tablet 400 mg, oral liquid 200 mg/5 mL (p)
	Mebendazole	P,S,T	Tablet 100 mg, oral liquid 100 mg/5 mL (p)
10.	**Anti-infective medicines: Antifilarial**		
	Albendazole	P,S,T	Tablet 400 mg, oral liquid 200 mg/5 mL (p)
	Diethylcarbamazine (DEC)	P,S,T	Tablet 50 mg, 100 mg, oral liquid 120 mg/5 mL (p)
	Ivermectin	P,S,T	Tablet 6, 12 mg
11.	**Antibacterials: Beta-lactam medicines**		
	Amoxicillin	P,S,T	Capsule 250 mg, capsule 500 mg, oral liquid 125, 250, 500, 1000 mg/5 mL
	Amoxicillin + Clavulanic acid	P,S,T	Tablet 500 mg + 125 mg, oral liquid 200, 125 mg + 28.5 mg, 31.25/5 mL
	Amoxicillin + Clavulanic acid	S,T	Powder for Injection 500 mg,1g + 100, 200 mg
	Benzylpenicillin	P,S,T	Powder for injection 5, 10 lac units
	Cefadroxil	P,S,T	Tablet 500 mg, 100 mg, oral liquid 125 mg/5 mL (p)
	Cefazolin	P,S,T	Powder for injection 500 mg, 1000 mg
	Cefixime	S,T	Tablet 200 mg, 400 mg, oral liquid 50 mg/5 mL,100 mg/5 mL (p)
	Cefotaxime	S,T	Powder for injection 250 mg, 500, injection 1000 mg
	Ceftazidime	S,T	Powder for injection 250 mg, 1000 mg
	Cefuroxime	P,S,T	Tablet 500 mg, oral liquid 125 mg/5 mL (p) injection 1500 mg
	Ceftriaxone	S,T	Powder for injection 250 mg, 500 mg, 1000 mg, 2000 mg
	Cloxacillin	P,S,T	Capsule 250 mg, 500 mg, oral liquid 125 mg/5 mL (p), powder for injection 250 mg

Sr. No.	Medicine	Level of healthcare	Dosage form(s) and strength(s)
	Piperacillin + Tazobactam	T	Powder for injection 1000, 2000, 4000 mg + 125, 250, 250 mg
	Meropenem	T	Powder for injection 500 mg + 1000 mg
	Azithromycin	P,S,T	Tablet 250, 500 mg
	Ciprofloxacin	P,S,T	Tablet 250 mg, 500 mg, oral liquid 250 mg/5 mL (p) injection 200 mg/ 100 mL
	Clarithromycin	S,T	Tablet 250 mg, 500 mg, oral liquid 125 mg/5 mL (p)
	Clindamycin	P,S,T	Capsule 150 mg, 300 mg injection 150 mg/mL
	Co-trimoxazole: Sulfamethoxazole + Trimethoprim	P,S,T	Tablet 400 mg + 80 mg
	Doxycycline	P,S,T	Capsule 100 mg, dry syrup 50 mg/5 mL (p) power for injection 100 mg
	Gentamicin	P,S,T	Injection 10 mg/mL, 40 mg/mL
	Metronidazole	P,S,T	Tablet 200 mg, 400 mg, oral liquid 200 mg/5 mL (p) injection 500 mg/100 mL
12.	**Antileprosy medicines**		
	Clofazimine	P,S,T	Capsule 50 mg, 100 mg
	Dapsone	P,S,T	Tablet 50 mg, 100 mg
	Rifampicin	P,S,T	Capsule 150 mg, 300 mg
13.	**Antituberculosis medicines**		
	Amikacin	S,T	Injection 100 mg/mL, 250, 500 mg/mL
	Bedaquiline	T	Tablet 100 mg
	Clarithromycin	S,T	Tablet 250, 500 mg, 750 mg
	Clofazimine	S,T	Capsule 50 mg, 100 mg
	Cycloserine	S,T	Capsule 125, 250 mg
	Delamanid	T	Tablet 50 mg
	Ethambutol	P,S,T	Tablet 200 mg, 400 mg, 600 mg, 800 mg
	Ethionamide	S,T	Tablet 125 mg, 250 mg
	Isoniazid	P,S,T	Tablet 100, 300 mg, oral liquid 50 mg/5 mL
	Levofloxacin	P,S,T	Tablet 250 mg, 500 mg, 750 mg
	Linezolid	P,S,T	Tablet 300 mg, 600 mg

Sr. No.	Medicine	Level of healthcare	Dosage form(s) and strength(s)
	Moxifloxacin	P,S,T	Tablet 400 mg
	Pyrazinamide	P,S,T	Tablet 500 mg, 750 mg, 1000 mg, 1500 mg, oral liquid 250 mg/5 mL (p)
	Rifampicin	P,S,T	Capsule 150 mg, 300 mg, 450 mg, 600 mg, oral liquid 100 mg/5 mL (p)
14.	**Antifungal medicines**		
	Amphotericin B	S,T	Liposomal amphotericin B—injection 50 mg/vial
	Clotrimazole	P,S,T	Pessary 100 mg
	Fluconazole	P,S,T	Tablet 50 mg, 100,150, 200, 400 mg, oral liquid 50 mg/5 mL (p)
	Itraconazole	S,T	Capsule 100 mg, 200 mg, oral liquid 10 mg/mL
	Mupirocin	P,S,T	Ointment 2%
	Terbinafine	P,S,T	Cream 1%
	Antiviral medicines: Antiherpes medicines		
	Acyclovir	P,S,T	Tablet 200, 400, 800 mg
15.	**Medicines used in the management of HIV**		
	Nucleoside reverse transcriptase inhibitors		
	Abacavir + Lamivudine	S,T	Tablet 60 mg, 600 + 30 mg
	Lamivudine	S,T	Tablet 100 mg, 150 mg
	Tenofovir + Lamivudine	S,T	Tablet 300 mg + 300 mg
	Tenofovir + Lamivudine + Dolutegravir	P,S,T	Tablet 300 mg + 300 mg + 50 mg
	Tenofovir + Lamivudine + Efavirenz	S,T	Tablet 300 mg + 300 mg + 600 mg
	Zidovudine + Lamivudine	S,T	Tablet 60, 300 mg + 30, 150 mg
	Non-nucleoside reverse transcriptase ihibitors		
	Efavirenz	S,T	Tablet 200, 600 mg
	Nevirapine	P,S,T	Tablet 200 mg
	Integrase inhibitors		
	Dolutegravir	S,T	Tablet 50 mg
	Raltegravir	S,T	Tablet 400 mg
	Protease inhibitors		
	Atazanavir + Ritonavir	S,T	Tablet 300 mg + tablet 100 mg

Sr. No.	Medicine	Level of healthcare	Dosage form(s) and strength(s)
	Darunavir + Ritonavir	S,T	Tablet 600 mg + tablet 100 mg
	Lopinavir + Ritonavir	S,T	Tablet 100, 200 mg + 25, 50 mg, oral liquid 80 mg + 20 mg/mL
	Medicines used in hepatitis B and hepatitis C		
	Daclatasvir	S,T	Tablet 30 mg, 60 mg
	Entecavir	S,T	Tablet 0.5 mg, 1 mg, oral liquid 0.05 mg/mL
	Ribavirin	S,T	Capsule 200 mg
	Sofosbuvir	S,T	Tablet 400 mg
	Tenofovir	S,T	Tablet 25 mg
	Tenofovir	S,T	Tablet 300 mg
	Medicines for amoebiasis		
	Metronidazole	P,S,T	Tablet 200 mg, 400 mg, injection 500 mg/100 mL, oral liquid 200 mg/5 mL
	Antimalarial medicines		
	Artemether + Lumefantrine	P,S,T	Tablet 80 mg + 480 mg
	Artesunate	P,S,T	Powder for injection 60 mg, 120 mg
	Artesunate + Sulfadoxine - Pyrimethamine	P,S,T	1 Tablet 100, 200 mg, + 1 tablet (750 mg + 37.5 mg)
	Chloroquine	P,S,T	Tablet 150 mg, oral liquid 50 mg/5 mL
	Clindamycin	P,S,T	Capsule 150 mg, 300 mg
	Primaquine	P,S,T	Tablet 7.5 mg, 15 mg
	Antineoplastic medicines		
	5-Fluorouracil	T	Injection 250 mg/5 mL
	6-Mercaptopurine	T	Tablet 50 mg
	Actinomycin D	T	Powder for injection 0.5 mg
	All-trans retinoic acid	T	Capsule 10 mg
	Bendamustine hydrochloride	T	Injection 25 mg/vial injection 100 mg/vial
	Bleomycin	T	Powder for injection 15 units
	Bortezomib	T	Powder for injection 2 mg
	Calcium folinate	T	Tablet 15 mg, injection 3 mg/mL
	Capecitabine	T	Tablet 500 mg
	Carboplatin	T	Injection 10 mg/mL

Sr. No.	Medicine	Level of healthcare	Dosage form(s) and strength(s)
	Chlorambucil	T	Tablet 2 mg, tablet 5 mg
	Cisplatin	T	Injection 1 mg/mL
	Cyclophosphamide	T	Tablet 50 mg, powder for injection 500 mg
	Cytosine arabinoside	T	Injection 100, 1000, 500 mg/vial
	Dacarbazine	T	Powder for injection 200 mg, powder for injection 500 mg
	Daunorubicin	T	Injection 5 mg/mL
	Docetaxel	T	Powder for injection 20, 80 mg
	Doxorubicin	T	Injection 2 mg/mL
	Etoposide	T	Capsule 50 mg, injection 20 mg/mL
	Gefitinib	T	Tablet 250 mg
	Methotrexate	S,T	Tablet 2.5, 5, 10 mg, injection 50 mg/mL
	Paclitaxel	T	Injection 30 mg/5 mL injection 100 mg/16.7 mL
	Rituximab	T	Injection 10 mg/mL
	Temozolomide	T	Capsule 20 mg,100, 250 mg
	Thalidomide	T	Capsule 50, 100 mg
	Trastuzumab	T	Injection 440 mg/50 mL
	Antianemia medicines		
	Erythropoietin	S,T	Injection 2000, 10000 IU/mL
	Ferrous salts Iron dextran	P,S,T	Injection 50 mg/mL
	Ferrous salt + Folic acid	P,S,T	Tablet 45, 100, mg elemental iron + 400, 500 µg, oral liquid 20 mg elemental iron + 100 µg/mL
	Folic acid	P,S,T	Tablet 1, 5 mg
	Hydroxocobalamin	P,S,T	Injection 1 mg/mL
	Iron sucrose	S,T	Injection 20 mg/mL
	Medicines affecting coagulation		
	Enoxaparin	S,T	Injection 40 mg/0.4 mL, 60 mg/0.6 mL
	Heparin	S,T	Injection 1000 IU/mL, 5000 IU/mL
	Phytomenadione (Vitamin K1)	P,S,T	Tablet 10 mg, injection 10 mg/mL
	Protamine sulfate	S,T	Injection 10 mg/mL

Sr. No.	*Medicine*	*Level of healthcare*	*Dosage form(s) and strength(s)*
	Tranexamic acid	P,S,T	Tablet 500 mg, injection 100 mg/mL
	Warfarin	S,T	Tablet 1 mg, 2, 3, 5 mg
	Antiplatelet and antithrombotic medicines		
	Acetylsalicylic acid	P,S,T	Conventional/effervescent/ dispersible/enteric coated tablets 75, 150, 325 mg
	Clopidogrel	P,S,T	Tablet 75 mg, 150 mg
	Dabigatran	S, T	Tablet 110 mg, 150 mg
	Enoxaparin	S,T	Injection 40, 60 mg/0.4, 0.6 mL
	Heparin	S,T	Injection 1000 IU/mL, 5000 IU/mL
	Streptokinase	S,T	Injection 750,000 IU, 15,00,000 IU
	Tenecteplase	S,T	Injection 30 mg/vial, 40 mg/vial
	Cardiovascular medicines		
	Diltiazem	P,S,T	Tablet 30, 60 mg, modified release tablet 180 mg
	Glyceryl trinitrate	P,S,T	Sublingual tablet 0.5 mg, injection 5 mg/mL
	Isosorbide dinitrate	P,S,T	Tablet 5 mg, 10 mg
	Metoprolol	P,S,T	Tablet 25, 50 mg, 100 mg, modified release tablet 100 mg
	Antiarrhythmic medicines		
	Adenosine	S,T	Injection 3 mg/mL
	Amiodarone	S,T	Tablet 100 mg, 200 mg, injection 50 mg/mL
	Digoxin	S,T	Tablet 0.25 mg, oral liquid 0.05 mg/ mL, injection 0.25 mg/mL
	Esmolol	S,T	Injection 10 mg/mL
	Lignocaine	S,T	Injection 2%
	Verapamil	S,T	Tablet 40, 80 mg, injection 2.5 mg/mL
	Antihypertensive medicines		
	Amlodipine	P,S,T	Tablet 2.5 mg, 5 mg, 10 mg
	Enalapril	P,S,T	Tablet 2.5 mg, 5 mg
	Hydrochlorothiazide	P,S,T	Tablet 12.5 mg, 25 mg
	Labetalol	P,S,T	Tablet 50 mg, 100 mg
	Ramipril	P,S,T	Tablet 2.5 mg, 5 mg
	Sodium nitroprusside	S, T	Injection 10 mg/mL
	Telmisartan	P,S,T	Tablet 20 mg, 40 mg, 80 mg

Sr. No.	*Medicine*	*Level of healthcare*	*Dosage form(s) and strength(s)*
	Medicines used in shock and heart failure		
	Dobutamine	S,T	Injection 50 mq/mL
	Dopamine	S,T	Injection 40 mg/mL
	Noradrenaline	S,T	Injection 2 mg/mL
	Spironolactone	P,S,T	Tablet 25, 50 mg
	Diuretics		
	Furosemide	P,S,T	Tab 40 mg, oral liquid 10 mg/mL, injection 10 mg/ mL
	Hydrochlorothiazide	P,S,T	Tablet 25, 50 mg
	Mannitol	P,S,T	Injection 10%, 20%
	Spironolactone	P,S,T	Tablet 25, 50 mg
	Gastrointestinal medicines		
	Omeprazole	P,S,T	Capsule 10, 20, 40 mg, powder for oral liquid 20 mg
	Pantoprazole	S,T	Injection 40 mg
	Antiemetics		
	Domperidone	P,S,T	Tablet 10 mg, oral liquid 1 mg/mL
	Metoclopramide	P,S,T	Tablet 10 mg, injection 5 mg/mL
	Ondansetron	S,T	Tablet 4 mg, oral liquid 2 mg/5 mL (p), Injection 2 mg/mL
	Antispasmodic medicines		
	Dicyclomine	P,S,T	Tablet 10 mg, oral solution 10 mg/5 mL, injection 10 mg/ mL
	Hyoscine butyl bromide	P,S,T	Tablet 100 mg, injection 20 mg/mL
	Laxatives		
	Bisacodyl	P,S,T	Tablet 5 mg, suppository 5 mg
	Ispaghula	P,S,T	Granules/husk/powder
	Lactulose	S,T	Oral liquid 10 g/15 mL
	Medicines used in diarrhea		
	Oral rehydration salts	P,S,T	As licensed
	Zinc sulfate	P,S,T	Dispersible tablet 20 mg
	Hormones, other endocrine medicines and contraceptives		
	Dexamethasone	S,T	Tablet 0.5 mg, injection 4 mg/mL
	Fludrocortisone	S,T	Tablet 0.1 mg
	Hydrocortisone	P,S,T	Tablet 5 mg, 10 mg, 20 mg, powder for injection 100 mg

Sr. No.	Medicine	Level of healthcare	Dosage form(s) and strength(s)
	Prednisolone	P,S,T	Tablet 5, 10, 20 mg, oral liquid 5, 15 mg/5 mL
	Hormonal contraceptives		
	Ethinylestradiol + Levonorgestrel	P,S,T	Tablet 0.03 mg + tablet 0.15 mg
	Levonorgestrel	P,S,T	Tablet 0.75, 1.5 mg
	Ormeloxifene (centchroman)	P,S,T	Tablet 30 mg
	Intrauterine devices		
	Hormone releasing IUD	T	Contains 52 mg of levonorgestrel
	IUD containing Copper	P,S,T	As licensed
	Medicines used in diabetes mellitus		
	Insulins and other antidiabetic agents		
	Glimepiride	P,S,T	Tablet 1, 2 mg
	Insulin (soluble)	P,S,T	Injection 40 IU/mL
	Insulin intermediate acting (NPH)	P,S,T	Injection 40 IU/mL
	Insulin glargine	P,S,T	Injection 100 IU/mL
	Insulin premix injection 30:70 (Regular: NPH)	P,S,T	Injection 40 IU/mL
	Metformin	P,S,T	Tablet 500, 1000 mg modified release tablet 1000 mg
	Teneligliptin	P,S,T	Tablet 20 mg
	Ovulation inducers		
	Clomiphene citrate	T	Tablet 50, 100 mg
	Human chorionic gonadotropin	S,T	Injection 2000 IU, 5000 IU, 10000 IU
	Medroxyprogesterone acetate	P,S,T	Tablet 5, 10 mg, injection 150 mg/mL
	Norethisterone	P,S,T	Tablet 5 mg
	Thyroid and antithyroid medicines		
	Carbimazole	P,S,T	Tablet 5, 10, 20 mg
	Levothyroxine	P,S,T	Tablet 12.5 μg to 150 μg
	Sera and immunoglobulins		
	Anti-rabies immunoglobulin	P,S,T	As licensed

Sr. No.	Medicine	Level of healthcare	Dosage form(s) and strength(s)
	Anti-tetanus immunoglobulin	P,S,T	As licensed
	Anti-D immunoglobulin	S,T	As licensed
	Diphtheria antitoxin	P,S,T	As licensed
	Hepatitis B immunoglobulin	S,T	As licensed
	Human normal immunoglobulin	T	As licensed
	Snake venom antiserum	P,S,T	Soluble/liquid polyvalent—As licensed
	For universal immunization		
	BCG vaccine	P,S,T	As licensed
	DPT+ Hib+ Hep B vaccine	P,S,T	As licensed
	DPT vaccine	P,S,T	As licensed
	Hepatitis B vaccine	P,S,T	As licensed
	Japanese encephalitis vaccine	P,S,T	As licensed
	Measles vaccine	P,S,T	As licensed
	Oral poliomyelitis vaccine	P,S,T	As licensed
	Rotavirus vaccine	P,S,T	As licensed
	Tetanus toxoid	P,S,T	As licensed
	Antiglaucoma medicines		
	Acetazolamide	P,S,T	Tablet 250 mg
	Latanoprost	P,S,T	Drops 0.005%
	Pilocarpine	P,S,T	Drops 2%, 4%
	Timolol	P,S,T	Drops 0.25%, 0.5%
	Mydriatics		
	Atropine	P,S,T	Drops 1%
	Homatropine	P,S,T	Drops 2%
	Phenylephrine	P,S,T	Drops 5%, 10%
	Tropicamide	P,S,T	Drops 1%
	Oxytocics and abortifacient		
	Dinoprostone	S,T	Tablet 0.5 mg, gel 0.5 mg
	Methylergometrine	P,S,T	Tablet 0.125 mg, injection 0.2 mg/mL

13 CHAPTER

Fixed Dose Combinations

CHEMOTHERAPY

1. **Inj ampicillin (1 g) + Sulbactam (500 mg)/1.5 g vial**
2. **Amoxicillin (250 mg) + Clavulanic acid (125 mg) tablet**
3. **Cefpodoxime (100 mg/200 mg) + Clavulanic acid (62.5/125 mg) tablet**
4. **Cefepime (250 mg) + Tazobactam (31.25 mg) injection (additional strength)**

   Beta lactamases are a family of enzymes which inactivate β-lactam antibiotics by opening the β-lactam ring. Hence, beta-lactam antibiotics get destroyed by this enzyme. Three inhibitors of this enzyme clavulanic acid, sulbactam and tazobactam are available for clinical use.

   Clavulanic acid/sulbactam/tazobactam have no antibacterial activity of their own. It inhibits a wide variety (class II to class V) of beta-lactamases produced by both gram-positive and gram-negative bacteria. They are 'progressive' inhibitors. Their binding with beta-lactamase is reversible initially but becomes covalent later. Inhibition increases with time. They are also called 'suicide' inhibitors, they get inactivated after binding to the enzyme.

   Hence, they destroy the defense mechanism of the bacteria and protect amoxicillin/cefpodoxime/cefepime/ampicillin from degradation by lactamase enzymes. Hence, it reestablishes the activity of the above antibiotics against various lactamase-producing microorganisms (S. aureus, H. influenzae, gonorrheal, Proteus, E. coli, Klebsiella, Salmonella, etc.).

   Indications:
   - Skin and soft tissue infections
   - Intra-abdominal gynecological sepsis
   - Urinary and respiratory tract infections
   - Gonorrhea.
5. **Tab Trimethoprim (80 mg) + Sulfamethoxazole (400 mg)**
6. **Tab Pyrimethamine (25 mg) + Sulfadoxine (500 mg)**

Rationale for combination

PABA taken up by bacteria
↓Folate synthetase (FS)
DHFA
↓Dihydrofolate reductase (DHFR)
Folic acid

PABA—Para-amino benzoic acid
DHFA—Dihydro folic acid
FS is inhibited by Sulfonamides (sulfamethoxazole, sulfadoxine)
DHFR is inhibited by Trimethoprim or Pyrimethamine

The combination produces a sequential block in bacterial folate metabolism. Individually both sulfonamides and trimethoprim are bacteriostatic, but the combination becomes bactericidal against most organisms.

Among the sulfonamides: Sulfamethoxazole is preferred because it has same t½ (10 hrs.) as trimethoprim.

Indications:
- Lower urinary tract infections
- Bacterial dysentery and diarrhoea
- Prophylaxis and treatment of pneumocystis carinii infection.
- Respiratory tract infections.

The combination of Pyrimethamine and Sulfadoxine is used in P. Falciparum Malaria along with artesunate.

7. **Benzoic acid (3%) + Salicylic acid ointment (WHO) (6%)**
   Rationale:
   - Benzoic acid is antifungal and antibacterial in an acidic medium. Salicylic acid is keratolytic in action, removes the infected tissue and promotes the penetration of Benzoic acid into the lesion.

   Indications:
   - Superficial fungal (dermatophytic)/ringworm/tinea infections.
8. **Rifampicin-300 mg+INH-200 mg Tablet**
9. **Rifampicin-450 mg+INH-300 mg Tablet**
10. **Rifampicin-600 mg+INH-300 mg Tablet**
    Rationale:
    - Both INH and Rifampicin are bactericidal to M. tubercle bacilli. Combination of these two drugs is synergistic. These two drugs are given along with ethambutol and pyrazinamide in the initial phase, so the duration of the therapy is shortened.
    - Use of a single drug results in the emergence of resistance strains, and relapse in almost 75% of the patients. The combination of the above decreases resistance to the tubercle bacilli.
    - Both are given as single doses daily, before breakfast, so compliance is better.

- Both eliminate fast multiplying bacilli so the response and symptomatic relief is evident within 2–4 months.

Dose:

One tablet daily ½ hour before breakfast.

**Pyridoxine (10 mg/day) has to be added because it prevents the peripheral neuritis produced by INH.

Indications:

Tuberculosis (In the initial and in the maintenance phase)

11. **Imipenem 50 mg + cilastatin 50 mg vial**

 Rationale:

 - Imipenem is a potent and broad-spectrum β-lactam antibiotic, but it is rapidly hydrolyzed by the enzyme dehydropeptidase I located on the brush border of renal tubular cells. Combination with cilastatin, which is a reversible inhibitor of dehydropeptidase enzyme prevents its destruction thus prolonging the duration of action of imipenem.
 - They have same t½ (1 hour). Newer carbapenems, such as meropenem, faropenem, doripenem and ertapenem are not hydrolyzed by renal dehydropeptidase so do not need to be combined with cilastatin.

 Indications:

 Serious hospital-acquired respiratory, urinary, abdominal, pelvic, skin and soft tissue infections including those in neutropenic, cancer and AIDS patients.

12. **Neomycin sulfate (5 mg) + Polymyxin B 5000 IU ointment**

 Neomycin is an aminoglycoside effective mainly against gram-negative bacteria but *Pseudomonas* and *Streptococcus* are not sensitive.

 Polymyxin B is effective against both gram-negative bacteria and *Pseudomonas, Salmonella* and *Shigella*. Combination of the antibiotics broadens the spectrum of action.

 Indications:

 - Skin infections, folliculitis, furunculosis, otitis externa
 - To prevent infection of abrasions, wounds and cuts

13. **Bacitracin 250 U + Neomycin 5 mg + Sulfacetamide 60 mg/g powder, skin ointment, eye ointment**

 - Bacitracin is active mainly against gram-positive organisms (both cocci and bacilli). *Neisseria, H. influenzae* and a few other bacteria are also affected. It is a bactericidal drug and is not absorbed orally.
 - Neomycin is an aminoglycoside effective mainly against gram-negative bacteria but *Pseudomonas* and *Streptococcus* are not sensitive. Combination of the antibiotics broadens the spectrum of action.

 Indications:

 Use is restricted to topical application for infected wounds, ulcers, and eye infections—generally in combination with neomycin, polymyxin, etc. It does not penetrate intact skin and, therefore, is of little value in furunculosis, boils, carbuncles, etc.

14. **Adapalene 0.1% + Clindamycin phosphate 3% ointment**
    - Adapalene is a synthetic tretinoin-like drug which binds directly to the nuclear retinoic acid receptor and modulates keratinization and differentiation of follicular cells. It has keratolytic and comedolytic properties. It also exerts anti-inflammatory action; comedone formation is suppressed.
    - Clindamycin is an antibiotic effective against *P. acne*. A combination of the two provides both keratolytic and antibacterial effects.
15. **Tab metronidazole (400 mg) + Diloxanide furoate (500 mg) + Simethicone (100 mg)**
    - Metronidazole is an antibiotic and also an amoebicide. It is effective for both intestinal and extraintestinal amoebiasis. The antibacterial mechanism is by damaging the DNA.
    - Diloxanide is a highly effective luminal amoebicide which directly kills trophozoites responsible for the production of cysts. Diloxanide is a weaker amoebicide with no systemic antiamoebic activity. It is less effective in invasive amoebic dysentery, because of poor tissue amoebicidal action. It is given after or along with metronidazole to eradicate cysts, to finish the luminal phase.
    - Metronidazole + diloxanide should be taken with food but at the same time every day.
    - This combination may cause dizziness. It is advised not to drive or do anything that requires mental focus, and avoid consuming alcohol.
16. **Tinidazole (600 mg) + Norfloxacin (400 mg)**
17. **Satranidazole (300 mg) + Ofloxacin (200 mg) tablet**
18. **Ornidazole + Ofloxacin 2 mg 5 mg per mL infusion**
19. **Tab Tinidazole (600 mg) + Norfloxacin (400 mg)**

    Rationale:
    - Ornidazole/satranidazole/tinidazole are effective against *Entamoeba* histolytica (which causes amoebic dysentery), giardia lamblia, and anaerobes.
    - Fluoroquinolones (norfloxacin, ofloxacin) are effective against *E. coli*, *Salmonella*, and *Shigella*, which cause bacterial/bacillary diarrhea. This combination is effective, especially against diarrhea of mixed origin.

    Indications:
    - Diarrhea and dysentery of mixed origin (amoebic, protozoan or bacterial origin).
    - Bowel preparation prior to surgery, appendicitis, ulcerative colitis.

    Dose: Twice daily for 5–7 days.
20. **Artemether 40 mg/80 mg + Lumefantrine 240 mg/480 mg tablets**
    - Artemether used alone is quick-acting, reduces the parasite load rapidly and kills >95% of plasmodia (*P. falciparum*). It has a shorter duration of action, leaving a small number of malarial parasites

to cause recrudescence. Lumefantrine (high efficacy erythrocytic schizontocide) being long-acting, will eliminate the remaining plasmodia, decreasing the problem of recrudescence.
- Overall gametocyte population is reduced decreasing the transmission rate.
- *Advantages of this combination:*
  - » Rapid clinical and parasitological cure
  - » High cure rates (>95%)and low recrudescence rate
  - » Decreased parasitic resistance
  - » Good tolerability profile
- This combination is used as a part of ACT (Artemisinin combination therapy) therapy in the treatment of *P. falciparum* malaria. It is given along with fatty food which enhances mainly lumefantrine absorption to ensure adequate blood levels.
- The combination should not be given to the patient receiving QTc prolonging drugs (Artemether prolongs QTc). Should be avoided in 1st trimester of pregnancy.

21. **Cefixime 100 mg/200 mg + Ofloxacin 100 mg**
    - Cefixime (Third generation cephalosporin) inhibits cell wall synthesis.
    - Ofloxacin is a fluoroquinolone that inhibits the DNA gyrase enzyme. Both are bactericidal. Improved efficacy with complete clearance of pathogens can be considered because of different modes of action.

    Advantages:
    - Combination also decreases resistance
    - Provides a broad spectrum of actions with maximum coverage
    - Well tolerated with an acceptable safety profile

    Indications:
    - Typhoid fever
    - Severe respiratory tract infection
    - Serious skin and soft tissue infections
    - Complicated urinary tract infection
    - Pyrexia of unknown origin (PUO)

22. **Ritonavir—33.3 mg + Lopinavir—133.3 mg**
    - HIV-1 protease cleaves both structural and functional proteins from precursor viral polypeptide strands and plays an essential role in the viral life cycle. Inhibition of the protease produces immature, non-infectious virions. PIs (Protease inhibitors) act at the late step of the viral cycle, they are effective in newly and chronically infected cells. PIs are atazanavir, indinavir
    - Nelfinavir, saquinavir, ritonavir, saquinavir, lopinavir, fosamprenavir, darunavir.
    - Lopinavir has poor oral bioavailability and extensive biotransformation. Lopinavir has a t1/2 life of 6 hours requiring a large tablet load roughly (6–18 tablets) to be taken daily for years. Therefore, patients' acceptability and compliance are very low.

- Ritonavir is a potent inhibitor of the enzyme CYP3A4 responsible for lopinavir metabolism.
- Ritonavir in low and subtherapeutic doses reduces high first-pass metabolism and improves bioavailability of Lopinavir. Ritonavir by slowing systemic metabolism decreases clearance of lopinavir thereby prolonging the duration of action of Lopinavir. This boosted PI regimen permits the reduction in the number/frequency of the tablets to be taken each day. Low-dose Ritonavir can be combined with all PIs except Nelfinavir.

Indications:

- Used in combination with 2 NRTIs or 1 NRTI + 1 NNRTI. However, they are avoided as a First line regimen. Most guidelines WHO and NACO preserve them for failure cases.

CARDIOVASCULAR SYSTEM

1. **Spironolactone (250 mg)/Amiloride (5 mg) + Hydrochlorothiazide (5 mg) tablet**
2. **Furosemide (20, 40 mg) + Spironolactone(50 mg) or Amiloride (5 mg) or Triamterene (50 mg) tablet**

   Rationale:
   - Hydrochlorothiazide is a medium efficacy diuretic.
   - Furosemide is a high efficacy diuretic. Both hydrochlorothiazide/ Furosemide cause hypokalemia as a side effect, which is counteracted by the K-sparing diuretics (spironolactone/amiloride/triamterene).

   Indications:
   » Mild-to-moderate hypertension
   » Edema due to congestive cardiac failure, hepatic cirrhosis.
3. **Atorvastatin (40 mg) + Ezetimibe (10 mg) tablet (addl. strength)**

   Rationale:
   - Statins inhibit enzyme HMG-CoA reductase therefore inhibiting conversion to H mg COA to mevalonate to cholesterol.
   - H mg COA

     ↓ H mg COA reductase X inhibited by statins

     Mevalonate

     ↓

     Cholesterol
   - Ezetimibe inhibits intestinal absorption of cholesterol and phytosterols by interfering with specific CH transporter protein (NPC1L1) in the intestinal mucosa. This causes compensatory increase in hepatic cholesterol synthesis. This enhanced cholesterol synthesis is blocked by statins. Hence, the combination will bring a better fall in cholesterol levels.

   Use:

   Primary and secondary hyperlipidemias.

4. **Aspirin (75 mg) + Clopidogrel (75 mg)**
   - TXA2 is generated by platelets which activates platelet aggregation. Platelets are exposed to aspirin in the portal circulation before it is deacetylated during first pass in the liver. Low dose aspirin inhibits irreversibly the COX and TX—synthase enzyme in platelets, thereby decreasing TXA2 in platelets. Also because platelets cannot synthesize fresh enzyme (have no nuclei), TXA2 formation is suppressed at very low doses until fresh platelets are formed. Thus, aspirin-induced prolongation of bleeding time lasts for 5–7 days.
   - Clopidogrel alters surface receptors (Gi-coupled P2Y12) on the platelets and inhibits fibrinogen-induced platelet aggregation. Because both have different mechanisms, additive antiplatelet action is obtained.

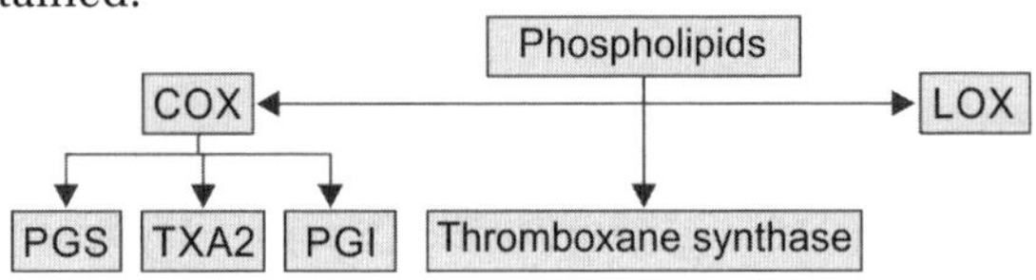

   Use:
   1. Prophylaxis in post-MI cases to prevent reinfarction.
   2. Prosthetic heart valves, arteriovenous shunts.

   Adverse effect: Bleeding

5. **Tab Aspirin (75 mg) + Dipyridamole (60 mg)**
   Rationale: Aspirin acts by inhibiting the cyclooxygenase and TX-synthetase irreversibly thus inhibiting platelet aggregation.
   - Dipyridamole inhibits the phosphodiesterase, which increases the cAMP which in turn potentiates prostacyclins interfering with platelet aggregation.
   - A combination of the two shows additive antiplatelet action.

   Indications:
   - Primary and secondary prevention of myocardial infarction.
   - Life-long therapy in patients of angina, myocardial infarction, hypertension.

6. **Losartan 25 μg + Amlodipine 5 mg tablets**
   - Losartan is an ARB (angiotensin receptor blocker) and amlodipine is a calcium channel blocker. Both have different mechanisms of action and a combination of the two will have an additive anti-hypertensive effect.
   - Amlodipine has a side effect of peripheral edema. This occurs as a result of the predominant arterial vasodilation of calcium channel blockers with little effect on the venous system. The arterial dilation increases capillary pressure and causes capillary leak syndrome and peripheral edema.
   - ARBs and angiotensin-converting enzyme (ACE) inhibitors cause arterial and venous dilation. By opening the venous system, pressures

in the capillaries decrease and there is an associated decrease in the edema.
- Thus, the combination of an ACE inhibitor and a dihydropyridine calcium channel blocker may result in less peripheral edema than that which occurs with the same dose of the calcium channel blocker given as a monotherapy.
- Both have long duration of action and can be given once daily. Compliance with once-a-day agents is greater than that with drugs taken more frequently.

7. **Enalapril (10 mg) + Hydrochlorothiazide (25 mg)**

   Rationale:
   - Enalapril is an angiotensin-converting enzyme inhibitor and Hydrochlorothiazide is a medium-efficacy diuretic. Both have a different mechanisms of action and a combination of two will have an additive antihypertensive effect.
   - Hydrochlorothiazide produces hypokalemia, which is counteracted by ACE inhibitors.
   - ACE inhibitors and hydrochlorothiazide both reduce left ventricular hypertrophy.
   - Tolerance to the antihypertensive effect of ACE inhibitors is prevented by the use of hydrochlorothiazide.

   Indications:
   - Patient of hypertension with CCF
   - Moderate to severe hypertension

8. **Atenolol (50 mg) + Hydrochlorothiazide (25 mg)**

   Rationale:

   Atenolol is a β-blocker and hydrochlorothiazide is thiazide diuretic. Both antihypertensives work via different pharmacological mechanisms, therefore when drugs addressing different BP-regulating pathways are combined, additive fall will be seen.
   - Thiazides causing diuresis indirectly activating the renin–angiotensin system (RAS). β-blockers, angiotensin-converting enzyme inhibitors, and angiotensin receptor blockers inhibit RAS work better in combination.

   Indications:
   - Patient of hypertension with CCF
   - Moderate to severe hypertension

9. **Nifedipine (20 mg) SR)/Amlodipine (5 mg) + Enalapril (5 mg)/ Lisinopril (5 mg)/Ramipril 2.5 mg)**
   - Nifedipine/amlodipine are calcium channel blockers (CCBs). Enalapril/lisinopril/ramipril are angiotensin converting enzyme (ACE) inhibitors. Both are well established antihypertensives and widely used in monotherapy. Combination of two antihypertensives with different mechanisms of action will provide an additive fall in BP.

- CCBs are vasodilatory and tend to increase plasma renin, therefore combination with an ACE inhibitor which inhibits the RAAS will counter the above effect.

Indications:

- Patient of hypertension with CCF
- Moderate to severe hypertension

10. **S(-) Amlodipine 2.5 mg + Atenolol 25, 50 mg**
    - Young people or those with high plasma renin activity are sensitive to β-blocker (Atenolol).
    - Amlodipine is a CCB. Both are well established antihypertensives and widely used in monotherapy. A combination therapy with additive effect would be superior as both are with different mechanism of action. Combination will work in most types of hypertension in terms of blood pressure reduction and prevention of end-organ damage.
    - Amlodipine does not change SA node function or AV node conduction in contrast to nifedipine which cause reflex tachycardia. Atenolol causes bradycardia hence combination with nifedipine neutralize each others side effect on heart rate.
    - In clinical studies in which amlodipine was administered in combination with beta-blockers to patients with either hypertension or angina, no adverse effects on electrocardiographic parameters were observed.

    Indications:

    - Moderate to severe hypertension
    - Prophylaxis of angina

11. **Telmisartan 40 mg, + Amlodipine besylate BP equivalent to Amlodipine 5 mg**
    - Telmisartan is a ARB (angiotensin receptor blocker. Amlodipine is a (CCB) calcium channel blocker. Both ARB and dihydropyridine CCB (amlodipine) are well established and widely used in monotherapy. Combination of two antihypertensives with different mechanisms of action will provide an additive fall in BP.
    - Combination will achieve tight blood pressure (BP) control because of the high efficacy and long half-life of each drug.
    - Both have long duration of action can be given once daily. Compliance with once-a-day agents is greater than that with drugs taken more frequently.
    - Calcium antagonists are vasodilatory and tend to increase plasma renin, therefore combination with an ARB which inhibits the RAAS will counter the above effect.

    Indications:

    - Patient of hypertension with CCF
    - Moderate to severe hypertension

12. **Sacubitril 49 mg + Valsartan 51 mg**
    - Endogenous ANP, BNP produce vasodilation and diuresis. They are destroyed by an enzyme neprilysin. Sacubitril is an orally active neprilysin inhibitor which prevents the degradation of endogenous ANP, BNP and other vasodilator peptides, producing vasodilatation, natriuresis and diuresis.
    - Angiotensin II receptor blockers (ARBs) are powerful vasodilators reduces both preload and afterload. It reduces cardiac workload and also decreases effects of aldosterone in the body.
    - Sacubitril combined with the ARB valsartan has been recently approved for use in advanced heart failure to decrease the incidence of death and acute decompensation.
13. **Nebivolol 5 mg + HCTZ 12.5 mg**
    - Nebivolol is a third generation β blocker. In addition to β receptor blockade, it activates endothelial nitric oxide (NO) synthase and enhances NO production. It thus causes vasodilatation and has the potential to improve endothelial function, which may delay atherosclerosis. Absence of deleterious effect on plasma lipids and on carbohydrate metabolism is another advantage.
    - HCTZ (hydrochlorothiazide) is a medium efficacy diuretic but at low doses it has an antihypertensive action.
    - The combination of NEB + HCTZ synergistically reduces systolic blood pressure compared with either monotherapy.

    Indications:

    Moderate hypertension
14. **Indapamide (SR) 1.5 mg + Nebivolol 5 mg**
    - Nebivolol is third generation β-blocker, because, in addition to β-receptor blockade, it activates endothelial nitric oxide (NO) synthase and enhances NO production. It causes vasodilatation and has the potential to improve endothelial function, which may delay atherosclerosis. Absence of deleterious effect on plasma lipids and on carbohydrate metabolism is another advantage.
    - Nebivolol is effective in mild-to-moderate hypertension and is associated with favorable metabolic effects.
    - Indapamide is a thiazide-like diuretic, has dual mechanism (diuretic action in distal tubule and direct vascular effect). Indapamide SR also protects against hypertensive target organ damage in heart and kidney with favourable metabolic profile.
    - Indapamide indirectly activates the renin–angiotensin system (RAS). β-blockers inhibits RAS work better in combination.

    Indications:
    - Moderate hypertension
15. **Atorvastatin 10 mg + Fenofibrate 160 mg**
    - Atorvastatin is Statin which inhibit enzyme H mg COA reductase therefore blocking conversion to H mg COA to mevalonate to cholesterol.

- Fenofibrate activates lipoprotein lipase degrading VLDL thus decreasing circulating triglycerides. It activates PPR α which increases fatty acid oxidation.
- Mixed hyperlipidemia is a major cause of coronary artery disease. Monotherapy with statins is considered the gold standard for treatment of mixed hyperlipidemia. But greater benefit may be expected by combination therapy. Combination may allow lower doses of statins and less adverse effects.

Indications:

Hyperlipidemia

16. **Amlodipine 10 mg/5 mg/5 mg/5 mg/2.5 mg + Olmesartan 40 mg/40 mg/20 mg/5 mg/5 mg + Hydrochlorothiazide IP 25 mg/12.5 mg/12.5 mg/12.5 mg/12.5 mg tablet**
    - Olmesartan is an ARB (angiotensin receptor blocker) and amlodipine is a CCB. Hydrochlorothiazide (25 mg/12.5 mg) is medium efficacy diuretic with antihypertensive action.
    - All have different mechanism of actions and combination of the three have additive antihypertensive effect.

    Indications:

    Moderate/severe hypertension
17. **Tranexamic acid BP-250 mg + Ethamsylate BP-250 mg**
    - Ethamsylate is a synthetic hemostatic drug used to reduce blood loss in many surgeries—obstetric, orthopedic, and urologic surgeries. Ethamsylate restores endothelial resistance and activation of platelet adhesiveness, thus minimizing capillary bleeding.
    - Tranexamic acid has an antifibrinolytic action that competitively inhibits the activation of plasminogen to plasmin, which is responsible for the degradation of fibrin. The combination of the two drugs will give better hemostatic effect.

    Indications:

    Epistaxis, menorrhagia, postoperative hemorrhage, tooth extraction.
18. **Ferrous ascorbate + Folic acid suspension (equivalent to elemental iron 30 mg + 550 μg per 5 mL)**
    - Ferrous ascorbate an oral iron salt has an excellent positive effect on hemoglobin value, it is postulated to have vasodilating property and superior tolerability. Folic acid will supply the required folate to correct megaloblastic anemia.

    Indications:

    Anemia

CENTRAL NERVOUS SYSTEM

1. **Tab L dopa (100/250 mg) + Carbidopa 10/25 mg)**

    Rationale:

    - Levodopa is precursor of dopamine. Levodopa is a prodrug, given alone it gets rapidly decarboxylated in peripheral tissues to dopamine. This peripherally formed dopamine cannot cross the blood brain

barrier. Therefore only 1–2% of administered levodopa crosses to the brain, is taken up by the surviving dopaminergic neurons, and is converted to dopamine.
- Carbidopa and benserazide are extra cerebral dopa decarboxylase inhibitors; they do not cross the blood brain barrier (BBB) and prevent peripheral decarboxylation of levodopa and make more of it available to cross the blood brain barrier.

Indications:

Parkinson's disease

2. **Pregabalin SR 75 mg/150 mg + Methylcobalamin 750 μg capsules**
   - Pregabalin (GABA analogue), is considered as one of the first-line drugs for the treatment of central and peripheral neuropathy. It blocks Ca^{2+} influx into nerve terminals, reducing excitatory transmitter release. It brings rapid pain relief.
   - Methylcobalamin is an essential element in the synthesis of the myelin sheath and in the maintenance of nerve function. The myelin sheath provides insulation to the nerve and aids in the proper and rapid conduction of impulses along the nerve. Deficiency of vitamin B_{12} results in damage to the myelin sheath. It helps to restore the function of the nerve in neuropathy.
   - Pregabalin has the limitation of having a short half-life (5–6.5 hours), which necessitates frequent administration of the drug and this might reduce patient compliance, especially when used for long-term therapy. Pregabalin SR may be a good option to overcome above mentioned limitation.

   Indications:
   - Diabetic neuropathy
   - Post herpetic neuralgia
   - Fibromyalgia
   - Complex regional pain syndrome
3. **Ketoprofen 50 mg/100 mg + Thiocolchicoside 4 mg/8 mg tablets**
4. **Aceclofenac IP (sustained released pellets) 200 mg/200 mg + Thiocolchicoside IP (sustained released pellets) 8 mg/16 mg capsules.**
5. **Diclofenac sod (50 mg)/Ibuprofen (400 mg) + Carisoprodol (175 mg)/ Chlorzoxazone (500 mg)/Methocarbamol (350 mg)/Chlormezanone (250 mg)/Tizanidine (2 mg)**
6. **Etoricoxib 60 mg + Thiocolchicoside 8 mg tablets**
7. **Tolperisone Hcl IP 150 mg + Diclofenac IP 50 mg tablets**
8. **Diclofenac sodium (50 mg) + Tizanidine (2 mg) tablets**

   Rationale:
   - Diclofenac, paracetamol, ibuprofen are NSAIDs which reduces musculoskeletal and somatic pain. NSAIDs blocks COX enzyme thereby inhibiting the formation of prostaglandins. They have strong anti-inflammatory and analgesic action.

- Carisoprodol, chlorzoxazone, methocarbamol and chlormezanone, thiocolchicoside, tolperisone, tizanidine are centrally acting skeletal muscle relaxants. They selectively depresses spinal and supraspinal polysynaptic reflexes involved in regulation of muscle tone. They have no effect on neuromuscular transmission (unlike dTc and succinylcholine) and on muscle fibers (unlike dantrolene). The above FDC is used in pain associated with spasm of the skeletal muscles.

Indications:

- Torticollis, lumbago, backache, neuralgias, sprains, tearing of ligaments and tendons, dislocations, fibrositis, bursitis.

9. **Diclofenac potassium 50 mg + Serratiopeptidase (as enteric coated pellets) 15 mg capsules**
   - Diclofenac sodium is a NSAID with analgesic/anti-inflammatory properties. It inhibits cyclooxygenase enzyme thus inhibiting synthesis of prostaglandin.
   - Serratiopeptidase, a proteolytic enzyme causes hydrolysis of histamine, bradykinin and serotonin. It has analgesic, anti-inflammatory and fibrinolytic effect. Serratiopeptidase reduces capillary permeability induced by above mediators; breaks down abnormal exudates facilitates the absorption of decomposed products through blood and lymphatics. Thus, Serratiopeptidase promotes wound healing and repair. Individually they act by different mechanisms and combination gives additive analgesic and anti-inflammatory action.

   Indications:
   - Arthritis, sinusitis, bronchitis, fibrocystic breast disease, and carpal tunnel syndrome, muscle pain, tooth and joint pain,

10. **Ketorolac IP 4.00 mg + Olopatadine Hcl equivalent to Olopatadine 1.00 mg Ophthalmic solution**
    - Ketorolac is a (NSAID) inhibits cyclooxygenase, thus inhibiting synthesis of prostaglandins. Prostaglandin D_2 is among the newly synthesized mediators released by mast cells following antigen stimulation, and inhibition of the production of this mediator can decrease the signs and symptoms of allergic conjunctivitis. It is used as additive drugs to reduce the conjunctival hyperemia.
    - Olopatadine inhibits the release of preformed and newly synthesized inflammatory mediators from mast cells and also has antihistaminic properties towards H1 receptors. Its dual activity is an advantage and the drug may be used both as a therapeutic and prophylactic agent, relieves itching and redness rendering the drug superior in terms of clinical effectiveness, rapid onset and length of duration of action .
    - Combination of olopatadine and ketorolac has faster recovery in hyperemia and itching for the management of allergic conjunctivitis.

GASTROINTESTINAL SYSTEM

1. **Each 5 mL contains 10 mg Oxethazaine in Alumina gel-containing Aluminum hydroxide (Al(OH)3) 291 mg, Magnesium hydroxide (mg(OH)2) 98 mg**

   Rationale:
   - Oxethazaine is potent surface analgesic used to relieve pain associated with peptic ulcer disease. Aluminum hydroxide and magnesium hydroxide are non systemic antacids. Magnesium hydroxide is an efficacious antacid with fast onset of action. Aluminum hydroxide is weak and slow-acting antacid, so the combination yields dual antacid benefit.
   - Magnesium salts are laxative while aluminum salts are constipating so combination may annul each other's side effect and the bowel movement is least affected. Aluminum salts tend to delay gastric emptying, and magnesium salts tend to hasten it so gastric emptying is least affected.
   - Though both are non-systemic antacid combination reduces dose of individual components; systemic toxicity is all the more minimized.

   Indications:

   Hyperacidity, gastritis, reflux esophagitis, dyspepsia.

2. **Levosulpiride (SR) 75 mg + Rabeprazole sodium IP (EC pellets) 20 mg capsule**
   - Rabeprazole sodium suppresses gastric acid secretion by the specific inhibition of the H^+/K^+-ATPase enzyme (proton pump). The effect is dose-related and leads to inhibition of both basal and stimulated acid secretion.
   - Levosulpiride is a prokinetic agent. Dopamine (acting through D_2 receptors) is an inhibitory transmitter in the git. It delays gastric emptying causing gastric dilatation and lower esophageal sphincter relaxation. Levosulpiride blocks D_2 receptors and has an opposite effect—hastening gastric emptying and enhancing LES tone.

   Indications:

   Gastroesophageal reflux disease (GERD)

3. **Cinnarizine 20 mg + Domperidone 15 mg**
   - Cinnarizine is a H1 antihistamine having additional antimuscarinic, anti-5HT, sedative and vasodilator properties. It modulates Ca^{2+} fluxes and attenuates vasoconstrictor action of many endogenous mediators. The antivertigo property may be due to calcium channel blockade.
   - Cinnarizine inhibits vestibular sensory nuclei in the inner ear, suppresses post rotatory labyrinthine reflexes, possibly by reducing stimulated influx of Ca^{2+} from endolymph into the vestibular sensory cells.
   - Domperidone is an anti-emetic acts by blocking D_2 receptors in CTZ.

   Indications:

   Méniére's disease treatment of motion sickness and nausea and vomiting.

4. ***Lacticaseibacillus rhamnosus* 1 billion cells + *Saccharomyces boulardii* 125 mg + Zinc enriched yeast 20 mg sachets and capsules**
   - *Lactobacillus* is a gram-positive, lactic acid-producing bacterium (probiotic) positively changes the intestinal flora, inhibits the growth of pathogenic bacteria, promotes adequate digestion, stimulates local immune function and increase resistance to infection.
   - *Saccharomyces boulardii* alters the composition of the gut flora and inhibits the action of pathogenic microorganisms. It produces lactic acid, hydrogen peroxide and acetic acid that increase the acidity of the intestine and inhibit the reproduction of many harmful bacteria. It also produces bacteriocins, which act as natural antibiotics. It helps in the synthesis of vitamin B_1, vitamin B_2, vitamin B_6, pantothenic acid and nicotinic acid.
   - The rationale for the beneficial effect of zinc supplementation is based on the depletion of zinc due to diarrhea and the deleterious effects of zinc deficiency on the immune system, leading to more severe enteric infections.
   - Zinc improves absorption of water and electrolytes by the intestines, regeneration of gut epithelium or the restoration of its function, increased levels of enterocytic brush-border enzymes, and enhanced immunologic mechanisms for the clearance of infection, including cellular immunity and higher levels of secretory antibodies.
   - Since zinc and probiotics work via different mechanisms, it is possible that adding both would have a synergistic effect.

   Indications:

   Acute diarrhea in children.

ENDOCRINE SYSTEM

1. **Glimepiride 1 mg, 2 mg + Metformin Hcl IP-500 mg in SR form**
2. **Glibenclamide 2.5, 5 mg + Metformin-400, 500 mg**
   - Glimepiride, glibenclamide, glipizide are sulfonylureas. They bind to a specific 'sulfonylurea receptor' (SUR1) located on the pancreatic β and release insulin.

     It has an extrapancreatic action where they sensitize the target tissues (especially liver) to the action of insulin.
   - Biguanides does not cause insulin release, metformin activates AMP-dependent protein kinase (AMPK). It suppresses hepatic gluconeogenesis and glucose output from liver. It also enhances insulin-mediated glucose uptake and disposal in skeletal muscle and fat. Metformin interferes with mitochondrial respiratory chain and promotes peripheral glucose utilization through anaerobic glycolysis.
   - Because of their complementary mechanisms of action, combination therapy with sulfonylurea and metformin is rational. Combination therapy with a sulfonylurea and metformin is potentially effective

in maintaining glycemic control and avoiding of insulin for a mean duration of 7.9 years.

Indication:

Diabetes not responding to metformin.

3. **Vildagliptin 50 mg/50 mg/50 mg + Metformin Hcl 500 mg + 850 mg + 1000 mg**
4. **Metformin 500/850/1000 mg + Sitagliptin phosphate 50/50/50 mg**
5. **Sitagliptin (As phosphate) 50 mg + Metformin Hcl 500 mg/1000 mg**
   - Metformin a biguanides acts by flowing mechanisms: It does not cause insulin release.
   - Metformin activates AMP-dependent protein kinase (AMPK). It suppresses hepatic gluconeogenesis and glucose output from liver. It also enhances insulin-mediated glucose uptake and disposal in skeletal muscle and fat. Metformin interferes with mitochondrial respiratory chain and promotes peripheral glucose utilization through anaerobic glycolysis.
   - Metformin reduces intestinal absorption of glucose and reduces blood glucose levels (fasting and postprandial). It also decreases weight thereby improves insulin resistance. Metformin is the first-line and commonly used pharmacological drug for patients with Type 2 diabetes mellitus.
   - Alogliptin, anagliptin, linagliptin, saxagliptin, sitagliptin, teneligliptin and vildagliptin are gliptins. On oral consumption of food, incretinssuch as glucagon-like peptide 1 (GLP1) and (GIP) are released. They act on pancreas and release insulin. However GIP has a short half life (7 min), (2 min) GLP-1. This is because they are destroyed by enzyme DPP-4. Gliptins are active inhibitors of this enzyme thereby prolonging duration of action of incretins and therefore longer release of insulin. Blood sugar lowering efficacy is moderate compared to that of SUs. The HbA1c lowering achieved by gliptins are almost equivalent to that with metformin. It carries low risk of hypoglycaemia because GLP-1evokes little insulin release at normal plasma glucose levels.
   - The combination of a DPP-4 inhibitor with metformin allows a broad and complementary spectrum of antidiabetic actions. This combination does not increase the risk of hypoglycaemia nor does it promote weight gain, an adverse effect of various other oral antidiabetic combinations.

   Indication:

   Diabetes not responding to metformin
6. **Metformin SR 500 mg/500 mg + Gliclazide SR 60 mg/30 mg + Pioglitazone 15 mg/15 mg**
7. **Gliclazide 40/80 mg + Metformin 500 mg + Pioglitazone 15 mg**
   - Biguanides does not cause insulin release (NOT AN INSULIN SECRETAGOGUE), infact it is an INSULINOMIMETIC. Metformin

activates AMP-dependent protein kinase (AMPK) in the cells. It suppresses hepatic gluconeogenesis and glucose output from liver. It also enhances insulin-mediated glucose uptake and disposal in skeletal muscle and fat. Metformin interferes with mitochondrial respiratory chain and promotes peripheral glucose utilization through anaerobic glycolysis. Metformin reduces intestinal absorption of glucose and reduces blood glucose levels (fasting and postprandial). Decreases weight thereby improves insulin resistance.

- Pioglitazone is selective agonist for the nuclear peroxisome proliferator-activated receptor γ (PPARγ) expressed in fat cells, muscle and some other cells. Pioglitazone enhances the transcription of several insulin responsive genes and reverses insulin resistance by enhancing GLUT4 expression and translocation. Entry of glucose into muscle and fat is improved. Entry of glucose into muscle and fat is improved. Hepatic gluconeogenesis is also suppressed. Activation of genes regulating fatty acid metabolism and lipogenesis in adipose tissue also contributes to the insulin sensitizing action.
- Thus, metformin and pioglitazone are well-known insulin-sensitizing agents (counter insulin resistance) that act through different mechanisms.
- Glimepiride, glibenclamide, glipizide are sulfonylureas. They bind to a specific 'sulfonylurea receptor' (SUR1) located on the pancreatic β cell membrane and provoke a brisk release of insulin. They have highest efficacy after insulin in controlling blood sugars.
- Combined pharmacological therapy of above three drugs acting via different pathways gives an additive effect.

Indication:

Uncontrolled diabetes

8. **Pioglitazone 15 mg + Metformin (OD) 500 mg**
   - Metformin and pioglitazone are well-known insulin-sensitizing agents that act through different mechanisms. Metformin reduces blood glucose levels predominantly by improving hepatic and peripheral tissue sensitivity to insulin.
   - Pioglitazone is selective agonists for the nuclear peroxisome proliferator-activated receptor γ (PPARγ) expressed in fat cells, muscle and some other cells. Pioglitazone enhances the transcription of several insulin-responsive genes and reverses insulin resistance by enhancing GLUT4 expression and translocation. Entry of glucose into muscle and fat is improved. Entry of glucose into muscle and fat is improved. Hepatic gluconeogenesis is also suppressed. Activation of genes regulating fatty acid metabolism and lipogenesis in adipose tissue also contributes to the insulin-sensitizing action.
   - Pioglitazone/metformin fixed-dose formulation combines two insulin sensitizers.

Indication:

Type 2 diabetes mellitus who are intolerant or not adequately controlled with metformin monotherapy.

9. **Diacerein 50 mg + Glucosamine sulfate (pCGS)**
   - Patented crystalline glucosamine sulfate (pCGS) is found naturally in the human body, acting as one of the building blocks of cartilage and a precursor for glycosaminoglycan, a major component of joint cartilage.
   - Diacerein works by inhibiting interleukin-1, one of the first cytokines that induces fever, controls lymphocytes, increases the number of bone marrow cells, and causes degeneration of the bone joint.

   Indication:

   Symptomatic relief in mild to moderate knee osteoarthritis to relieve joint pain and delay joint destruction and cartilage loss.

10. **Levonorgestrel (0.15 mg)/Norethisterone (0.75 mg) + Ethinyl estradiol (30 µm)**
    - Progesterone (levonorgestrel/norethisterone) inhibits the frequency of LH secretory pulses while estrogen (ethinylestradiol) inhibits the FSH secretion. The combination of the two, inhibit the follicular development and the midcycle LH surge. So ovulation does not occur.
    - Progesterone produces thick cervical mucus difficult for sperm penetration. If by chance ovulation and fertilization occurs blastocyst fails to implant because endometrium is either hyperproliferative or hypersecretive or atrophic. In any case, it is out of phase with fertilization—not suitable for implantation.

    Indications:
    - Contraception in women. One tablet is taken daily for 21 days starting from 5th day of the menstrual cycle
    - Post-coital contraception
    - Endometriosis
    - Dysfunctional uterine bleeding
    - Serious adverse effects:
      - Venous thromboembolism especially in leg veins and pulmonary veins
      - Increase in the incidence of vaginal, cervical, and breast cancer
    - Advantages of use of OC pills:
      - Regularization of menstrual cycle
      - Decrease incidence of endometrial and ovarian carcinoma

RESPIRATORY SYSTEM

1. **Guaifenesin + Bromhexine or Acetylcysteine + Ambrolite or Carbocysteine cough syrup**
2. **Ambroxol Hcl 15 mg, Salbutamol 1 mg, Guaifenesin 50 mg, Menthol 1 mg**
3. **Ambroxol + Loratadine + Guaifenesin syrup (30 mg + 5 mg + 50 mg per 5 mL)**
4. **Ambroxol 30 mg + Terbutaline 2.5 mg + Guaifenesin 100 mg + Menthol 2.5 mg per 5 mL syrup**
   - Ambroxol, bromhexine, carbocysteine, N-acetyl cysteine (NAC) are mucoactive agents (mucolytic). Guaifenesin is a mucokinetic drug. Mucoactive drugs include expectorant, mucolytics and mucokinetics. Mucolytics have mucus-thinning activity, expectorants have cough-inducing property, and mucokinetics have cough transport facilitating action.
   - Bronchospasm can aggravate cough. Terbutaline and salbutamol are B_2 agonists relieving bronchospasm especially in bronchial hyperreactivity.

   Indications:

   Bronchiectasis, COPD, acute, and chronic bronchitis or simply to relieve symptoms of acute cough caused by RTI.

5. **Dextromethorphan 10 mg + Chlorpheniramine 2 mg per 5 mL liquid**
   - Dextromethorphan is a synthetic central NMDA (N-methyl D-aspartate) receptor antagonist which has an antitussive action. Dextromethorphan does not depress mucociliary function of the airway mucosa and is practically devoid of constipating action.
   - Chlorpheniramine affords relief in cough due to its sedative and anticholinergic action, but lack selectivity for the cough centre. They have no expectorant property, may even reduce secretions by anticholinergic action.

   Indications:

   Combination used in dry non-productive cough.

6. **Formoterol 6 μg/6 μg + Budesonide 100 μg/200 μg per actuation**
7. **Budesonide IP 1 mg/0.5 mg + Formoterol IP 20 μg/20 μg respirator suspension. (Additional strength)**
8. **Fluticasone 50 μg/125 mcg/250 μg + Salmeterol 5 μg/25 μg/25 μg powder for inhalation**
   - Budesonide, fluticasone propionate are inhaled corticosteroid (ICS). Formoterol is LABA (Long-acting B_2 agonist), has a quick onset bronchodilatory action. The anti-inflammatory properties of the ICS and the bronchodilatory effect of LABA plays complementary roles in reducing inflammation in the airways and improving lung function

with relief of symptoms related to bronchospasm. Formoterol has long duration of action make it effective for acute attack as well as for long term prophylaxis.
- The combination of ICS plus LABA for maintenance therapy is recommended in asthma treatment guidelines for moderate to severe asthma.

9. **Each 2.5 mL contains; Ipratropium bromide 500 µg, Salbutamol su sulfate equivalent to Salbutamol 2.5 mg respiratory suspension. (Additional strength)**
   - Salbutamol cause bronchodilatation through β2 receptor stimulation → increased cAMP formation in bronchial muscle cell → relaxation. It is the most effective and fastest acting bronchodilator.
   - Ipratropium bromide cause bronchodilatation by blocking M3 receptor mediated cholinergic constrictor tone. They act primarily in the larger airways. Anticholinergics are less efficacious than inhaled β_2 sympathomimetics in bronchial asthma. Combination of the above two will produce marked and long lasting bronchodilator effect because of additive effect.

   Indications:
   - Severe attack of asthma/COPD
   - Nebulized solution is used in refractory asthma
10. **Montelukast 10 mg + Olopatadine Hcl 5 mg tablets**
11. **Montelukast 5 mg + Levocetirizine dihydrochloride 2.5 mg dispersible tablet**
12. **Montelukast + Desloratadine (10 mg + 5 mg) tablets**
   - Montelukast (leukotriene antagonist) and desloratadine (antihistaminic) synergistically inhibit the allergen-induced early asthmatic response.
   - Histamine is a major mediator of allergic rhinitis via stimulation of H_1 receptor. Levocetirizine is a nonsedating, oral antihistamine that is widely used in alleviating early-phase symptoms of allergic rhinitis, including sneezing, nasal itchiness, and rhinorrhea. However, the effect of antihistamine on nasal obstruction is minimal.
   - Many mediators in rhinitis and asthma contribute to airway hyperreactivity and repetitive symptoms, including wheezing, dyspnea, chest tightness, and coughing. Amongst these, leukotrienes are one of the important mediators responsible for upper (rhinitis) and lower (asthma) airway diseases.
   - Leukotrienes produce airway edema, smooth muscle contraction, and inflammatory cell infiltration. In addition, leukotrienes induce increased blood flow and mucus oversecretion, which elicits nasal obstruction in allergic rhinitis. Montelukast (leukotriene antagonist) effectively relieves above symptoms. It also reduces daytime and nighttime nasal (i.e., late-phase) symptoms of patients with rhinitis.

- Combination gives improved efficacy with early and late phase reactant.

Indications:

Allergic rhinitis.

AUTONOMIC NERVOUS SYSTEM

1. **Inj Lignocaine Hcl 2% I.P + Epinephrine (1 in 100,00) USP multiple dose vial**
   - Adrenaline is a vasoconstrictor, therefore the following advantages are seen on combination with local anesthetics (LAs).
   - Prolongs duration of action of LAs by decreasing their rate of removal from the local site into the circulation. Contact time of the LA with the nerve fiber is prolonged thereby enhancing the intensity of nerve block
   - Reduces systemic toxicity of LAs—rate of systemic absorption is reduced and metabolism keeps the plasma concentration lower.
   - Provides a more bloodless field for surgery.
   - *Limitations of the combination are:* Increased chance of subsequent local tissue edema and necrosis as well as delayed wound healing by reducing oxygen supply and enhancing oxygen consumption in the affected area.
   - Hence, combination contraindicated in end arteries. (Tip of the feet, toes, fingers, penis, pinna).
   - May raise BP and promote arrhythmia hence contraindicated in hypertensives.
2. **Drotaverine hydrochloride 80 mg + Mefenamic acid 250 mg**
   - Drotaverine hydrochloride, is a potent antispasmodic which acts directly on the smooth muscles by inhibiting phosphodiesterase and is devoid of any anticholinergic side effects.
   - Mefenamic acid (NSAID) inhibits cyclooxygenase enzyme thereby inhibiting prostaglandin synthesis. It has a strong anti-inflammatory and analgesic action.
   - Fixed dose combination of drotaverine with mefenamic acid will give additive effect.

   Indications:

   Abdominal pain, functional bowel disorders, dysmenorrhea (menstrual cramps) and menorrhagia, heavy bleeding during periods, renal colic pain, and pain after surgery and menstrual pain.
3. **Finasteride 5 mg + Tamsulosin 0.04 mg (as modified release pellets)**
   - The α-blockers includes alfuzosin, doxazosin, silodosin, tamsulosin, and terazosin.
   - Tamsulosin is a uroselective $\alpha_{1A/}\alpha_{1D}$ blocker which relaxes the bladder trigone and sphincter, improving the voiding of urine.

- Tamsulosin has an advantage as it does not cause significant changes in BP or HR. It has minimal action α_{1B} (present on vascular smooth muscles) hence no postural hypotension.
- The 5α reductase inhibitors are dutasteride and finasteride. Finasteride is a competitive inhibitor of the enzyme 5α-reductase which converts testosterone into the more active DHT responsible for androgen action in many tissues (prostatic hyperplasia). It primarily reduces the static component of obstruction, while α_1 blockers overcome the dynamic component.

Indications:

Mild-to-moderate benign hypertrophy of prostate.

14 CHAPTER

Experimental Pharmacology

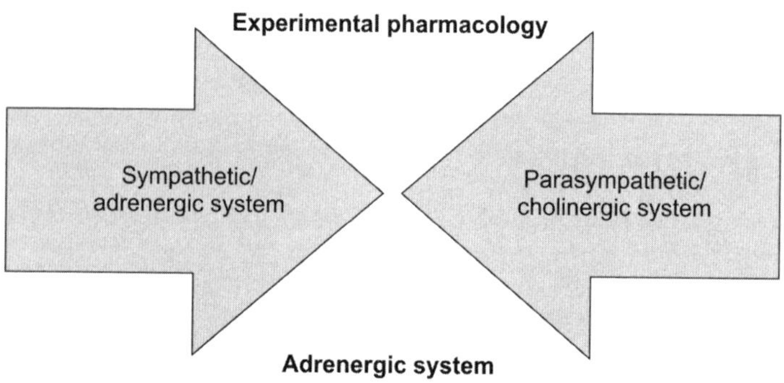

ADRENERGIC SYSTEM

Need to know location and action when receptors are present and what happens on stimulation

- α_1: Site—vascular smooth vessel of blood vessels
  Action: Blood vessel—
  - When the α_1 receptor on vascular smooth muscle (VSM) of blood vessels is **stimulated**

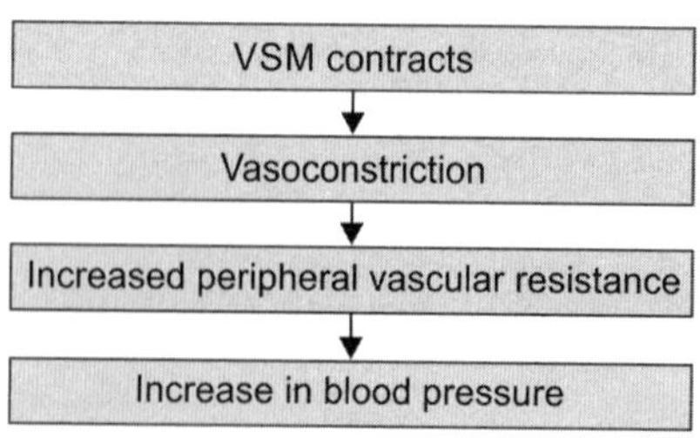

- β_1: Site—heart
  - SA node
  - AV node
  - Atrioventricular muscle of myocardium

Action:

Stimulation of β1 receptor
↓
Increase in heart rate
↓
Increase in conduction
↓
Increase in oxygen consumption
↓
Increase in blood pressure

- β_2: Smooth muscles—vascular smooth muscle, bronchial uterine.

Stimulation of β receptor
↓
Relaxation of VSM
↓
Vasodilation
↓
Decrease in peripheral vascular resistanc
↓
Decrease in blood pressure

Noradrenaline (Stimulates α_1, α_2 and 1 but not β_2)
Adrenaline (Stimulates α_1, α_2, β_1 and β_2)

1. **Effect of adrenaline on blood pressure**

   Adrenaline acts on α_1, β_1 and β_2

   In standard dose:

   Initial marked rise in blood pressure because of activation of α_1 and β_1 receptors followed by slight fall because of β2 response which is long-lasting **(Fig. 14.1)**.

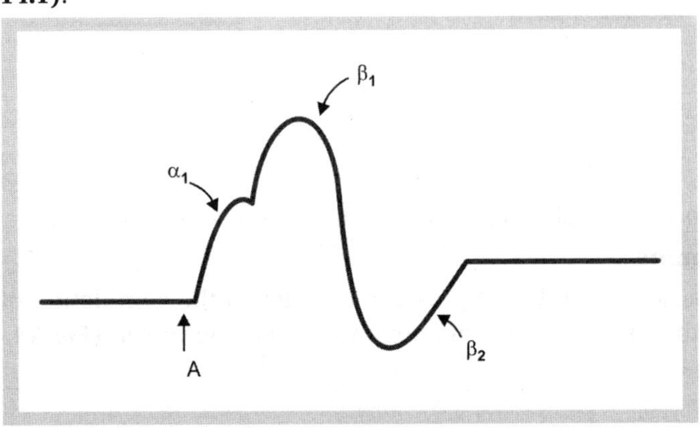

Fig. 14.1: Graphical representation of effects of adrenaline on blood pressure.

2. **Noradrenaline**

Acts on α_1 receptors. No effect on β_2 receptor.
Only a sharp rise in blood pressure but no fall is seen because there is no β_2 action **(Fig. 14.2)**.

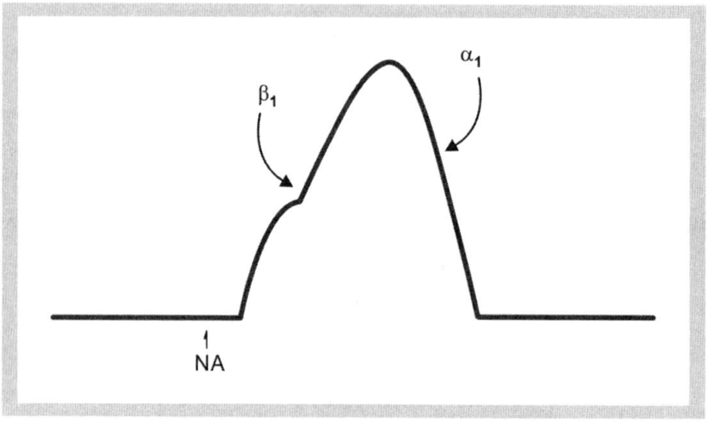

Fig. 14.2: Graphical representation of effects of noradrenaline on blood pressure.

3. **Isoprenaline**

It is a more selective agonist for the β_2 receptor. An initial slight rise (β_1) followed by a sustained fall (β_2) is seen. Long-lasting fall because it is resistant to degradation by MAO enzyme **(Fig. 14.3)**.

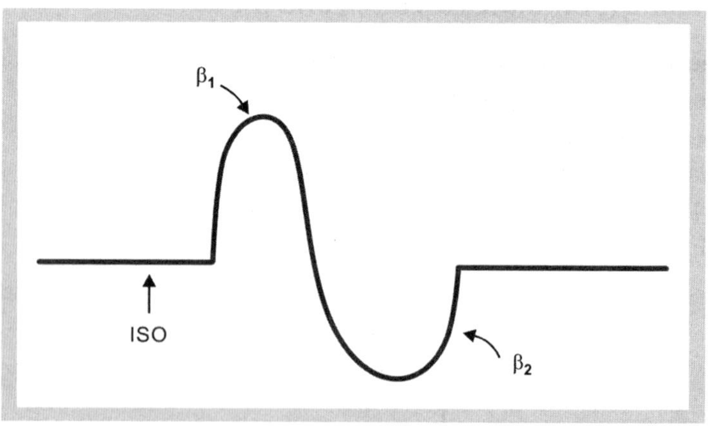

Fig. 14.3: Graphical representation of effects of isoprenaline on blood pressure.

4. **Histamine**

It causes a fall in blood pressure because of the stimulation of the H1 receptor on the vascular smooth muscle of blood vessels **(Fig. 14.4)**.

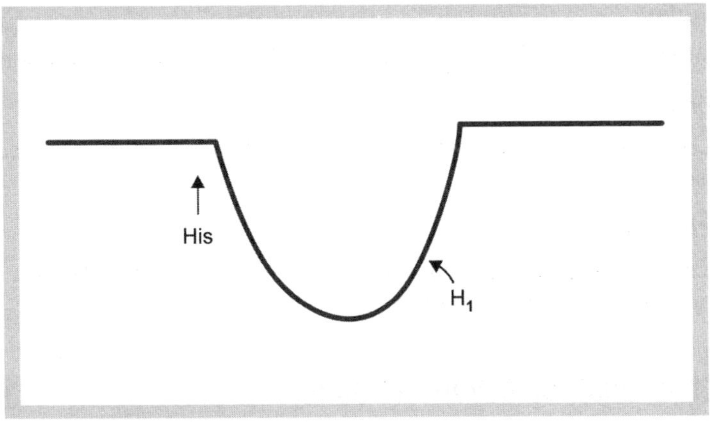

Fig. 14.4: Graphical representation of effects of histamine on blood pressure.

5. **Acetylcholine**

   Sharp and short-lasting fall in blood pressure (M3) (endothelial cells) receptor action. It is degraded by acetylcholinesterase enzyme **(Fig. 14.5)**.

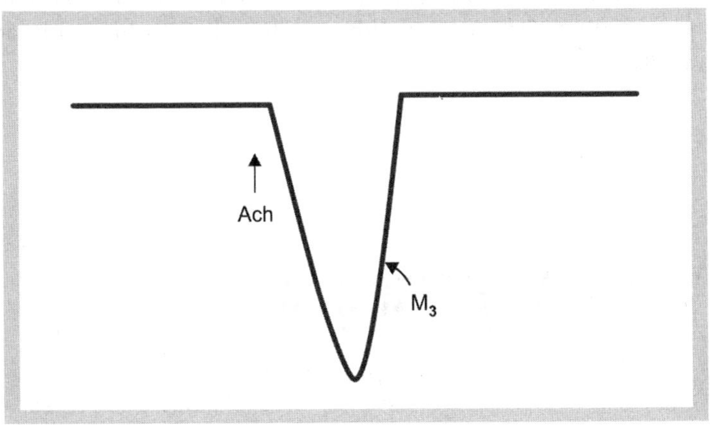

Fig. 14.5: Graphical representation of effects of acetylcholine on blood pressure.

Effect on Respiration

Adrenaline

Adrenaline increases the amplitude of respiration and there is transient apnea. Increased amplitude is B_2, mediated bronchodilation because of high BP. Transient apnea is because of reflex respiratory center inhibition.

Noradrenaline

Noradrenaline causes transient apnea but no change in amplitude. Noradrenaline has no effect on the B receptor. Transient apnea is because of reflex respiratory center inhibition.

Isoprenaline

Predominant β_2 action hence shows increased amplitude of respiration (β_2)

Histamine

It reduces amplitude because of bronchospasm. This is H1 receptor-mediated response.

Acetylcholine

It reduces amplitude because of bronchospasm. This is the effect on the M receptor in bronchial smooth muscles.

EFFECT OF DRUGS ON BLOOD PRESSURE

1. **Dales vasomotor reversal**

   There is a rapid rise in blood pressure ($\alpha 1$) when adrenaline is given intravenously followed by a fall (B_2). α blocker (Prazosin) is administered. Adrenaline is repeated. Only a fall in BP is seen because $\alpha 1$ action is blocked. This is a reversal of the previous response: initially rise later fall. This phenomenon is not seen with noradrenaline (it has no B_2 action) **(Fig. 14.6)**.

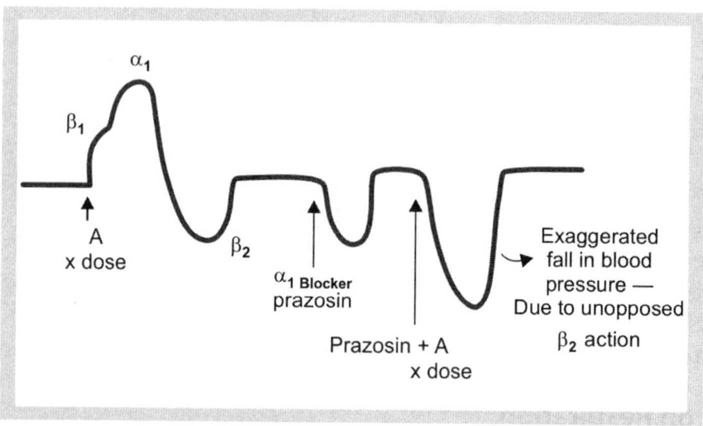

Fig. 14.6: Graphical representation of Dales vasomotor reversal.

2. **Nicotinic action of acetylcholine**

   Acetylcholine administration leads to a fall in blood pressure. Atropine is administered to block the muscarinic receptors. Acetylcholine is re-administered. There is no response (Followed by that acetylcholine is administered in higher doses (1000 times more). There is a sharp rise in blood pressure. This is because of the activation of nicotinic receptors situated in the autonomic ganglia and adrenal medulla **(Fig. 14.7)**.

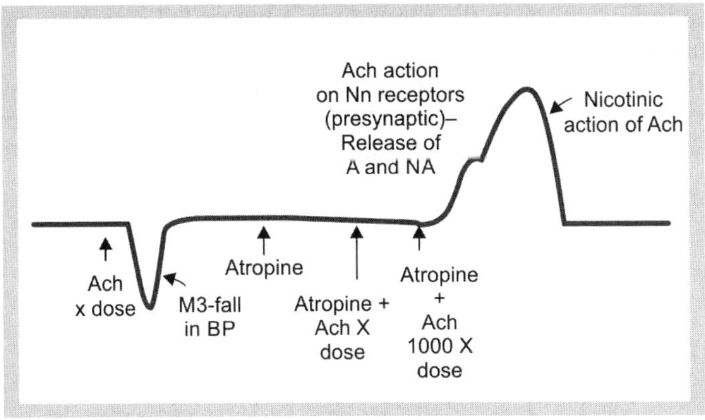

Fig. 14.7: Graphical representation of nicotinic action of acetylcholine.

3. **Potentiation**

It means one drug enhances the effect of another drug. two types—adrenergic and cholinergic potentiation.

a. **Pressor (adrenergic)**: This is shown with noradrenaline and ephedrine. Adrenaline is given. There is a rise in blood pressure. Once the blood pressure touches the baseline, ephedrine is administered. It also shows a rise in blood pressure.

Adrenaline is repeated in the same dose after ephedrine and shows a higher rise in blood pressure previous response. Ephedrine has a potentiated adrenaline response.

The reason is ephedrine is indirectly acting sympathomimetic, facilitating the release of adrenaline at post-ganglionic sympathetic nerve endings **(Fig. 14.8)**.

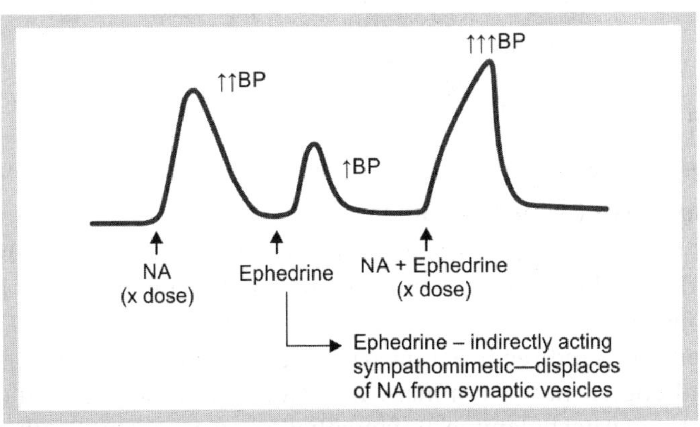

Fig. 14.8: Graphical representation of potentiation (pressor).

b. **Depressor (cholinergic)**: This is shown with acetylcholine (Ach) and physostigmine. After Ach administration, there is a sharp fall (V-shaped fall) in BP. Next physostigmine is administered which also causes a fall in BP.

Re-administer Ach in the same dose. A bigger fall is seen as compared to before.

The effect of Ach on blood pressure is facilitated by physostigmine. Physostigmine, a reversible anticholinesterase prevents the degradation of acetylcholine. Thus, increasing Ach levels **(Figs. 14.9A and B)**.

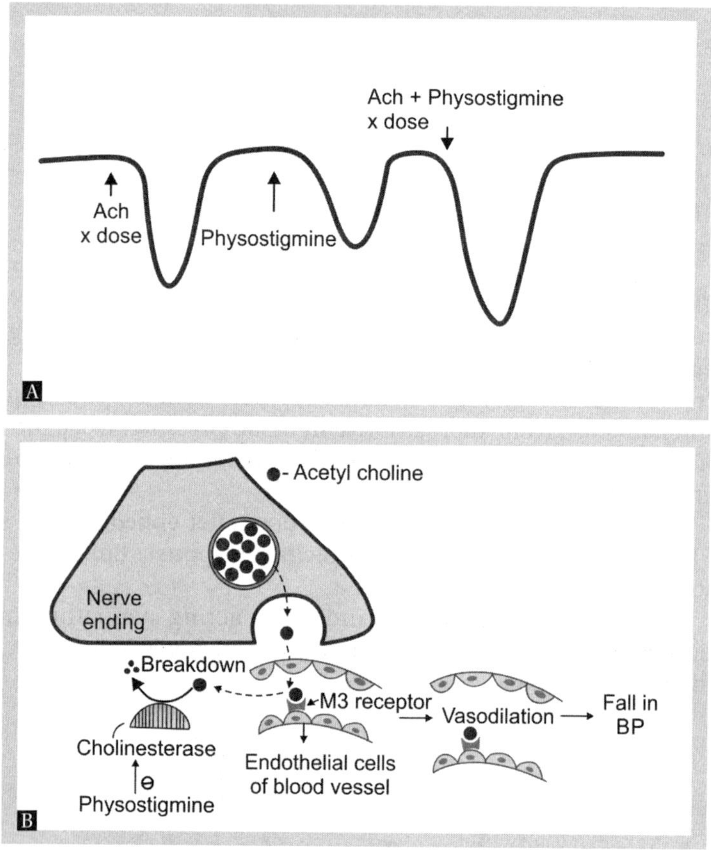

Figs. 14.9A and B: Graphical representation of potentiation (depressor).

4. **Tachyphylaxis (acute tolerance)**

When tyramine is administered frequently at short intervals in the same doses. The pressure response reduces. This phenomenon is called tachyphylaxis.

Tyramine is indirectly acting sympathomimetic acts by releasing NA from adrenergic nerve terminals. When administered quickly, it depletes the stores of catecholamine at sympathetic nerve endings. Synthesis does not happen as fast as depletion, hence response falls.

This phenomenon is seen with other indirectly acting sympathomimetics (ephedrine amphetamine tyramine) **(Figs. 14.10A and B)**.

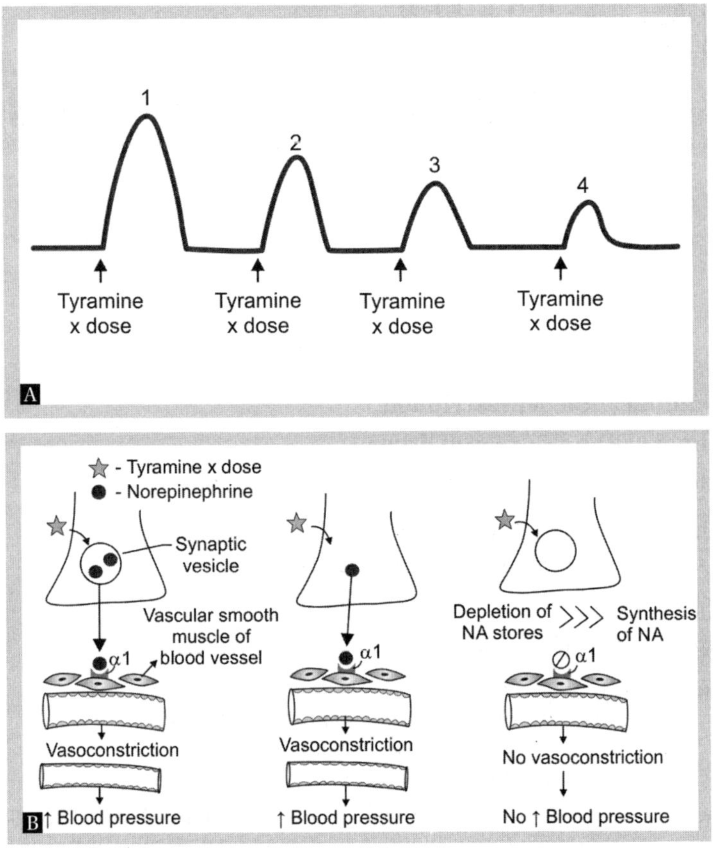

Figs. 14.10A and B: Graphical representation of tachyphylaxis.

15 CHAPTER
Communication of Prescription

A. Communication of prescription

B. Optimal use and storage of drugs

C. Optimizing medication adherence in chronic illness

7-R framework and the 7 Rs stand for respect, reason/s, regimen, risks, revisit instructions, and revision, reassurance statements.

Content	*Item*
Respect	Greet the patient
Reason	Explain the disease Explain the reason for prescribing the medication 1. Explain what will happen if untreated 2. How this medication helps?
Regimen	State the drug regimen (drug name, dose, frequency, and duration) State special instructions (in relation to food, storage, and dose missed as applicable)
Risks	State adverse effects/precautions/contraindications
Revisit	State routine or emergency follow up due to disease, or drug side effects
Revision	Ensures understanding
Ressurance	Empathises with patient

GASTROINTESTINAL SYSTEM

Communicate the following prescription to the patient, **for duodenal ulcer**.

Rx:
Kit containing:
Tab Lansoprazole 30 mg one tablet twice daily
Cap Amoxicillin 1000 mg one tablet twice daily
Tab Clarithromycin 500 mg one tablet twice daily
The kit is to be taken for 2 weeks.

To continue with Lansoprazole 20 mg one tablet daily before breakfast for 4 weeks.
To follow up later after 4 weeks.

Dr ABC
Reg. No.:

Respect: Greet the patient and ask the patient in which language he/she is comfortable. Introduce yourself as a treating physician.

Reason: You have been diagnosed as peptic ulcer. A peptic ulcer is a sore on the lining of your stomach, small intestine or esophagus. A peptic ulcer in the stomach is called a gastric ulcer. A duodenal ulcer is a peptic ulcer that develops in the first part of the small intestine (duodenum). Increase acid and reduced mucus is the reason for the ulcer. The symptoms, such as pain and burning sensation, which you are having because of the ulcer. Leaving ulcer untreated will cause your lining to become thinner and cause a hole in stomach giving to more complications.

You have been prescribed a drug named Lansoprazole which will control your acidity. Some action will start immediately but control of full symptoms will almost take 4–5 days. If Lansoprazole alone is prescribed for 2 weeks the ulcer may relapse because of a microorganism *H. pylori* which causes it. Therefore, along with Lansoprazole you have been prescribed an antibiotic regimen which will kill *H. pylori* and completely cure your ulcer.

- **Regimen**: Lansoprazole dose is 30 mg which you have to take half hour before food.
  - Along with the above drug you have been prescribed amoxycillin (strength: 1000 mg), clarithromycin 500 mg in the kit. These two are antibiotics which will kill the microorganism responsible for ulcer. These two have to be taken along with Lansoprazole half an hour before food. The complete course is to be taken for 14 days.
  - Store the kit in cool and dry place.
- **Risks**: You may experience side effects, such as diarrhea, skin rash, nausea, dizziness. If any of above side effect persist for long or are severe in intensity you can contact me.
- **Revisit**: Follow-up after 14 days, but if the acidity is not getting controlled within 1 week you can revisit.
- **Revision**:
  - Ask him if everything is clear.
  - Ask him if he has any questions.
  - Ask him to repeat the most relevant points.
  - Repeat if the patient has forgotten and revise.

Ressurance: Do not worry, if you take the regimen properly then ulcer will heal completely and it would not recur.

Cardiovascular System

1. **A 57-year-old male with presents to OPD with exertional chest pain. Physical examination shows a blood pressure of 152/90 mm Hg but is otherwise unremarkable. Physical examination shows a blood pressure of 152/90 mm Hg but is otherwise unremarkable. The ECG is normal. Write a prescription for acute angina pectoris.**

   Rx:
   - Tab Isosorbide dinitrate 5 mg one tablet sublingually kept under the tongue (sublingual) until every 5 minutes, till maximum of 10 minutes
   - Tab Aspirin 325 mg and tab clopidogrel 300 mg start.

     Once the acute attack subsides

     Tab Isosorbide dinitrate 5 mg one tablet thrice daily.
   - Tab Aspirin 75 mg and tab clopidogrel 75 mg stat. One tablet daily.

     Follow-up after 15 days.

   Non-pharmacological treatment
   - No smoking or alcohol
   - Moderate exercise
   - Weight reduction

   Dr ABC

   Reg. No.:

- **Respect:** Greet the patient and ask the patient in which language he/she is comfortable
  - Introduce yourself as a treating physician
  - Explain the diagnosis and prognosis of angina
  - You have been diagnosed with a condition called hypertension
- **Reason**: I am prescribing you a tablet, isosorbide dinitrate of 5 mg strength. This tablet works by widening veins, bringing less blood back to the heart from the rest of the body thus reducing the strain on the heart and increasing the blood supply to the heart muscles
  - You may have been prescribed clopidogrel/aspirin to help stabilize the clot if formed and will prevent further blood clots from forming to reduce the risk of heart attack, stroke or death because you have suffered a severe type of chest pain called angina.
- **Regimen**: This tablet, isosorbide dinitrate of 5 mg strength has to be kept under the tongue (sublingual) every 5 minutes, till a maximum of 10 minutes for acute attack (at the time of chest pain). This drug also has to be taken on a regular basis to prevent acute attacks. After the pain subsides you will have to take the drug isosorbide dinitrate with the strength of 5 mg, one tablet three times a day. This will prevent the acute chest pain from coming recurrently.
  - Tab clopidogrel/aspirin of 75/75 mg strength has to be taken one tablet once a day after food.
  - When you are taking the above drug on a regular basis, the timing of intake is very important for this drug. You can take this drug at the same

time every day. Do not chew, break or crush the tablet before you swallow If you take this drug at frequent intervals, it may not work as expected.

- Try to take the tablets at the same times of day each day, as this will help you to remember to take your doses regularly. If you forget to take a dose at your usual time, take it when you remember. However, if it is nearly time to take your next dose when you remember, then leave out the forgotten dose and take your next dose when it is due. Do not take two doses together to make up for a missed dose.
- Store out of the reach and sight of children. Keep it at room temperature. in a cool place, away from direct sunlight

❖ **Risks**: Because of the isosorbide dinitrate you may experience headache and flushing for 1–2 weeks, it will subside with time. You may experience light-headedness on standing, especially just after rising from a lying or seated position. So get up slowly.

- Do not take this along with any medicine for erectile dysfunction as it can produce a dangerous fall in your blood pressure.
- Aspirin and clopidogrel which will prevent clots may increase the risk of bleeding and gastric irritation. If you experience abnormal bruising or bleeding—abnormal nose bleeds—bloody or black bowel motions—or red or purple blotches on your skin, please inform us immediately.

❖ **Revisit:** Please revisit after two weeks for further evaluation and dose adjustment if required.

❖ **Revision:** Repeat if the patient has forgotten and revise. Reassure the patient Ask him to everything is clear. Ask him if he has any questions. Ask him to repeat the most relevant points.

❖ **Ressurance:** Reassure the patient. If you take these medications properly then the risk of getting heart attack and chest pain is very low.

2. Mathura a 35-year-old executive is diagnosed with essential hypertension. The average BP from 3 consecutive readings is 158/100 mm Hg. Prescribe suitable drugs for this patient.

Rx:

Tab Enalapril 5 mg once daily

Non-pharmacological treatment

- Salt and water restriction
- Weight reduction with regular exercise
- to quit smoking if smoker
- Reduce alcohol intake

Follow up after 15 days for evaluation and dose adjustment, if necessary.

Dr ABC
Reg. No.:

Respect: Greet the patient and ask the patient in which language he/she is comfortable

- Introduce yourself as a treating physician
- Explain the diagnosis and prognosis of angina
- You have been diagnosed with a condition called angina where there is chest pain due to reduced oxygen supply to your heart muscles

Reason: You have been diagnosed with hypertension, a condition where your blood pressure remains high. If left untreated it can lead to heart disease and kidney problems. I am prescribing you a tablet called enalapril which will keep your blood pressure under control. This medicine works by widening your blood vessels. This lowers your blood pressure. The medicine usually starts to work within an hour and the effect lasts for at least 24 hours. Some people may require several weeks of treatment until the best effect on your blood pressure is seen.

Regimen: Take one tablet of enalapril 5 mg every day once in the morning after food. Do not chew, break or crush the tablet before you swallow

- Try to take the tablets at the same times of day each day, as this will help you to remember to take your doses regularly. If you forget to take a dose at your usual time, take it when you remember. However, if it is nearly time to take your next dose when you remember, then leave out the forgotten dose and take your next dose when it is due. Do not take two doses together to make up for a missed dose.
- Store out of the reach and sight of children. Keep it at room temperature, in a cool place, away from direct sunlight.

Risk:

- When you start taking this medicine you may feel faint or dizzy. If this happens, it will help to lie down. This is caused by your blood pressure lowering. It should improve as you continue to take the medicine. If you are worried, please talk to me.
- If you notice any of the following—swelling of your face, lips, tongue or throat which may cause difficulty in breathing or swallowing—swelling of your hands, feet or ankles, dry cough, dizziness or skin rash which might occur in some patients, you need to report immediately.
- Do not stop medication on your own, as hypertension requires long-term treatment and stopping the treatment will result in complications.
- Reduce the amount of salt intake up to 2 grams per day in your food. Avoid pickles, papads or noodles. Have a diet rich in vegetables, fruits, legumes, nuts, whole grains, fish, polyunsaturated fatty acids. Minimize consumption of processed meat, refined carbohydrates, and sweetened beverages.
- Do regular exercise of mild to moderate intensity (150 minutes/week approx.). Avoid smoking and alcohol consumption. Have adequate sleep. All this will regulate your BP.
- Maintain a diary recording of your blood pressure either at home or in the nearest healthcare facility for the next one month.

Revisit: please revisit after two weeks for further evaluation and dose adjustment if required.

Revision: Repeat if the patient has forgotten and revise. Reassure the patient. Ask him to everything is clear. Ask him if he has any questions. Ask him to repeat the most relevant points.

Reassurance: Taking this medicine regularly and keeping your blood in control will prevent complications of hypertension.

CENTRAL NERVOUS SYSTEM

1. **A 20-year-old female Ms Kala, experiences seizures characterized by sudden loss of consciousness and then rigidity of the body for a few minutes. This is followed by jerking of the body musculature that lasts for 3–5 minutes followed by a state of flaccidity. Immediately after the seizure, she recovers consciousness but remains in a confused state. Prescribe suitable drug(s) for this patient. (Generalized tonic clonic seizures, i.e., GTCS)**

   Rx:

   Tab Phenytoin sodium 100 mg one tablet thrice daily after food for 15 days
   To follow-up after 15 days for evaluation and dose adjustment, if necessary.

   Dr ABC
   Reg. No.:

Respect: Greet the patient and ask the patient in which language he/she is comfortable

- Introduce yourself as a treating physician
- Explain the diagnosis and prognosis of generalized tonic-clonic seizure.
- You have been diagnosed with generalized tonic-clonic seizure (GTCS). A seizure is a short episode of symptoms caused by a burst of abnormal electrical activity in your brain.

Reason: I am prescribing you tablet phenytoin at the dose of 100 mg which works by stabilizing the electrical activity of your brain, which prevents occurrence of seizures. You need to take it every day regularly to control seizures.

Regimen: Take one tablet three times a day after food regularly. Try to take your doses of phenytoin at the same times each day. This will help you to avoid missing any doses.

- If you forget to take a dose, take it as soon as you remember unless it is nearly time for your next dose, in which case leave out the missed dose. Do not take two doses together to make up for a missed dose. Keep this medication in the container it came in, tightly closed, and out of reach of children. Store it at room temperature.
- Do not change the brand of the medicine on your own. As it can cause variations in drug levels leading to enhanced toxicity or reduced effectiveness.

Risk: Some common adverse effects seen with this drug are dizziness, increased sleepiness, change in taste, gum hypertrophy, increased male-pattern hair growth in females, coarsening of facial features and acne.

- Take good care for your teeth, gums, and mouth during your treatment with phenytoin. It is very important that you care for your mouth properly to decrease the risk of gum damage caused by phenytoin.
- At toxic doses, it affects your brain and ear-balancing components causing dizziness, double vision, and imbalance. Report immediately, if you develop any of the above symptoms.
- Do not stop the drug even if you do not have seizures for a long time. Stopping the drug suddenly can aggravate seizures.
- Do not take any other drug along with phenytoin, because they can interact with it. Please consult a doctor before taking them.
- If you take birth control pills along while on phenytoin, the contraceptive action may be lost. Use alternate methods of contraception. Avoid pregnancy while on phenytoin as it can harm the fetus.

Revisit: Please revisit after two weeks for further evaluation and dose adjustment if required.

Revision: Repeat if the patient has forgotten and revise. Reassure the patient. Ask him to everything is clear. Ask him if he has any questions. Ask him to repeat the most relevant points.

Reassurance: Reassure the patient. If you take the above drug properly you will lead a seizure free life.

2. Prescribe for a patient 26-year-old female with diagnosis of petit-mal epilepsy.

Rx:

Tab Sodium valproate 200 mg one tablet three times a day after food.
To follow up after 15 days for evaluation and dose adjustment, if necessary.

Dr ABC
Reg. No.:

Respect: Greet the patient and ask the patient in which language he/she is comfortable

- Introduce yourself as a treating physician
- Explain the diagnosis and prognosis of petit-mal epilepsy.
- You have been diagnosed with petit-mal epilepsy. A seizure is a short episode of symptoms caused by a burst of abnormal electrical activity in your brain.

Reason: I am prescribing you tablet sodium valproate at the dose of 200 mg which works by stabilizing the electrical activity of your brain, which prevents occurrence of seizures. You need to take it every day regularly to control seizures.

Regimen: I am prescribing you a tablet called valproate that works by stabilizing the electrical activity of your brain, which prevents the seizures from occurring.

- You need to take tablet valproate 200 mg three times a day every day after food.
- Try to take your doses of valproate at the same time each day. This will help you to avoid missing any doses.
- If you forget to take a dose, take it as soon as you remember unless it is nearly time for your next dose, in which case leave out the missed dose. Do not take two doses together to make up for a missed dose.
- Do not take any other drug along with phenytoin, because they can interact with it. Please consult a doctor before taking them.
- Do not change the brand of the medicine on your own

Risk: Common side-effects you may experience are loss of appetite, vomiting, heartburn, drowsiness, loss of balance and shakiness. You may experience blisters with skin detachment (blistering, peeling or bleeding on any part of your skin which is a part of allergic reaction. You need to inform immediately.

- Long-term use of valproate may cause weight gain and metabolic adverse effects. Maintain a healthy lifestyle. Eat a balanced diet, and do regular exercise.
- You should immediately report if you experience abdominal pain, dark urine or jaundice which are suggestive of liver problems.
- Do not stop the drug even if you do not have seizures for a long time. Stopping the drug suddenly can aggravate seizures.
- Avoid pregnancy while on valproate as it can cause fetal anomalies.

Revisit: Please revisit after two weeks for further evaluation with LFT reports and dose adjustment, if required.

Revision: Repeat if the patient has forgotten and revise. Reassure the patient. Ask him to everything is clear. Ask him if he has any questions. Ask him to repeat the most relevant points.

Reassurance: Reassure the patient. If you take the above drug properly you will lead a seizure free life.

RESPIRATORY SYSTEM

1. **Prescribe for a 22-year-old girl Miss Rani with h/o dyspnea and wheeze for at least 2 times during the night in a month. On examination, her PEF was >80%. She was diagnosed to have mild persistent asthma. Prescribe suitable drugs for this patient.**

   Rx:

   - Formoterol (6 μg per puff) + Budesonide (100 μg/puff) MDI 2 puffs twice a day through a spacer.

- One additional inhalation can be used as needed in response to symptoms. No more than 6 inhalations should be taken on any single occasion.
- Patient instructed to gargle, following use of inhaled corticosteroids to prevent topical side effects.
- To follow up after a month for clinical evaluation and assessment of response.

Dr ABC
Reg. No.:

Respect: Greet the patient and ask the patient in which language he/she is comfortable. Introduce yourself as a treating physician.

Explain the diagnosis and prognosis of bronchial asthma. Bronchial asthma is a medical condition which causes the airways of the lungs to narrow and swell. Due to this, the airways produce excess mucus making it hard to breathe, which results in coughing, shortness of breath, and wheezing. The disease is chronic and interferes with daily work.

Reason: To treat this condition, I have prescribed some drugs in the form of a metered dose inhaler (MDI). Formoterol fumarate belongs to a group of medicines called 'long-acting beta 2 receptor agonists' or 'bronchodilators'. It works by relaxing the muscles in your airways. This helps you to breathe more easily. Budesonide belongs to a group of medicines called 'corticosteroids'. It works by reducing and preventing swelling and inflammation in your lungs.

Regimen: This device is called metered dose inhaler which will deliver the drug directly to your lung. It has a mouthpiece and drug canister which can be pressed to deliver the drug. You should hold the MDI vertically. Now gently shake the MDI for 3–4 times. Now breathe out gently and keep the mouthpiece of MDI between the upper and lower front teeth and seal with lips. Press the canister once while taking the breath. Try to hold your breath for at least 10 seconds. Before you breathe out, release your finger from the counter and remove the inhaler from your mouth.

Keep the inhaler upright. Then breathe out slowly. To take another inhalation, shake the inhaler well for at least 5 seconds and repeat steps. Replace the mouthpiece cover.

You have to take 2 puffs twice a day through a spacer. One additional inhalation can be used as needed in response to symptoms. No more than 6 inhalations should be taken on any single occasion.

Rinse your mouth with water after your daily morning and evening doses and spit it out. It will help to remove the drug deposited in the throat and prevent unwanted side effects.

Please always have an extra fully loaded canister with you in case of emergency use. You can check the remaining medicine in the canister by viewing the dose counter or you can use calendar methods.

If you forget to take a dose, take it as soon as you remember. However, if it is nearly time for your next dose, skip the missed dose. Do not take a double dose to make up for a forgotten dose.

Risk: You may experience palpitations (awareness of your heart beating), trembling or shaking. If these effects occur, they are usually mild and usually disappear as you continue to use the inhaler.

You can get thrush (a fungal infection) in the mouth. This is less likely if you rinse your mouth out with water after using your inhaler. Other adverse events are mild sore throat, coughing and a hoarse voice. There is also a pamphlet along with this inhaler.

Revisit: Please revisit after two weeks for further evaluation and dose adjustment if required.

Revision: Repeat if the patient has forgotten and revise. Reassure the patient. Ask him if everything is clear. Ask him if he has any questions. Ask him to repeat the most relevant points. Ask the patient to demonstrate the usage of MDI.

Reassurance: Reassure the patient that proper use of devices with drugs will lead to improved quality of life.

HEMOPOIETIC SYSTEM

1. **A 23-year-old patient Mrs Mahalakshmi, was found be slightly anemic on routine check up. Her hemoglobin was found to be 10 g/dL. Prescribe suitable drug(s) for this patient.**

   Rx

   Tab Ferrous sulfate 200 mg twice a day for 30 days
   To follow up after one month to estimate Hb levels.

Dr ABC
Reg. No.:

Respect: Greet the patient and ask the patient in which language he/she is comfortable. Introduce yourself as a treating physician. Explain the diagnosis and prognosis of anemia.

Reason: Anemia is a condition in which the body does not have enough healthy red blood cells. Red blood cells provide oxygen to body tissues.

Bone marrow needs iron to make hemoglobin. Without enough iron, the body can not make enough hemoglobin for red blood cells. Most of your symptoms of anemia, such as tiredness, weakness, shortness of breath, and pale or yellowish skin are due to it.

Regimen: Ferrous sulfate tablets belong to a group of medicines called iron supplements. These medicines work by replacing body iron. Iron is a mineral that the body needs to produce red blood cells. You have to take one tablet twice a day. This drug works better if you take it on an empty stomach. You may take this drug with food if it causes an upset stomach. Some foods, such as eggs, dairy products, coffee, and tea and antacids may make this drug not work as well as it slow absorption. Taking this with fruit juice will increase its absorption. Swallow the tablets whole with water. Do not suck, chew or keep the tablet in your mouth, after food to reduce gastrointestinal side effects.

Store at room temperature protected from light. Store in a dry place. Do not store in a bathroom. Keep all drugs in a safe place. Keep all drugs out of the reach of children and pets. Throw away unused or expired drugs.

Risks: Even though it may be rare of you signs of an allergic reaction, such as rash; please contact me immediately. The most common adverse effect seen are constipation, diarrhea, stomach pain, upset stomach, throwing up, or decreased appetite, change in color of stool to green. Stomach cramps and staining of the mouth, teeth, or fillings.

Revisit: To follow up after one month with Hb levels

Revision: If the patient has forgotten and revise. Reassure the patient. Ask her to everything is clear. Ask her if he has any questions. Ask her to repeat the most relevant points.

Reassurance: Reassure the patient that treatment of anemia will lead to improve her symptoms.

Endocrine

2. **A 35-year-old male patient presents to the medicine OPD with a history of increased thirst, increased frequency of urination and unexplained loss of weight. His random blood sugar was 280 mg%. He was diagnosed to have type II DM. Prescribe suitable drug(s) for this patient.**

   Rx:
   Tab Metformin 500 SR mg one tablet after meals once daily for 15 days
   To follow up after 15 days for dose adjustment depending upon glycemic control.

Dr ABC
Reg. No.:

Reason: Diabetes is a chronic (long-lasting) health condition that affects how your body turns food into energy. With diabetes, your body does not make enough insulin or cannot use it as well as it should. Over time, that can cause serious health problems, such as **heart disease, vision loss, and kidney** disease. There is not a cure yet for diabetes, but losing weight, eating healthy food, and being active and taking prescribed drugs can really help.

You have been prescribed metformin tablets to help with your diabetes. Metformin improves your blood glucose control and enables the insulin produced by your pancreas to work more efficiently. The role of insulin is to help your cells to take in glucose and convert it to energy. Metformin works by allowing glucose to enter your cells (reducing insulin resistance) and by slowing down the release of glucose stored in your liver. You should not experience any weight gain from taking metformin and it may help protect your heart.

Regimen: You have been started on metformin 500 SR mg tablets, one tablet twice a day after food. Swallow your metformin tablets whole with water. Do not chew them. If you miss a dose of metformin, skip the missed dose and take the next dose at the usual time. Do not take 2 doses to make up for a forgotten dose.

Risks: Metformin is very well tolerated. However, as with all medications, there are some potential side effects, including stomach-ache, diarrhea, and nausea (feeling sick). These side effects are common when first start taking metformin, but they tend to settle down after a few weeks.

Metformin can cause vitamin B_{12} deficiency by reducing vitamin B_{12} absorption in the gastrointestinal tract.

Metformin has been associated with a rare condition called 'lactic acidosis.' 'Lactic acidosis' is associated with the build-up of acids in your blood and is most commonly seen in people admitted with severe illness and/or infection.

You should stop taking metformin if you become very unwell, especially if you have vomiting and/or diarrhea or are not eating and drinking. The risk of 'lactic acidosis' is increased if your kidneys and liver does not work well.

There is no problems of hypoglycemia with metformin as with other antidiabetic drugs.

Treatment for diabetes is usually for life.

If you stop taking metformin suddenly, your blood sugar levels will go up and your diabetes will get worse. Keep this medication in the container it came in, tightly closed, and out of reach of children. Store it at room temperature.

Revisit: Please revisit after two weeks for further evaluation and dose adjustment, if required.

Revision: Repeat if the patient has forgotten and revise. Reassure the patient. Ask him to everything is clear. Ask him if he has any questions. Ask him to repeat the most relevant points.

Reassurance: Reassure the patient that control of blood sugars will decrease long term complications of diabetes.

ENDOCRINE SYSTEM

1. **A 21-year-old married women requires contraception to postpone pregnancy. Prescribe a suitable method of contraception for her.**

   Rx:

   Fixed dose combination of tab ethinyl estradiol + levonorgestrel (20 µg + 0.1 mg) 1 tablet daily beginning on the 5th day of menstruation for next 21 days followed by a 7 day inert pink/peach tablet. Next course should be started on 5th day of next menstrual cycle.

   Dr ABC
   Reg. No.:

Reason: I am prescribing these birth control pills as a method of contraception since you are planning to avoid pregnancy for one year. The combined oral contraceptive pill is often just called "the pill".

It contains synthetic female hormones oestrogen and progesterone, which are produced naturally in the ovaries. If sperm reaches an egg (ovum), pregnancy can happen. Contraception tries to stop this happening usually by keeping the egg and sperm apart or by stopping the release of an egg (ovulation).

When taken correctly, the pill is over 99% effective at preventing pregnancy. This means that fewer than 1 in 100 who use the combined pill as contraception will get pregnant in 1 year.

Regimen:

You start by taking the first white pill beginning on day 5 of your menstrual bleeding phase. During this first cycle of medication, you should take one white tablet daily and then 7 pink inert tablets for twenty-eight (28) consecutive days.

Withdrawal bleeding usually occurs within 3 days following the last white tablet and may not have finished before the next pack is started.

You are to begin the subsequent course on next day after last pink tablet, i.e., start taking the white tablets on the next day after ingestion of the last pink tablet, regardless of whether or not a menstrual period has occurred or is still in progress.

You should follow the same dosing schedule—21 days on white tablets followed by 7 days on pink tablets.

If in any cycle, you start tablets later than the proper day, you should protect herself against pregnancy by using a non-hormonal back-up method of birth control until you has taken a white tablet daily for 7 consecutive days.

You can continue the same as long as if you wish to avoid conception.

It is important that you take these pills every day without fail to provide effective contraception. You could get pregnant if you do not do this, or if you miss a pill, or vomit or have severe diarrhea.

Suppose, if you miss a pill one day, and then take the missed pill as soon as you remember or take the missed pill along with the next dose. However, if two or more pills are missed, then take only the most recently missed pill and continue from the next dose in the usual time.

In such situations, you need to use back-up contraception (e.g., condoms) or avoid intercourse until hormonal pills have been taken for 7 consecutive days.

In addition to birth control, this will also reduce blood loss during periods. Some medicines may make the pill less effective. Check with me or any other doctor if you get prescribed any other tablets. This pill only protects you from pregnancy. To avoid sexually transmitted infections including chlamydia, gonorrhea and HIV, it is important to use condoms as well.

Risks: You may experience minor side effects include mood swings, nausea, breast tenderness and headaches—these usually settle down in a few months.

There is no evidence that the pill will make you gain weight.

Research suggests that users of the pill appear to have a small increase in the risk of breast cancer and cervical cancer.

There is a very low risk of serious side effects, such as blood clots.

The combined pill is not suitable if you smoke or have diabetes, or if you have certain medical conditions as they may aggravate.

If spotting or breakthrough bleeding occurs, you are to continue on the same regimen. This type of bleeding is usually transient and without significance; however, if the bleeding is persistent or prolonged, then consult me.

Revisit: Please revisit after one month for further evaluation.

Revision: Repeat if the patient has forgotten and revise. Reassure the patient. Ask him to everything is clear. Ask him if he has any questions. Ask him to repeat the most relevant points.

Reassurance: Reassure the patient that use of oral contraceptives in a correct and appropriate manner will prevent unwanted pregnancies.

CHEMOTHERAPY

1. Rajni, of 25-year-old comes to medicine OPD with the complaints of dry cough, loss of appetite and weight for the past one month. Detailed history reveals that she also has evening rise of temperature. Sputum examination reveals acid fast bacilli. Chest radiograph shows apical pulmonary infiltrates. Her current weight is 45 kg. Prescribe suitable drug therapy for this patient. (Tuberculosis)

Rx:

Tab Isoniazid (INH) 300 mg 1 tablet once daily for 2 months
Tab Rifampicin 600 mg 1 tablet once daily for 2 months
Tab Pyrazinamide 1500 mg 1 tablet once daily for 2 months
Tab Ethambutol 800 mg 1 tablets once daily for 2 months
This is followed by continuation phase:
Tab Isoniazid (INH) 300 mg 1 tablet once daily for 4 months
Tab Rifampicin 600 mg 1 tablet once daily for 4 months
Tab Ethambutol 800 mg 1 tablets once daily for 4 months
To follow up after 1 month for assessment and appearance of side effects.
Follow up after 2 weeks for evaluation.

Dr ABC
Reg. No.:

Reason: You have been diagnosed to have tuberculosis. Tuberculosis is an infectious disease that mainly affects the lungs, but it can also spread to other body parts, such as kidneys, brain, spine and bone marrow. This is a bacterial infection which can lead to serious complications if left untreated. Some of the bacterial grow rapidly but some very slowly inside the cells.

Hence, longer treatment duration, i.e., minimum of 6 months is required to get complete cure.

It is important that you take these medicines regularly every day. Your symptoms may improve before the infection is completely cured. But do not stop taking it without consulting as doing so may cause the infection to return or worsen. Your disease may cause more complications or you will develop resistance to the therapy. In that case, only few drugs are available to treat your disease and those drugs will produce more side effects.

The course of therapy takes a minimum of 6 months. For the first two months, I am prescribing you a Kit fixed-dose combination of four medicines (HRZE).

Regimen:

This Kit is a combination of four medicines—isoniazid, rifampicin, ethambutol and pyrazinamide which treat tuberculosis. Isoniazid works by preventing the TB bacteria from forming their own protective covering, while rifampicin inactivates a bacterial enzyme (RNA-polymerase) which is required by TB bacteria to make essential proteins and to reproduce. Together, they kill the bacteria and eradicate the infection. Ethambutol and pyrazinamide on the other hand, work by slowing the growth of these bacteria.

You will have to take it on an empty stomach 30 minutes before food or 2 hours after food and preferably at the same time every day. Swallow AKT-4 Kit 1's as a whole with water, do not crush or chew it. Try not to forget a dose, as this increases the risk of the bacteria becoming resistant to the medicine. If you miss a dose, take it as soon as possible. However, if it is almost time for your next dose, skip the missed dose and go back to your regular schedule. Do not double the dose.

Along with this, I am prescribing you a vitamin tablet which has to be taken daily at night to prevent nerve related side effects caused by these drugs.

Store in a cool and dry place away from sunlight. Avoid drinking alcohol while taking as this may increase the risk of side effects on the liver.

Depending on the sputum reports, your further course of treatment will be decided. In the second part of the treatment, even if your sputum result comes negative for TB, you will be given a combination of two tablets that have to be taken daily for the next 4 months for the reasons I explained. Take more fruits, vegetables and protein-rich diet which will improve your health.

Risks: The common adverse effects are **nausea, vomiting, rash, fever, dark colored urine, sweating, salivation, watery eyes, peripheral neuropathy:** (tingling and numbness of feet and hand, **increased liver enzymes, jaundice, increased uric acid level in blood, visual impairment, joint pain.**

It may discolor your urine, sweat, saliva and tears a reddish/orange color. This is normal and not harmful.

It may cause vitamin B_6 deficiency. You also prescibed vitamin B_6 supplements to help avoid potential problems associated with its deficiency, such as inflammation of the nerves (neuritis).

Please use a reliable contraceptive method (such as condoms or a diaphragm) to prevent pregnancy while you are taking this Kit as it may make hormonal contraceptives, such as the pill less effective.

Revisit: Please revisit after two weeks for further evaluation with LFT reports.

Rcvision: Repeat if the patient has forgotten and revise. Reassure the patient. Ask him to everything is clear. Ask him if he has any questions. Ask him to repeat the most relevant points.

Reassurance: Reassure the patient that use of drugs for TB in a correct and appropriate manner will provide complete cure.

2. **A 30-year-old Mr Muthu complains of lower abdominal pain, flatulence and occasional diarrhea. Stool culture showed *E. histolytica* and he was diagnosed to have mild intestinal amoebiasis. Prescribe suitable drug(s) for this patient.**

   Rx:
   Tab Metronidazole 400 mg thrice daily for 7 days
   Tab Diloxanide furoate 500 mg thrice daily for 10 days
   To follow up after 10 days for evaluation of response

Dr ABC
Reg. No.:

Reason: You have been diagnosed to have amoebic dysentery (watery stools containing blood and mucus)) which is a gut infection caused by a parasite.

Regimen: I am prescribing you antibiotic metronidazole at the dose of 400 mg. You must take this tablet three times a day for 5 days. This drug should be taken after food.

Do not skip the dose. If you miss a dose of this medicine, take it as soon as possible. However if it is almost time for your next dose, skip the missed dose and continue with the regular dosing schedule. DO NOT DOUBLE THE DOSES.

Complete the course of antibiotics even if your symptoms improve. If you do not complete the course, it may increase your risk of further infection that is resistant to antibiotics.

This medicine can cause loss of appetite, vomiting sensation, stomach upset, metallic taste, diarrhea, mouth or tongue irritation, numbness or tingling of hands or feet.

Risk:

You can get tingling sensation at periphery, (peripheral neuropathy), seizures, skin reactions. If you develop rash, itching, stuffy nose, fever or joint pain, report immediately.

- Avoid alcohol intake while you are taking metronidazole and for at least 3 days after you stop taking the drug, because it will produce serious side effects, such as dizziness, palpitations, sweating, etc.
- Maintain personal hygiene
- If your symptoms do not subside report back.

Revisit: Please revisit after 10 days for evaluation of response.

Revision: Repeat if the patient has forgotten and revise. Reassure the patient. Ask him to everything is clear. Ask him if he has any questions. Ask him to repeat the most relevant points.

Reassurance: Reassure the patient that use of drugs in a correct and appropriate manner will provide complete cure.

MALARIA

3. A 38-year-old patient Mr Govinda presented to your clinic with the complaints of periodic attacks of sequential chills, fever and sweating for the past three days. Peripheral blood smear examination reveals *P. falciparum* parasites. Prescribe suitable drug(s) for this patient.

Rx:

Fixed dose combination of Artemether 80 mg + Lumefantrine 480 mg one tablet twice a day for 3 days to be taken with fatty meal

- Tab Primaquine 45 mg single dose
- Follow up after 7 days

Dr ABC

Reg. No.:

Respect:

- Ask the patient in which language he is comfortable
- Introduce yourself as a treating physician
- Explain the diagnosis and prognosis of *P. falciparum* malaria.

Reason: You have been prescribed a tablet which contains a combination of two drugs artemether and lumefantrine. The two antimalarial drugs, artemether and lumefantrine in fixed dose, work together to kill the malaria parasite (a tiny organism that is found inside the red blood cells). In addition another tablet primaquine is also prescribed to you.

These drugs will kill the malarial parasite in the blood. You may get relief of fever by 2nd day but you need to complete the entire course so that all the malarial parasites in the blood are killed. Taking complete course is important otherwise malarial symptoms will reccur. Primaquine has action on sexual forms of malarial parasites, preventing transmission.

Regimen: The tablet contains combination of artemether and lumefantrine whose strength is 80 mg and 480 mg respectively. One tablet is to be taken twice a day after food for 3 days. Primaquine a single strength of 45 mg is to be taken on day one.

Risks

This combination is well tolerated by most patients but you may experience some GI side effects, such as nausea, vomiting, abdominal pain. Rarely itching, headache, dizziness can occur. Other side effects (>1 in every 10 patients treated) include palpitations, muscle pain, weakness, tiredness, sleep disorders.

If any of above side effect persist for long or are severe in intensity you can contact me.

You have to do investigation to rule out G6PD deficiency. This has to be done as primaquine can cause hemolysis of RBCs in G6PD deficient individuals.

Revisit: Follow up after 7 days, but if the fever does not subside by the 3rd day you can revisit.

Revision: Repeat if the patient has forgotten and revise. Reassure the patient. Ask him to everything is clear. Ask him if he has any questions. Ask him to repeat the most relevant points.

Reassurance: Reassure the patient that use of drugs in a correct and appropriate manner will provide complete cure.

4. **Mr Naresh, a company executive wanted to tour for 2 months in an area where malaria is endemic. He consulted the doctor. The doctor advised him to take a tablet once weekly.**

   Rx:

   Tab Atovaquone/Proguanil (250/100 mg) 1 tablet once daily with food starting 1 day before entering the endemic area, continued during the stay and for 7 days after leaving the endemic area.

Dr ABC

Reg. No.:

Reason: This medication contains 2 medicines—atovaquone and proguanil. It is used to prevent and treat malaria caused by mosquito bites in countries where malaria is common. Malaria parasites can enter the body through these mosquito bites, and then live in body tissues, such as red blood cells or the liver. This medication is used to kill the malaria parasites living inside red blood cells and other tissues. Both medications may be needed for a complete cure and to prevent the return of infection (relapse).

You have been prescribed a tablet which contains a combination of two drugs atovaquone/proguanil in a strength of 250 mg and 100 mg respectively. Take this tablet after food preferably on the same time of the day.

If you get infected by malarial parasite, the above drugs will kill them in the blood preventing the further multiplication.

Take this medication by mouth with food or a milky drink (such as whole milk, milkshake) that contains fat. If you vomit within 1 hour of taking a dose, repeat the dose. Swallow the tablet whole because of its bitter taste. Do not chew. If you have trouble swallowing tablets, this medication may be crushed and mixed with condensed milk. Take the entire mixture right away.

Start taking this tablet 2 days before travel to malaria endemic areas. It should be taken daily during your stay at the malarious area and continued for 7 days after leaving that area.

Also use mosquito repellent, mosquito nets, clothing covering the whole body, and staying in well-screened areas, especially from early night time until dawn. This will offer further protection from infective mosquitoes.

Risks: If you develop abdominal pain, nausea, vomiting, diarrhea, headache, dyspepsia, report to the nearest healthcare facility.

Revisit: Follow up after 7 days, but if the fever does not subside by the 3rd day you can revisit.

Revision: Repeat if the patient has forgotten and revise. Reassure the patient. Ask him to everything is clear. Ask him if he has any questions. Ask him to repeat the most relevant points. Explain advantages of use.

Reassurance: Reassure the patient that use of drugs in a correct and appropriate manner will provide complete cure.

Communication 2: Optimal use and storage of drugs:

1. Explain advantages of use
2. Check the purchased device for
3. Read the manufacturer manual
4. Demonstrate and explain the steps of use
5. Explain how to store
6. When to discard
7. How to clean the device
8. Need of adherence

Q. An elderly diabetic patient is discharged from hospital after an operation. She is advised to take insulin subcutaneously at home by insulin Pen. Communicate with patient regarding use and storage of insulin Pen.

1. **Explain advantages of use:**
   » Simpler to administer compared with a vial and syringe.
   » Deliver highly accurate doses using an insulin pen
   » The portable, discreet, and convenient nature
   » Small and thin needle sizes that reduce fear and pain
   » Memory features that recall the timing and amount of the previous dose
   » Easier storage and use
2. **Check the purchased device for**
   » Manufacturer date and expiry date
   » Retail price
   » Sealed packaging
3. **Read the manufacturer manual**
4. **Demonstrate and explain the steps of use**:

Here are the steps you will take:

1. Clean the skin with an alcohol pad. Let the alcohol air-dry.
2. Take the cover off the pen. You can see the insulin in the pen.
3. If you are using a cloudy insulin, gently roll the pen between your hands to mix the insulin.

4. Use alcohol to clean the end of the pen where the needle twists.
5. Peel back the cover on the needle. Screw the needle onto the pen. The needle should be snug but not too tight.
6. **To clear the air out of the pen:**
   - Remove the cap from the needle
   - Turn the dose dial to 2 units
   - Hold the pen so the needle is up in the air
   - Push the end of the pen in to clear the air
   - Watch the tip of the needle for a drop of insulin. You may need to do this more than once to see the drop of insulin on the needle.
7. To set your dose of insulin, turn the dial clockwise until you see the number for your insulin dose.
8. With one hand pinch and hold the skin at the site where you inject the pen. (You do not need to do this if you are using an 8 mm or smaller pen needle.)
9. Push the needle straight into the skin in a straight, quick motion. The needle should be all the way into the skin.
10. Using your thumb, push the end of the pen down slowly until the dial reads 0 (zero). Make sure the needle is all the way in the skin before pushing in the insulin.
11. If you used a pen needle larger than 8 mm let go of the pinch of skin.Wait a few seconds.
12. Pull the needle out.
13. Remove the needle from the pen. Throw it into the needle disposal container.

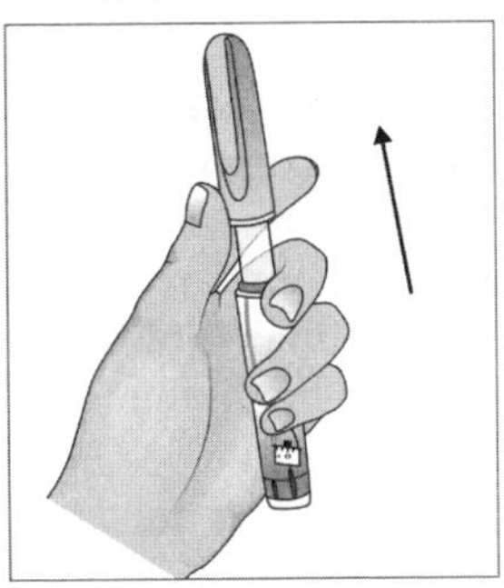

1, 2

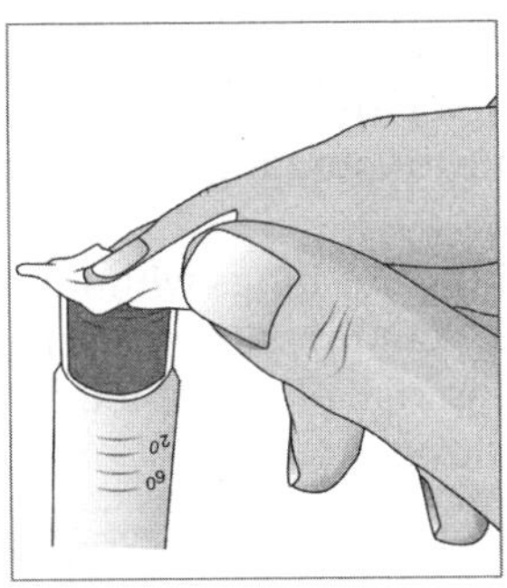

3, 4

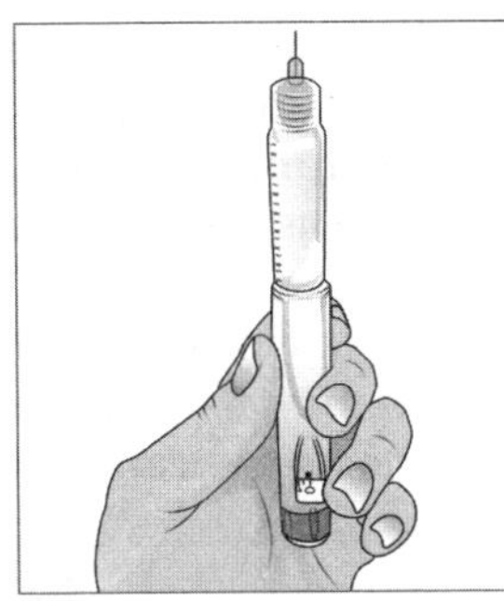

5

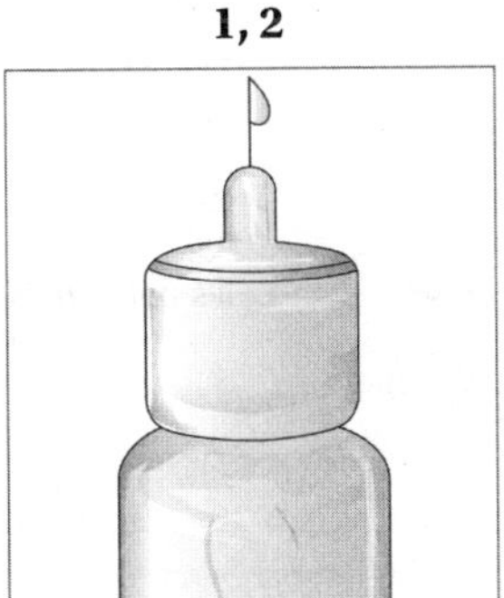

6

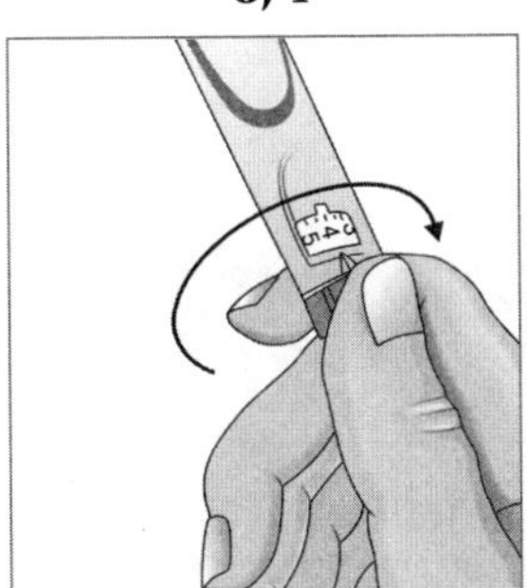

7

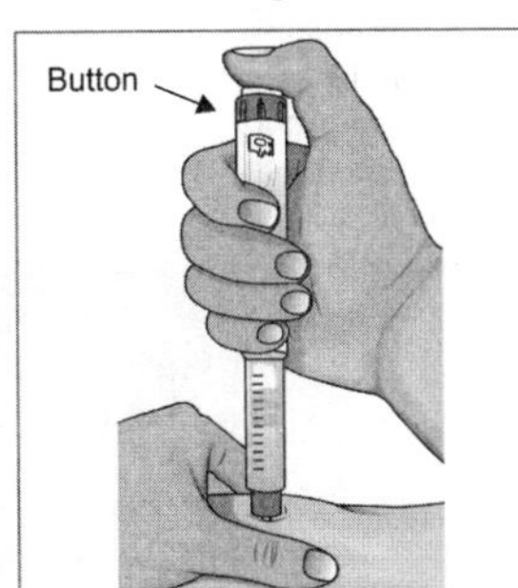

8

5. **Explain how to store**
   - Store unopened pens in the refrigerator. They will be good until the expiration date printed on the box. Write the date on the insulin pen when you first open it.
   - Store open insulin pens at room temperature. Avoid temperatures that are too hot or too cold. This can change how the insulin works.
   - Most pens are good for 28 days once opened.
   - Do not use insulin pens that have lumps, are discolored or have been frozen.
   - Place used pen needles and lancets for blood sugar testing in a hard plastic or metal container
6. **When to discard**

   Throw away pen/vials **after 28 days of use**, even if there is still insulin left.
7. **How to clean the device?**
   - Try not to expose your disposable pen to dust, dirt or liquid.
   - Do not try to pull your disposable pen apart to clean it.
   - If necessary, clean your disposable pen with a damp cloth, but do not wash, soak or lubricate it.
8. **Need of adherence—explain need to take insulin regularly to control blood sugars to prevent long term complications of diabetes.**

Q. A 18-year-old is diagnosed with asthma. He is prescribed an inhaler with spacer. Communicate with use him the use of spacer with the inhaler and storage of the device.

1. **Explain advantages of use:**

   Using a spacer with your pMDI or puffer inhaler can make it easier to get more of your medicine to your lungs where it is needed, compared with just using your inhaler.

   You can breathe it into your lungs without having to coordinate your breath with activating your pressurized metered dose inhaler (pMDI)

   It may also reduce the risk of side effects from your medicine (e.g., hoarseness and oral thrush).

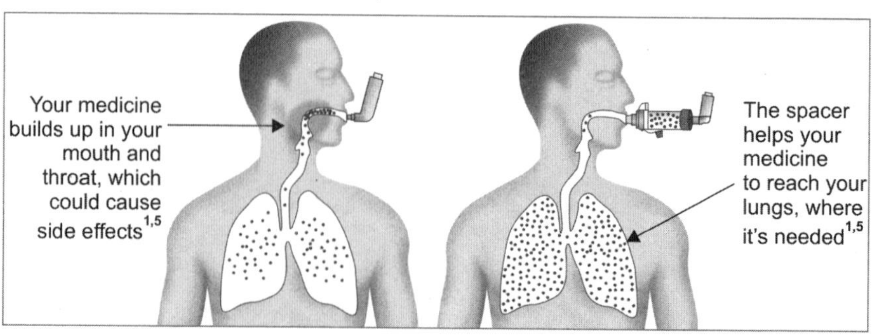

2. **Check the purchased device for:**
   » Manufacturer date and expiry date
   » Retail price
   » Sealed packaging
3. **Read the manufacturer manual**
4. **Demonstrate and explain the steps of use**

"Shake"

1. Remove the protective cap from the inhaler and from the mouthpiece of the spacer.
2. Insert inhaler into the spacer device. Shake the unit including the inhaler for a few seconds (to mix the contents of the inhaler)
3. Breathe out gently away from the spacer (to make room in your lungs to breathe in deeply)
4. Place the spacer mouthpiece into your mouth and form a seal (to prevent the drug escaping), ensure your tongue remains flat and does not obstruct the mouthpiece. Keep the inhaler canister in position.

"Breathe"

5. Press the canister down ONCE only and breathe in slowly and deeply through your mouth to fill your lungs. If you hear a whistling sound you are breathing in too quickly.

"Hold Breath"

6. Hold your breath for up to 10 seconds (to allow the drug to settle in your lungs), and then breathe out slowly away from the spacer.
7. For a second dose wait 30 seconds before repeating steps 2–6

Breathe in slowly!

8. Always rinse your mouth, gargle and spit out after using steroid inhalers (e.g., beclomethasone, budesonide, fluticasone

5. **Explain how to store**

   Do not leave your inhaler where it might get too hot or cold—for example, in your car or on a sunny windowsill. Keep your inhaler somewhere dry. Keeping your inhaler in a bathroom can make the medicine damp. Store all medicines safely, out of reach of children—

6. **When to discard.**

   You should replace your spacer at least every year, especially if you use it daily, but some may need to be replaced sooner.

7. **How to clean the device**

   Clean your spacer about once a month and after you have recovered from any cold or respiratory infection. Your spacer may become a bit cloudy over time, but it should not be moldy or brown.
   To clean your spacer:
   - Dismantle your spacer, if necessary
   - Wash all the parts in clean warm water with liquid dishwashing detergent

- Allow the parts to air dry without rinsing—drying with a cloth or paper towel can result in static building up on the inside of the spacer, which makes the medication stick to the sides
- Wipe the mouthpiece clean of detergent, if needed
- When completely dry, reassemble, if necessary

New spacers also need to be washed before you use them for the first time. If a new spacer has to be used immediately, you can 'prime' the spacer by firing at least multiple (at least 10) puffs into it to begin with to help reduce the static build-up inside. You can then take your medication dose as usual.

8. **Need of adherence**

Use of spacer will help drug delivery into lung which will improve the asthma.

Communication 3: Optimizing medication adherence in chronic illness.

Exercises:

1. **A patient diagnosed with rheumatoid arthritis was prescribed methotrexate. The patient reported in another hospital a few days later with fever and blood investigations showing pancytopenia. The patient deteriorated in the ICU and died a few days later. On taking the history of the patient, it was revealed the patient took methotrexate daily instead of taking it twice weekly resulting in this side effect. How should the treatment be explained to the patient to avoid such an incident in the future?**

   Answer: This tragic incident was mainly a result of miscommunication on the part of the healthcare provider. To avoid this, the physician must thoroughly explain the diagnosis, prognosis and treatment plan to the patient in a language that the patient is comfortable conversing in. All expected side effects of methotrexate must be explained to the patient and it must be stressed that the drug must be taken only two times a week.

   a. To make sure the patient understands, we can ask him/her to repeat the dosing schedule.
   b. The patient can be encouraged to set bi-weekly reminders to make sure no dose is missed.
   c. The consequence of taking the drug more than prescribed should be explained to the patient.
   We can encourage the patient to come for regular follow-ups.

2. **Viva question: What are the key points in the communication of patient- and medication-related strategies in patients suffering from end-stage renal disease?**

   Answer: Before interacting with the patient, the doctor should be aware of his own feelings about death and about interacting with terminally-ill patients.

   We have to make the patient feel positive about the prognosis and try to make them believe that dialysis will help them lead a better life.

The patient should be explained in simple terms that during dialysis:

d. A machine will receive blood from his body and will run it through a filter called a dialyzer that removes wastes and excess fluids.
e. The machine then will reintroduce the filtered blood back into the patient's body.
He/she should be asked to follow a good dietary plan from a dietician and eat kidney-friendly food, stay physically active, take all medications and supplements as prescribed, avoid smoking, and alcohol consumption and establish a good sleep routine.

3. **Viva question: You have decided to put a 24-year-old female going to get married, on oral contraceptives after having taken a history and done a physical examination. Give instructions on the use of this packet of contraceptive pills which contain low dose combination pills.**

Answer: I will inform her that tab norgestrel 0.3 mg + ethinyl estradiol 30 μg combination tablet is to be taken, starting on the 5th day of your menstrual cycle.
One tablet must be taken daily for 21 days followed by a gap of 7 days every month as long as the contraception is required.
If she misses a pill, she can take it the next day, and if she misses two pills an additional contraceptive cover may be required.
Additional methods of contraception for the first cycle are:
Barrier method—condom, diaphragm, vaginal rings—plastic rings that release hormones into the vagina to suppress ovulation.

4. **Viva question: What are the key points in the communication of patient- and medication-related strategies to improve adherence in HIV patients?**

Answer: We have to make the patient feel positive about the prognosis and make them believe that the emergence of highly effective anti-retroviral drug therapy has made HIV infections a chronic condition rather than a terminal disease. We have to help eliminate the stigma related to the disease and counsel the patient and his/her family accordingly.
Strategies to improve adherence in HIV patients:

a. Offer ART regimens that are highly effective; prescribe once daily or other simple regimens that reduce pill burden, dosing frequency, and dietary restrictions as much as possible.
b. Explain that treatment is well tolerated.
c. Prepare patients for the possibility of ART side effects and regularly evaluate and manage side effects if they arise.
d. Encourage patients to recruit friends and/or family members to help with adherence.

5. **Viva question: What are the key points in the communication of patient- and medication-related strategies to improve adherence in hypertensive patients:**

Answer: Strategies to improve adherence in hypertensive patients are—Choose a prescription in accordance with the patient's level of understanding and financial status. Preferably single drug therapy, in appropriate dosage form and with a simple dosage schedule. Ask the patient to repeat what he/she has understood about the treatment.

Explain the complications of hypertension and the need for proper compliance. Encourage the patient to speak out about his suffering and educate them regarding the adverse effects of the drug.

Encourage the patient to come for regular follow-ups Methods to avoid missing doses:

a. Reminders, alarms and diaries can be used to ensure that the drug is taken daily without fail.
b. Taking medication can be coupled with a daily habit.
c. To maintain a drug passport to tick into after taking medication/ use pill boxes.

16 CHAPTER

Pharmacoeconomics

APPLICATIONS

1. **Physician**
   - Knowing the cost burden of treatment can help in making clinical decisions, chose P-drugs
   - Prescribing cost-effective drugs can improve patient compliance and adherence to treatment
2. **Healthcare providers and administrators:** Cost-analysis helps healthcare providers be better informed about the services they provide
3. **Pharmaceutical companies:** Pharmacoeconomics guide pricing of medicines and keep the market competitive
4. **Government/Private sector**
   - Pharmacoeconomics plays a key role in guiding healthcare policies: Economic clinical humanistic outcomes (ECHO)
   - Preparing essential medicine list (EML)
   - Deciding reimbursement
   - Avoid lack of adherence, reduced physician visits, and need for emergency care

Types

1. Cost-benefit analysis
2. Cost-utility analysis
3. Cost-effectiveness analysis
4. Cost-minimization analysis

Cost-effectiveness Plane

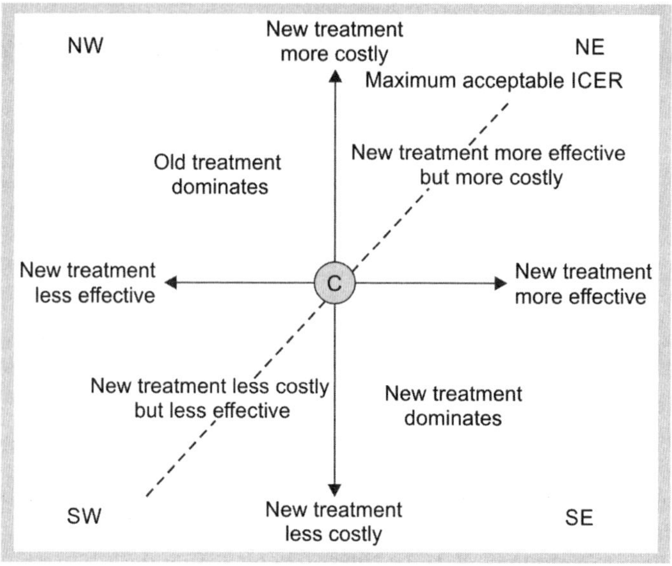

Exercise 1

In acute musculoskeletal disorders (tendinitis, bursitis, painful post-operative conditions, rheumatoid arthritis), one among the following drugs is used. The cost per unit of each drug is provided.

Drug name	COST (₹)/UNIT (MG)	Dose(mg)/frequency
Acetaminophen	0.50/500	1000/QID
Aspirin	0.25/350	1050/TID
Ibuprofen	1.00/600	600/TID
Indomethacin	1.00/25	25/TID
Diclofenac	0.75/50	50/TID

Questions:

1. To which group does the above mentioned drugs belong?
2. Work out the cost for each drug.
3. Which drug causes the least gastrointestinal adverse effect as anti-inflammatory agent?

Drug/dose/frequency	*Cost/unit*	*Total cost (₹/day*
Acetaminophen: 1000 mg × 2	0.5/500 = 1/1000	2 × 1 = 2
Aspirin: 1050 mg × 3	0.25/350 = 0.75/1050	3 × 0.75 = 2.25
Ibuprofen: 600 mg × 3	1/600	3 × 1 = 3
Indomethacin: 25 mg × 3	1/25	3 × 1 = 3
Diclofenac: 50 mg × 4	0.75/50	4 × 0.75 = 3

- **Group:** NSAIDs
- **Least GIT side effects:** Acetaminophen AKA paracetamol

Exercise 2

Mr X is suffering from uncomplicated chlamydial urethritis. The cost of various regimen is given below:

Schedule A: Cap Doxycycline 100 mg bd × 7 days

Schedule B: Tab Azithromycin 1 g single dose × 3 days

Schedule C: Cap Amoxicillin 500 mg tds × 7 days

Price: Cap Doxycycline 100 mg—₹ 4.00
Tab Azithromycin 500 mg—₹ 17.50
Cab Amoxicillin 500 mg—₹ 6.50

Questions:

1. Work out the cost for each schedule.
2. Which therapy will you suggest? Why?
3. If a pregnant woman is suffering from uncomplicated chlamydial urethritis which therapy will you select? Why?

Schedule: Drug, dose	*Frequency and days*	*Cost/unit*	*Total cost of treatment*
A: Doxycycline 100 mg	2 × 7	4/1000 mg	4 × 2 × 7 = 56
B: Azithromycin 1000 mg	1 × 3	17.5/500 mg —35/1000 mg	35 × 1 × 3 = 105
C: Amoxicillin 500 mg	3 × 7	6.5/500 mg	6.5 × 3 × 7 = 136.5

- **Preferences**
  - Doxycycline—based on cost
  - In pregnancy, doxycycline is contraindicated due to risk of impairment of the skeletal development of the fetus. Penicillin group of drugs are safe, so amoxycillin is preferred.

Exercise 3

A 60-year-old diabetic male came to skin OPD with itchy patches in abdomen. He was diagnosed as tinea corporis and was started on antifungal drugs.

Schedule A: Tab Griseofulvin 250 mg BD for 4 weeks

Schedule B: Tab Fluconazole 150 mg once a week for 4 weeks

Schedule C: Tab Terbinafine 250 mg OD for 4 weeks

Price : Tab Griseofulvin 250 mg—₹ 2.60/250 mg tab
Tab Fluconazole 150 mg—₹ 28.00/150 mg tab
Tab Terbinafine 250 mg—₹ 20.00/250 mg tab

Questions:

1. Work out the cost for each schedule.
2. Which schedule is economical?
3. Among the schedule drugs which is not effective against T versicolor?

Schedule: Drug, dose	*No. of tablets*	*Cost/unit*	*Cost of treatment*
A: Griseofulvin 250 mg	2 × 4 × 7	2.6/250 mg	2.6 × 2 × 4 × 7 = 145.60
B: Fluconazole 150 mg	1 × 4	28/150 mg	28 × 1 × 4 = 112
C: Terbinafine 250 mg	1 × 4 × 7	20/250 mg	20 × 3 × 7 = 420

- Schedule A is most economical
- However, griseofulvin is ineffective in T versicolor.

Exercise 4

A 60-year-old male a known case of cirrhotic liver with pedal edema and ascites was planned to be treated with diuretics.

Schedule A: Tab Furosemide 40 mg OD/morning for 5 days

Schedule B: Tab Torsemide 20 mg OD/morning for 5 days

Schedule C: Tab Frusemide 20 mg + T spironolactone 50 mg BD for 5 days

Price: Tab Frusemide 40 mg; ₹ 2.00/unit
Tab Torsemide 20 mg; ₹ 3.75/unit
Tab Frusemide 20 mg + T spironolactone 50 mg; ₹ 4.00/unit

Questions:

1. Work out the cost for each schedule.
2. Which schedule is economical?
3. Which schedule is suitable to this patient? Justify.

Schedule: Drug, dose	*No. of tablets*	*Cost/unit*	*Cost of treatment*
A: Furosemide 40 mg	1 × 5	2.00	1 × 5 × 2 = 10
B: Torsemide 20 mg	1 × 5	3.75	1 × 5 × 3.75 = 18.75
C: Furosemide 20 mg + spironolactone 50 mg	2 × 5	4	2 × 5 × 4 = 40

- Schedule A is most economical
- Schedule C is most suitable since spironolactone will counteract the hypokalemia caused by furosemide.

Exercise 5

An adolescent boy attending medicine OPD with complaints of running nose and sneezing for 3 days. He was diagnosed to have allergic rhinitis. Select an appropriate regimen for management.

Regimen A: Tab Astemizole 10 mg od × 5 days

Regimen B: Tab Chlorpheniramine 25 mg od × 5 days

Regimen C: Tab Cetirizine 10 mg od × 5 days

Cost of drugs:

Tab Astemizole 10 mg ₹ 10.50/10 tab
Tab Chlorpheniramine 25 mg ₹ 4.50/10 tab
Tab Cetirizine 10 mg ₹ 25.00/10 tab

Regimen: Drug, dose	*No. of tablets*	*Cost*	*Cost of treatment*
A: Astemizole: 10 mg	1 × 5	10.50/10 tab = 5.25/5 tab	52.5
B: Chlorpheniramine: 20 mg	1 × 5	4.50/10 tab = 2.25/5 tab	22.5
C: Cetirizine: 250 mg	1 × 5	25/10 tab = 12.5/5 tab	125

- Chlorpheniramine is a first-generation antihistamine which causes sedation
- Cetirizine is a second-generation antihistamine with less sedation associated with it and can be preferred.

Exercise 6

Bipin aged 45 years visited a government hospital OPD, was prescribed generic tablet Paracetamol 500 mg TDS for three days, for the treatment of flu. His friend Gopal also had similar symptoms for flu, for which he was prescribed tablet DEF (Paracetamol) 500 mg tds for three days by a private practitioner. Fever subsided after one hour of tablet intake in both cases. (Generic Paracetamol 500 mg—₹ 5.40/tab, Tab DEF 500 mg—₹ 9.50/10 tab)

a. Calculate the cost of drugs prescribed by the government hospital and private clinic.
b. Identify to which pharmacoeconomic evaluation method this belongs to with explanation.

Brand	*No. of tablets*	*Cost/tab*	*Cost of treatment*
Generic PCM 500 mg	3 × 3	5.40	48.6
DEF 500 mg	3 × 3	9.50	85.5

Cost—minimization analysis

Exercise 7

According to the survey done by the gastroenterology department of a tertiary care hospital eradication of *H. pylori* revealed that around 124 patients (group 1) were administered XYZ Kit (Lansoprazole 30 mg two caps + Amoxycillin 750 mg two tabs + Clarithromycin 250 mg two tabs) twice daily for two weeks. Another group 2 of 124 patients were administered ABC Kit (Omeprazole 20 mg two caps + Amoxycillin 750 mg two tabs + Tinidazole 500 mg two tabs) twice daily for two weeks. After one month, in group 1 gastric mucosal biopsy showed absence of *H. pylori* in 117 patients whereas group 2 showed absence of *H. pylori* in 95 patients. (XYZ Kit—₹89.70, ABC Kit—₹33.)

a. What is the percentage of eradication of *H. pylori* in group 1 and 2?
b. Calculate the incremental cost-effective ratio.

Regimen: Drug, dose	***No. of patients cured***	***% of patients with -ve biopsy***	***Cost of treatment***
XYZ Kit ($n = 124$)	117	117/124 = 94.35%	89.7
ABC Kit ($n = 124$)	95	95/124 = 76.61%	33
Difference	22	17.74	56.7

4

$$ICER = Cost_{XYZ} \text{-} Cost_{ABC} / Effect\ \%_{XYZ} - Effect\ \%_{ABC}$$

$$= 56.7/17.74$$

$$= 3.196$$

17 CHAPTER

Medical Ethics

Short Notes

1. Healthcare as a right.
2. Bioethics.
3. Communication: Empathy.
4. Informed consent.
5. Optimal storage of medicine.
6. Medication adherence.
7. Cost of treatment vis a vis patient compliance.
8. Drug dependence—prevention and management.
9. Educating patients about various aspects of drug use.
10. Over-the-counter drugs.
11. Ethical and legal aspects of prescription writing.

HEALTHCARE AS A RIGHT

1. Definition
2. Key aspects of the right to health
3. Core components of the right to health
4. Violations of human rights in health
5. WHO response
6. Obligations on states and responsibilities towards the right to health
7. Agencies working on health and human rights

1. Definition

Enjoyment of the highest attainable standard of health is one of the fundamental rights of every human being without distinction of race, religion, political belief, economic or social condition. The right to health is a **fundamental part of human rights** and of understanding of a life in dignity

2. Key Aspects of the Right to Health

- **The right to health is an inclusive right:** Right to health is not only access to health care and the building of hospitals but also includes the following, such as safe drinking water and adequate sanitation; safe food; adequate nutrition and housing; healthy working and environmental conditions; health-related education and information; gender equality.

- **The right to health contains freedoms:** The right to be free from non-consensual medical treatment, such as medical experiments and research or forced sterilization.
- **The right to health contains entitlements:** Access to essential medicines; maternal, child and reproductive health; equal and timely access to basic health service.
- Health services, goods and facilities must be provided to all without any discrimination.
- All services, goods and facilities must be available, accessible, acceptable and of good quality.

3. Core Components of the Right to Health

Right to Health (Article 12) was defined in General Comment 14 of the Committee on Economic, Social and Cultural Rights.

Availability

Refers to the need for a sufficient quantity of functioning public health and healthcare facilities, goods and services, as well as programs for all.

Accessibility

- Requires that health facilities, goods, and services must be accessible to everyone:
  - Access to essential medicines;
  - Maternal, child and reproductive health;
  - Equal and timely access to basic health services.
- Accessibility has four overlapping dimensions: non-discrimination, physical accessibility, economic accessibility (affordability), and information accessibility.

Acceptability

Acceptability requires that health facilities, goods, services and programs are people-centered and cater for the specific needs of diverse population groups in accordance with international standards of medical ethics for confidentiality and informed consent.

Quality

Facilities, goods, and services must be scientifically and medically approved. Quality is a key component of Universal Health Coverage, and includes the experience as well as the perception of health care. Quality health services should be:

- **Safe**—avoiding injuries to people for whom the care is intended;
- **Effective**—providing evidence-based healthcare services to those who need them;

- **People-centered**—providing care that responds to individual preferences, needs and values;
- **Timely**—reducing waiting times and sometimes harmful delays;
- **Equitable**—providing care that does not vary in quality on account of gender, ethnicity, geographic location, and socioeconomic status;
- **Integrated**—providing care that makes available the full range of health services throughout the life course;
- **Efficient**—maximizing the benefit of available resources and avoiding waste

4. Violations of Human Rights in Health

Mental ill health is still given inadequate attention in public health, violations of human rights not only contribute to and exacerbate poor health but for many, including people with disabilities, indigenous populations, women living with HIV, sex workers, people who use drugs, transgender and intersex people.

5. WHO (World Health Organization) Response

WHO has made a commitment to mainstream human rights into healthcare programs and policies on national and regional levels.

WHO has been actively strengthening its role in **providing technical, intellectual, and political leadership** on the right to health including:

- Strengthening the capacity of WHO and its **Member States to integrate a human rights-based approach to health**;
- Advancing the **right to health in international law and international development processes**; and
- **Advocating for health-related human rights**, including the right to health.

6. Obligations on States and Responsibilities Towards the Right to Health

The government has the primary obligation to protect and promote human rights.

General Obligations

Three types of obligations:

1. The obligation to **respect**: The obligation to respect requires states to refrain from interfering directly OR indirectly with the right to health.
2. The obligation to **protect**: The obligation to protect requires states to prevent third parties from interfering with the right to health.
3. The obligation to **fulfil**: The obligation to fulfil requires states to adopt appropriate legislative, administrative, budgetary, judicial, promotional and other measures to fully realize the right to health.

7. Agencies Working on Health and Human Rights

- United Nations, agencies, in particular, UNICEF
- Joint United Nations Programme on HIV/AIDS (UNAIDS)
- United Nations Population Fund (UNFPA)
- WHO

BIOETHICS

1. Definition
2. Pillars:
   - Autonomy
   - Beneficence
   - Non-maleficence
   - Confidentiality
   - Justice
   - Conflict of interest
3. Education

1. Definition

Bioethics (ethics—way of life) is commonly understood to refer to the ethical implications and applications of the health-related life sciences.

2. Pillars of Medical Ethics

- **Autonomy:**
  - The right **of competent adults to make informed decisions about their own medical care**.
  - Respecting the principle of autonomy obliges the physician to disclose medical information and treatment options that are necessary for the patient to exercise self-determination and supports informed consent, truth-telling, and confidentiality.
- **Beneficence:**
  - The obligation of the physician **to act for the benefit of the patient** and supports moral rules to protect and defend the right of others, prevent harm, remove conditions that will cause harm, help persons with disabilities, and rescue persons in danger
  - *Non-maleficence:* The obligation of a physician **not to harm the patient**. This supports several moral rules—do not kill, do not cause pain or suffering, do not incapacitate, do not cause offence, and do not deprive others of the goods of life.
  - *Justice:* Fair, equitable, and appropriate treatment of persons. The one that is most pertinent to clinical ethics is **distributive justice.** Distributive justice refers to the **fair, equitable, and appropriate distribution of healthcare resources.**
- **Confidentiality:**
  - The physician is obligated **not to disclose confidential information given by a patient** to another party without the patient's authorization.
  - An obvious exception (with implied patient authorization) is the sharing necessary of medical information for the care of the patient from the primary physician to consultants and other healthcare teams.
- **Conflict of interest:** Treatment **should not be influenced by any person or money.**

Bioethics is taught in courses at the undergraduate and graduate level in different academic disciplines or programs, such as philosophy, medicine, law, social sciences. It has become a requirement for professional accreditation in many health professional programs.

COMMUNICATION

1. **Definitions:** Empathy, compassion, sympathy
2. Benefits of employing empathy in healthcare
3. **Methods to develop empathy:** Verbal and nonverbal

E **EYE CONTACT**
M **MUSCLE OF FACIAL EXPRESSION**
P **POSTURE**
A **AFFECT**
T **TONE OF VOICE**
H **HEARING THE PATIENT**
Y **YOUR RESPONSE**

Definitions

- **Empathy** is the ability to **understand** and share other people's feelings: Empathy in healthcare is—"the act of correctly acknowledging the emotional state of another without experiencing that state oneself."
- **Compassion** is closer to empathy than sympathy is, but they are still quite different.
  - Derived from Latin, compassion means **"to suffer with.**"
  - Compassion usually involves a desire or drive to alleviate the suffering of the other person.
  - However, the intellectual understanding of the other person's emotions may be missing with compassion.
- **Sympathy** is an emotional response to the suffering of another person: It is when you realize and understand that something bad has happened to someone else and you imagine that pain.

Clinical empathy consists of four important dimensions:
- **Affective empathy:** The ability to understand a patient's emotions.
- **Cognitive empathy:** The ability to understand the patient's mental state and intellectual ability to identify the patient's thinking in response to his/her current situation.
- **Behavioral empathy:** The ability (of the doctor) to respond appropriately to all those emotional perspectives of the patient.
- **Somatic empathy:** The ability (of the doctor) to express a physical reaction in response to the patient's emotional and mental state.

Empathy is conveyed through verbal and nonverbal expression. Checklist for nonverbal methods to improve empathy.

Empathy		Better Communication	
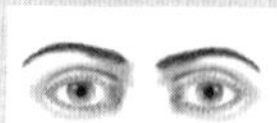	E	**Eye Contact**	Making meaningful eye contact
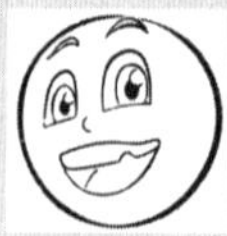	M	**Muscle of Facial Expression**	Decoding facial expressions, specifically fear detection
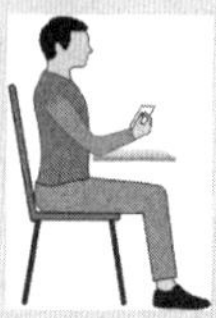	P	**Posture**	Posture is a powerful signal of positive and negative emotions, independent of facial expressions *For example,* sitting down with patients at eye level conveys both interest in and time for patients
	A	**Affect**	Conscious assessment of patients' affective states crucial for improved patient satisfaction, increased adherence, and lower anxiety
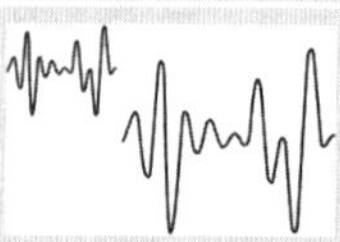	T	**Tone of Voice**	Tones conveying warmth and anxiety about a patient's condition conveys interest
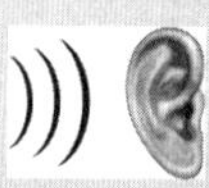	H	**Hearing the Whole Patient**	Hear the "whole patient" by placing the nonverbal signals into the context of the patient's narrative and social world
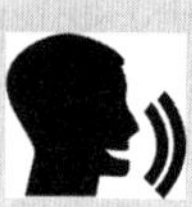	Y	**Your Response**	Should be empathetic. Be aware of your own body language, facial expression, attitude, words, tone, and voice modulation

Benefits of Employing Empathy in Healthcare:

- Better patient outcomes
- Increases adherence to treatment plans
- Builds trusting relationships (doctor–patient)
- Better patient satisfaction
- Reduce chances of medicolegal issues

INFORMED CONSENT

- Information about a particular treatment or test in order for the patient to decide whether or not she/he wishes to undergo a treatment or test. This process of understanding the risks and benefits of treatment is known as informed consent.

- Informed consent is an ethical and legal requirement for medical treatment. Informed consent is one of the nine core principles of the medical ethics. In practice, informed consent is a shared responsibility between patient and doctor.
- For many types of interactions (for example, a physical exam with your doctor), **implied consent** is assumed. For more invasive tests or for those tests or treatments with significant risks or alternatives, you will be asked to give **explicit (written) consent**.

Exceptions to the informed consent rule: An emergency in which medical care is needed immediately to prevent serious or irreversible harm.

Principles of Informed Consent

1. The patient must be **mentally competent** to give consent:
   - When participating in a clinical trial, undergoing a research experiment or receiving medical treatment, the patient must be able to make an informed consent. Thus, he must be of a **sound mind**.
   - He must also be of **legal age**—otherwise, his legal guardian must consent on his behalf.
2. The healthcare provider must disclose enough information for the patient to make an informed choice.
3. The patient must **indicate his understanding of the information** he received. The patient must acknowledge that he understands the in-depth information communicated to him regarding his treatment. The healthcare provider must judge that the patient understands the information.
4. The patient must freely authorize the treatment plan, usually with their signature.

In practice, procedures that are likely to require signed consent include:

- Treatment with high-risk medications, such as opioids
- Tests and medical interventions that go inside your body, such as endoscopy
- Childbirth interventions, such as forceps delivery or episiotomy
- Surgery
- Biopsy
- Medical implants
- Use of anesthesia
- Use of radiation
- Chemotherapy
- Blood transfusions
- Genetic testing
- Clinical trials involving human research subjects (including psychology research)
- Procedures involving medical students
- Certain vaccines
- Any transfer of your personal information

OPTIMAL STORAGE OF MEDICINE

1. Factors affecting the stability of medicine
2. Benefits of optimum storage
3. Various storage conditions

1. Factors Affecting the Stability of Medicine

The pharmacological properties of a medicine change (worsen) faster with exposure to:

- **Temperature:** With the increase in temperature (hastens decomposition)
- **Humidity:** With the increase in humidity (causes crust formation and microbiological growth)
- **Air:** With exposure to air, causes oxidation of the drug
- **Light:** With exposure to light, there is photogeneration of light-sensitive compounds (that is why some drugs are packed in amber color or lightproof containers)
- **Microbial contamination:** Makes it unsafe and increases decomposition

The physician must communicate regarding the correct storage conditions and the reasons for the same.

2. Benefits of Optimum Storage

- Assured efficacy of drugs
- Better treatment outcomes
- Prevents accidental intake by children/other relatives
- Cost-effective use of medicine reduces the need for repeated buying

3. Various Storage Conditions

At Home

Cool: Any temperature **between 8°C and 25°C** (Cool, dry and dark place). Antibiotics, LMWH, vitamins, etc., are stored in this condition.

Cold: Any temperature **not exceeding 8°C** and usually **between 2°C to 8°C.** A refrigerator is a cold place in which the temperature is maintained thermostatically.

Vaccines, toxins, antitoxins, adrenaline, parenteral antibiotics, insulin ophthalmic preparations

Room temperature: The temperature prevailing in a working area.

- Heat, air, light, and moisture may damage medicine.
- Store medicines in a dry place.
- Store in a dresser drawer or a kitchen cabinet away from the stove, sink, and any hot appliances, or in a storage box, on a shelf, or in a closet.
- Not in the bathroom cabinet.
- Take the cotton ball out of the medicine bottle. The cotton ball pulls moisture into the bottle.
- Ask the pharmacist about any specific storage instructions.

Keep children safe

- Always store medicine out of reach and out of sight of children.
- Store medicine in a cabinet with a child latch or lock.

Do not use the following damaged medicine

- Medicine that has changed color, texture, or smell, even if it has not expired
- Pills that stick together, are harder or softer than normal, or are cracked or chipped

Get rid of old medicines

- Check the expiration date on your medicine. Throw out medicines that are out of date.
- Do not keep old or unused medicine around. It goes bad and should not be used.
- Do not flush your medicine down the toilet. This is bad for the water supply.
- To throw away medicine in the trash, first mix medicine with something that ruins it, such as coffee grounds. Put the entire mixture in a sealed plastic bag.
- Unused medicines can be returned to the pharmacist.
- Use community "drug give back" programs if they are available.

Traveling with Medicine

- Do not keep medicine in the glove compartment of the car. Medicine can get too hot, cold, or wet there.
- If you are taking an aeroplane, keep medicines in the carry-on luggage.
- **To help with security at the airport:**
  - Keep medicine in the original bottles.
  - Ask the healthcare provider for a copy of all the prescriptions. It may be needed in case medicine is damaged or is over.
  - In case of having diabetes, the doctor may provide for a letter explaining diabetes and providing a list of all supplies. The patient can be allowed to carry her medicine, blood glucose meter, and lancet device on a plane.

MEDICATION ADHERENCE

1. Definition
2. Measurements of medication adherence
3. Improving adherence

Definition

- The WHO defines adherence as "the extent to which the person's behavior (including medication-taking) corresponds with agreed recommendations from a healthcare provider".
- It includes the initiation of the treatment, implementation of the prescribed regime, and discontinuation of the pharmacotherapy

Measurements of medication adherence are categorized by the WHO as:
- **Subjective measurements:** Patient's evaluation of their medication-taking behavior
- **Objective measurements:** Pill counts, electronic monitoring, secondary database analysis and biochemical measures

Reasons for Medication Nonadherence

Fear

Patients may be frightened of potential side effects. They may have also experienced previous side effects with the same or similar medicine.

Cost

A major barrier to adherence is often the cost of the medicine prescribed to the patient.

Misunderstanding

Nonadherence can also happen when a patient does not understand the need for the medicine, the nature of side effects or the time it takes to see results. This is especially true for patients with chronic illness.

Too Many Medications

When a patient has several different medicines prescribed with higher dosing frequency, the chances that they are nonadherent increase.

Lack of Symptoms

As stated above, nonadherence might occur when there is a lack of symptoms. Patients who do not feel any different when they start or stop their medicine might see no reason to take it.

Additionally, once a patient's condition is controlled, they may think the problem has been resolved and may discontinue using the medication.

Worry

If a patient is concerned about becoming dependent on a medicine, it can also lead to nonadherence.

Depression

Patients who are depressed are less likely to take their medications as prescribed.

Measures of adherence: Methods for assessing medication adherence: direct and indirect measures

1. **Direct measures:**
   - Identification and estimation of medicine or its metabolite in blood or urine.
   - Identification and estimation of the biological marker in blood or tissue.

Direct measures are the most confirming evidence of taking medicine. However not practical for routine clinical use or variations in metabolism may give biased results.

2. Indirect measures:

- *Patient questionnaires:* For example, Morisky scale questionnaire. (structured and validated 8-item assessment tool). It can be used easily in follow-up visits to measure non-adherence.
- *Self-reports:* It is easy, commonly used and often biased due to inaccurate patient recall. It is an optimistic overestimation that is usually reported by patients.
- *Pill counts:* Pill counts are easy to perform, but it does not give any clue about exact timing of medicine intake. It can be falsely changed by patients (e.g., pill dumping).
- *Rate of prescription refills/pharmacy refills:* It is a commonly used method. "Frequency of getting refilled vs. refills required", reflects the patient's adherence.
- Assessment of the patient's clinical response
- Electronic medication monitors
- Measurement of physiological markers. BP control
- *Patient diaries:* This method is used in clinical trials

Use the **SIMPLE method** to help improve medication adherence among your patients.

Simplify the Regimen

- Encourage patients to use adherence tools, such as day-of-the-week pill boxes or mobile apps.
- Work to match the action of taking medication with a patient's daily routine (e.g., meal time or bedtime, with other medications they already take properly)

Impart Knowledge

Write down prescription instructions clearly, and reinforce them verbally.

Provide websites for additional reading and information.

Modify Patients' Beliefs and Behavior

Provide positive reinforcement when patients take their medication successfully, and offer incentives if possible.

Talk to patients to understand and address their concerns or fears.

Provide Communication and Trust

- Allow patients to speak freely. Time is of the essence, but research shows that most patients will talk no longer than two minutes when given the opportunity.
- Use plain language when speaking with patients. Say, "Did you take all of your pills?" instead of using the word "adherence."

- Ask for patients' input when discussing recommendations and making decisions.
- Remind patients to contact your office with any questions.

Leave the Bias

- Understand the predictors of non-adherence and address them as needed with patients.
- Ask patients specific questions about attitudes, beliefs, and cultural norms related to taking medications.

Evaluate Adherence

Ask patients simply and directly whether they are sticking to their drug regimen.

Use a medication adherence scale—most are available online:
- Morisky-8 (MMAS-8)
- Morisky-4 (MMAS-4 or Medication Adherence Questionnaire)
- Medication Possession Ratio (MPR)
- Proportion of Days Covered (PDC)

COST OF TREATMENT VIS A VIS PATIENT COMPLIANCE

Introduction

- Cost of medicine (treatment) is one of the most important barriers of patient's compliance/adherence, especially in managing chronic disease, due to prolonged course of treatment, repeated doctor visit and investigations.
- Cost of treatment is more concern for patients belonging to low-income group or who are not covered by health insurance. physician should consider patient's economic condition during prescribing and treat the patient more cost-effectively.
- Research studies have shown that most of the physicians and patients wish to discuss about the cost of treatment and patients expect that the doctor should initiate such conversation. Patient may also feel embarrassed to talk about the financial inability to afford the cost of treatment.

Guide to Physician to Improve Cost Communications: **IDEA**

Inquire
D-discuss
E-educate
Act

Inquire

Physicians should initiate the discussion on cost-of-treatment routinely, as a part of history taking. Respectful and empathetic approach decreases patient embarrassment, and he/she will feel free to talk about his/her real financial hardship to afford medicine or cost of relevant tests.

Discuss

Discuss her/his condition or disease; current recommended treatment, rationale and evidence of such recommendation at the level of patient's understanding. Discuss about the possible alternative treatment options, their pros and cons; cost of all possible treatment option, etc. This type of discussion makes the patient confident in choosing their preferences and shared decision making. This reduces anxiety—improves adherence, treatment outcomes, satisfaction of the patient and also enhances physician-patient relationship.

Educate

- Educate them about risks of not receiving treatment; benefits of treatment; possible side effects of the drugs; benefits of adherence; how non-adherence may increase the total cost of the treatment, etc.
- **Educate the patient about the benefits of generic medicine:** Cost of the generic drugs are lesser than branded drugs, where the effective. ness is comparable,
- **Use drugs from National Essential Medicine List (NELM):** Try to choose drugs that are included in NELM,
- **If possible stores where those medicines will be available:** Various health insurances and health schemes that may provide economic benefit to the patient.
- **Up-to-date knowledge on all available treatment:** Physicians should always remain up-to-date regarding all available treatment regimen, generic and costs of such treatment.

Act

Start treatment as per agreed shared discission. Use low-cost generic drugs. Do not prescribe extravagantly, do not use/stop unnecessary or minimally beneficial medicines. Patients always prefer those physicians, who try to give solutions for non-medical problem also.

DRUG DEPENDENCE: PREVENTION AND MANAGEMENT

Definations of drug dependence: Physical psychological dependance, withdrawl syndome.

Prescription Drugs that Cause Dependence

- The drugs that are most commonly abused and have potential in producing drug dependence, are:

- *Opioids:* e.g., morphine, meperidine, tapentadol
- *Anxiolytics/sedatives and hypnotics:* Alprazolam, diazepam, lorazepam, nitrazepam, oxazepam, midazolam, etc.
- *CNS stimulants:* Methylphenidate, modafinil.

Precautions to be taken in Prescribing Drugs Likely to Produce Dependence

- Up-to-date knowledge about such drugs: 'Schedule X' Drugs (annexed list of Drugs and Cosmetics Act 1940', 'Drugs and Cosmetics Rules 1945); and those are listed in the 'Narcotic Drugs and Psychotropic Substances Act, 1985' are known to cause dependence or addiction.
- Rational prescribing: Prescribe these drugs rationally, avoid prescribing drugs that have dependence liability and only prescribe when the benefit of using such drug exceeds the extent of harm. Use safer alternative whenever possible (e.g., tramadol has least dependance amongst opioids).
- Optimal prescribing: Use these drugs optimally, with appropriate dose, regimen and duration.
- Practicing telemedicine: Prescribing drugs known to cause dependence or addiction, via telemedicine practice is considered as professional misconduct.
- Refill advice: Refill advice should be written appropriately in legible handwriting.
- Educate about optimal use: Patients should be educated regarding the use of drugs in accordance to prescribed treatment. Do not use in excess.
- Closely monitor adherence: Monitor patient adherence before changing (increasing) dose.
- Engage caregiver/relative: Engage relative of the patient in the treatment (supervised treatment), when there is a chance of abuse or dependence.
- Identify patients having potential for drug abuse

EDUCATING PATIENT ABOUT VARIOUS ASPECTS OF DRUG USE

- Why are you using this medicine: Communicate and educate the patient about the prescribed drugs, especially what is his/her need (disease or condition) and which drug is used to fulfill that need.
- Drug allergy: Alert and educate your patient about drug allergy. You should tell the patient to always make a note about those drugs causing allergic reaction and inform their physician during each visit.
- When starting a new medicine: Sometimes, patients having chronic illness know about their drugs as they are using them for longer time. Whenever a new drug is added to their existing treatment or a new drug is used to substitute their current treatment, educate the patient, why it is necessary to add on/substitution.
- How to access medicine in cost effective manner. Inform and educate patient about as generic drug and its benefit, where it is available.
- Check medicines during purchase
- How to store drugs

- Educate importance of adherence
- Educate about refill
- Educate about adverse events of the drug
- Educate about significance of concomitant drug intake
- Educate about how food affects absorption of the drug
- Educate about safe disposal of drugs
- Educate about informed use of OTC drugs

OVER-THE-COUNTER DRUGS

Over-the-counter (OTC) drugs are those drugs that are safe and effective for use by the general public without seeking treatment by a health professional (US-FDA). But the term "over-the-counter drugs" is legally undefined in Indian context. It is not mentioned in the Drugs and Cosmetics Act, 1940 or the Drugs and Cosmetics (D&C) Rules, 1945.

By terms of Rule 123, the drugs listed in Schedule K of the D&C Rules, 1945, do not need a license for sale by shop other than a chemist's shop.

Examples of some common **"Schedule K" Drugs**

- Aspirin tablets
- Paracetamol tablets
- Analgesic balms
- Antacid preparations
- Gripe water for use of infants
- Inhalers containing drugs for treatment of cold and nasal congestion
- Syrups, lozenges, pills and tablets for cough
- Liniments for external use
- Skin ointments and ointments for burns
- Absorbent cotton wool, bandages, absorbent gauze and adhesive plaster
- Castor oil, liquid paraffin and Epsom salt
- Eucalyptus oil
- Tincture iodine, tincture Benzoin Co and Mercurochrome solution in containers not exceeding 100 mL
- Tablets of iodochlorohydroxyquinoline 250 mg
- Contraceptives
- Cosmetics
- Ophthalmic ointments of the tetracycline group of drugs
- Hair fixers
- Tablets of chloroquine salts
- Preparations applied to human body for the purpose of repelling insects like mosquitoes
- Medicated dressings and bandages for first aid
- Oral rehydration salts
- White or yellow petroleum jelly IP (nonperfumed)

Advantages of OTC Medicines

- Direct and rapid access to the medicine without prescription
- Available at pharmacies as well as grocery stores
- No physician visits
- Decreases health care costs
- Promotes self-treatment for minor illness (such as fever, headache, etc.), decreases the burden of healthcare system

Disadvantages of OTC Medicines

- Self-medications may be dangerous, if diagnosis is incorrect, this minor symptom (say headache) may be cue for a more serious disease
- Increases chance of drug interactions with prescription medicine
- OTC medication may delay doctor's visit for a serious treatable disease
- Risk- benefit ratio is uncertain
- Illiteracy may be burden for safe and effective use of OTC drugs
- Inadequate labeling of OTC products—makes it difficult to use
- A cause of polypharmacy

Precautions with OTC Drugs

- Do not self-treat on the basis of assumption to avoid further complications. Be sure about diagnosis and then take OTC medicine.
- Read package insert (product labels) carefully, it will give all relevant information regarding the drug use including name, active ingredients, indications for use, usual dosage, when to stop using the medication or when to see a doctor, possible side effects and expiration dates.
- Do not use OTC medications for longer duration or at higher doses than recommended
- Always read warning and contraindication of its use. Contact physician, if any confusion.
- Inform your physician about your OTC medicine, to avoid unwanted drug interactions and adverse effects.
- Store OTC drugs as per manufacturers guideline.
- Check expiry date during and after purchase, and safely dispose which have expired.
- In pregnancy, breastfeeding and pediatric use, consult physician before taking OTC drugs.
- Know when not to take: Avoid alcohol, if taking antihistamines as OTC drugs because this may increase drowsiness, avoid laxative, if there is stomach pain, nausea or vomiting.

ETHICAL AND LEGAL ASPECTS OF PRESCRIPTION WRITING

Rational prescribing (use of drugs): It is the basis of ethical prescribing. The drugs should be medically and scientifically justified for patient's condition. So that benefit or treatment always outweighs the risk of harm.

Conflict of interest: Prescription should never be influenced by any person, material or money. Prescription should always be in the best interest of the patient.

Respect patients" autonomy, dignity, right, as well as moral, social and cultural belief: Physician should provide relevant information about disease and drugs that enable patients to make informed decisions.

Truth-telling: Physician should discuss about present condition (with patients or relatives) by telling the truth and being transparent (without exaggerating or minimizing), to help them in making shared decisions.

Remember and respect professional boundaries: Physician should always remember his her professional boundaries in terms of competence, credentials and privilege.

- Never hesitate to consult concerned specialist for patient's benefit.
- Never "refuse to treat a patient in case of medical emergency".
- Never "discriminate between patients based on gender, race, religion, caste, social, economic or cultural grounds".
- Always respect laws and regulations of country.

Managing prescription errors: Physicians are humans, and humans are supposed to make errors. disclose prescription errors and explain empathetically to the patient how the error has happened, way to come back from consequences and leam from it to ensure that the error does not happen again.

Prescribing off-label medicines: Physicians should usually prescribe medicines for labeled indications. Sometimes, it becomes necessary to prescribe drugs for unapproved indications (off' label use) for patient's benefit. The physician must give information to the patient about such use to take an informed decision.

Confidentiality of the patient: The physician is ethically and legally bound to keep the patient's information (medical and personal) confidential. That information can only be disclosed to court of law; or to the competent authority after verbal or written consent from the patient for their best interest.

Prescribing sports medicine: Clinicians should not prescribe medicines for enhancing an individual's performance in sport.

Legal Aspects of Prescribing

Generic drugs prescribing: Always try to prescribe drugs with their "generic* *non-proprietary"/pharmacological" name, Better avoid prescribing "branded" or "branded generic" drugs, before prescribing ensure the availability of those generic drugs. Educate patient about benefit of generic drugs. And inform where they are available.

Rational prescribing: Always prescribe rationally and optimally according to patient's need, Avoid overprescribing, under prescribing, inappropriate prescribing (all these are known as prescribing faults) and extravagant prescribing.

Definitive diagnosis/provisional diagnosis: Prescription should contain a diagnosis, followed by treatment.

Fixed-dose combinations: Always use approved FDC rationally.

Legible prescribing: Hand writing should be legible, or else use electronic gadgets for typed and printed prescription, to avoid misinterpretation.

Use **CAPITALS**: Preferably write in CAPITAL letters that will help to avoid misinterpretation of prescription.

- **Avoid prescription errors:** Try to avoid errors, those come from the act of writing (for example, mg vs meg; appropriate use of decimal)
- A prescription should mandatorily contain following details:
  - *Prescriber's details:* Doctors name, registration number, qualification, full address and other contact details (such as telephone number, email, WhatsApp, etc.), contact details during emergency symbol Rx which means "take thou" or "to take".
  - *Patient's details:* Name, age, gender address of the patient, height and weight.
- **Inscription:** Contains the name of the drugs, their dosage form and amount or strength of the drugs.
- **Subscription:** Instructions to pharmacist about the medicines to be dispersed.
- **Transcription (Signatura or Sig):** Contains instructions to the pharmacists and the patients regarding prescribed drug use.
- Prescriber's signature and date. The prescription must be signed and dated by the pro scriber to complete the document by his/her own hand.
- The physician should exhibit his degrees on prescription as recognized and accredited council.

18 CHAPTER

Demonstrating Techniques: Objective Structured Practical Examination (OSPE)

A. For Parenteral Injections

1. Demonstrate drug administration by IM route
2. Demonstrate drug administration by SC route
3. Demonstrate drug administration by intradermal route
4. Demonstrate drug administration by IV bolus route
5. Demonstrate IV drip setting
6. Demonstrate technique of aspirating drug from ampoule into syringe (page 30) Figure 3.1
7. Demonstrate technique of aspirating drug from vial into syringe (page 31) Figure 3.2
8. Demonstrate technique of dissolving dry medicine in vial and aspirate it into syringe (page 31)

B. For Oral Route (Dosage Forms Viva)

1. Reconstitute suspension for oral use page 12
2. Instruction for use of OC pills (Pages 265–6)

C. **For Topical Route (Dosage Forms Viva)**

1. Instructions for applying ointment: Page 15
2. Instructions for using suppositories: Page 16
3. Instructions for using rectal suppositories: Page 18
4. Instructions for using vaginal suppositories: Page 19
5. Procedure for using MDI: Pages 20–21, Page 274
6. Procedure for using spacer: Pages 20–21
7. Procedure for using spacer: Pages 20–21. Figure 2.9
8. Procedure for using rotahaler: Page 22. Figure 2.10
9. Procedure for instilling ear drops: Pages 22–23
10. Procedure for instilling eye drops: Pages 24–25
11. Procedure for instilling eye ointment: Page 25
12. Procedure for instilling nasal drops: Page 26
13. Procedure for instilling nasal spray: Page 26
14. Method of using transdermal patch: Page 27
15. Instructions for using insulin pen: Page 272

GENERAL INSTRUCTIONS TO BE FOLLOWED WHILE GIVING PARENTERAL INJECTIONS

BEFORE giving the injection:

1. Check the name of drug from prescription and expiry date of the medication
2. Introduce yourself to the patient, confirm the patient's identity and the drug to be administered. Explain the process of administering the injection in a language and manner the patient understands. Make the patient comfortable.
3. Ensure you have all your equipment ready as follows—spirit, gloves, alcohol wipe, disposable tourniquet, IV cannula, suitable plaster, syringe, saline.
4. During the preparation procedure, materials should be kept sterile. Wash your hands before preparing the injection and also after the procedure. Expose the area and disinfect the injection site with appropriate antiseptic-in an anticlockwise and outward direction. Take care not to prick yourself or somebody else during the procedure.

Aspirate the drug—as mentioned before: Figure 3.2. Page 31

Administer the injection—at the angle mentioned according to the route of Administration.

AFTER giving the injection

1. Check the patient's reaction and give additional reassurance, if necessary
2. Clean up, and dispose of waste safely. Do not recap the needle—the needle must be disposed of in a sturdy, puncture and leak-proof **sharps container** (white plastic container) immediately after use
3. Syringes (without needles) to be discarded in the **red-colored bag**; cotton swabs in the **yellow-colored bag**
4. Wash hands

Specific Instructions

Intramuscular

Before giving the injection: As mentioned above

In addn:

1. Uncover the area to be injected (deltoid, vastas lateralis, gluteus maximus).
2. Ask the patient to relax the muscle
3. Typical needle used is 22-25 gauge
4. Insert the needle at 90°, holding the syringe like a dart (*refer* to Figures 3.12, 3.13, 3.2 for location)
5. Aspirate briefly—if blood appears, withdraw the needle, replace it, and start again
6. Inject slowly
7. Withdraw the needle swiftly and put pressure on the injection site

Additional Information

- Advantages disadvantages of IM route: Page 36
- Site of IM injection Figures 3.13, 3.2, Page 37
- Examples of drug given by IM route: Page 37

Subcutaneous

Before giving the injection: As mentioned above

In addn:

1. Uncover the area to be injected (upper arm, upper thigh, anterior abdominal wall)
2. Use 25–26 gauge needle
3. Pinch the skin to get access to the subcutaneous space.
4. Insert the needle in the base of the skin fold at an angle of 30°–45°.
5. Aspirate briefly—if blood appears, withdraw the needle, replace it, and start again.
6. Inject slowly—0.5–2 mL.
7. Withdraw the needle swiftly and put pressure on the injection site.

Additional Information

- Advantages and disadvantages of SC route: Page 38
- Site of SC injection Table 3.2, Page 39,
- Examples of drug given by SC route: Page 38

Intradermal

1. Uncover the area to be injected (e.g., forearm)
2. *Stretch* the skin to make it taut
3. Insert the needle at an angle of 10°–15°, almost parallel to the taut skin
4. Aspirate briefly—if blood appears, withdraw the needle, replace it, and start again
5. Inject slowly (0.1 mL)
6. Withdraw the needle swiftly and put pressure on the injection site

Additional Information

- Advantages disadvantages intradermal route: Page 38
- Site of intradermal injection Table 3.2, Page 39
- Examples of drug given by intradermal route: Page 39

Intravenous: Bolus Injections

1. Position the arm so that it is comfortable for the patient and identify a vein
2. Apply the tourniquet and re-check the vein. Wait for the vein to swell
3. Insert the needle, bevel upwards at about 30°. Aspirate. Blood should come in the tip of the needle, If it does not come try again
4. Loosen tourniquet
5. Inject the drug slowly. Check for pain, hematoma

6. After complete injection of drug remove the needle fully. Press sterile cotton on to the opening. Secure with adhesive tape.
7. Check patient's reaction, give additional assurance

Additional Information

- IV versus bolus injection: Page 41
- Advantages disadvantages of IV route: Page 44
- Micro-dip and macro-drip: Page 45
- Types of IV fluids: Page 46

Intravenous: IV Drip Infusion

Primary IV Fluid Infusion
Most commonly used primary IV fluid bag contains 1,000 mL. They consist of various types of fluid, such as 0.9% normal saline, 0.45% (½) normal saline, lactated ringers solution, and dextrose (5%) preparations. It runs at consistent infusion rates for a prescribed period of time. For example, a continuous fluid infusion may be ordered at a rate of 125 mL/hour for 24 hours.

Secondary Fluid Infusion
Secondary IV fluid administration is usually an intermittent infusion that infuses at regular intervals (e.g., every 8 hours). This form of IV therapy usually contains medications that are supplied in a smaller infusion bag and mixed with a diluent fluid like saline (e.g., IV antibiotics). Many common preparations come in 25 to 100 mL bags.

IV Administration Equipment

Two types: Primary Tubing and Secondary Tubing.

Primary IV Administration Sets

Primary IV administration sets are used to infuse continuous or intermittent fluids or medications. It can be a macro-drip or micro-drip solution set.

A macro-drip infusion set delivers 10, 15, or 20 drops per milliliter, whereas a micro-drip infusion set delivers 60 drops per milliliter. The drop factor is located on the packaging of the IV tubing. Macro-drip sets are used for routine primary infusions for adults. Micro-drip IV tubing is used in pediatric or neonatal care where small amounts of fluids are administered over a long period of time.

Parts of primary IV administration sets (Fig. 3.14), Page 41.

Sterile spike: This part of the tubing must be kept sterile as you spike the IV fluid bag.

Drip chamber: The drip chamber allows air to rise out from a fluid so that it is not passed onto the patient. It is also used to calculate the rate at which fluid is administered by gravity (drops per minute). It should be kept ¼ to ½ full of solution.

Backcheck valve: A backcheck valve prevents fluid or medication from travelling up into the primary IV bag.

Access ports: Access ports are used to infuse secondary medications and to administer IV push medications. These may also be referred to as "Y ports."

Roller clamp: A roller clamp is used to regulate the speed, or stop, an infusion by gravity.

Secondary IV Administration Sets

Secondary IV administration sets are used to intermittently administer a secondary medication, such as an antibiotic, while the primary IV is also running. Secondary IV tubing is shorter in length than primary tubing and is connected to a primary line via an access port or an IV pump. The secondary infusion is hung above the primary infusion and connected at an access port.

Preparing an intravenous infusion:

Precautions before stating IV infusion: Point 1–8

1. Verify IV order against the physician order. Clarify any inconsistencies. Check the patient's chart for allergies. Check for color, clarity, expiration date, etc.
2. Know techniques for IV insertion, precautions, purpose of the IV administration, and medications if ordered.
3. Gather all equipment and bring to bedside.
4. Identify the patient. Ask the patient if allergic to any medication, iodine, or tape, as appropriate. If considering using an anesthetic (numbing) cream or 1% lidocaine injection, check for allergies for these substances as well.
5. Explain the need for the IV and procedure to patient.
6. Perform hand hygiene. If using an anesthetic cream, apply the anesthetic cream to a few potential insertion sites.
7. Prepare IV solution and tubing:
   a. Maintain strict aseptic technique when opening sterile packages and IV solution. Remove administration set from package.
   b. Clamp IV tubing, uncap spike on administration set, and insert into entry site on IV bag or bottle as manufacturer directs.
   c. Squeeze drip chamber and allow it to fill at least halfway.
   d. Remove cap at end of the IV tubing and while maintaining its sterility, open the IV tubing clamp, and allow fluid to move through tubing. Allow fluid to flow until all air bubbles have disappeared and the entire length of the tubing is primed (filled) with IV solution. Close clamp and recap end of tubing, maintaining sterility of the setup.
   e. If an electronic device is to be used, follow manufacturer's instructions for inserting tubing and setting infusion rate.
   f. Apply label if medication was added to container (pharmacy may have added medication and applied label). Label tubing with date and time that tubing was hung.
   g. Place time-tape on container and hang IV on pole.
8. Place patient in low Fowler's position in bed. Place protective towel or pad under patient's arm. Close the door to the room or pull the bedside curtain.

9. Provide emotional support as needed.
10. Select and palpate for an appropriate vein. Avoid an arm that has been compromised such as with presence of arterio venous fistula.
11. If the site is hairy and agency policy permits, clip a 2″ area around the intended site of entry.
12. Apply a tourniquet 3” to 4” above the venipuncture site to obstruct venous blood flow and distend the vein. Direct the ends of the tourniquet away from the site of entry. Make sure the radial pulse is still present.
13. Instruct the patient to hold the arm lower than the heart.
14. Put on clean gloves.
15. Cleanse insertion site with alcohol using a circular motion. Use a circular motion to move from the center outward.
16. Use the nondominant hand, placed about 1″ or 2″ below at the entry site, hold the skin taut against the vein. Avoid touching the prepared site. Ask the patient to remain still while performing the venipuncture.
17. Enter the skin gently, holding the catheter by the hub in your dominant hand, bevel side up, at a 10- to 15° angle. Catheter may be inserted from directly over the vein or the side of the vein. While following the course of the vein, advance the needle or catheter into the vein. A sensation of “give” can be felt when the needle enters the vein.
18. When blood returns through the lumen of the needle or the flashback chamber of the catheter, advance either device 1/8″ to 1/4″ farther into the vein. A catheter needs to be advanced until the hub is at the venipuncture site, but the exact technique depends on the type of device used.
19. Release the tourniquet as soon as possible. Quickly remove the protective cap from the IV tubing and attach the tubing to the catheter or needle. Stabilize the catheter or needle with your non-dominant hand.
20. Start the flow of solution promptly by releasing the clamp on the tubing. Examine the tissue around the entry site for signs of infiltration.
21. Secure the catheter with narrow non-allergenic tape (1/2″), placed sticky side up under the hub and crossed over the top of the hub.
22. Place sterile dressing over venipuncture site. Apply tape to dressing if necessary. Loop the tubing near the site of entry, and anchor to dressing.
23. Label the IV dressing with the date, time, site, and type and size of catheter used for the infusion on the tape anchoring the tubing.
24. Remove all equipment and dispose of properly. Remove gloves and perform hand hygiene.
25. Anchor arm to an arm board for support if necessary, or apply a site protector or tube-shaped mesh netting over the insertion site. Explain to patient the purpose of the arm board and the importance of safeguarding the site when using the extremity.
26. Adjust the rate of solution flow according to the amount prescribed, or follow manufacturer’s directions for adjusting flow rate on infusion pump.
27. Document procedure and patient’s response. Chart time, site, device used, and solution.

28. Return to check flow rate and observe IV site for infiltration 30 minutes after starting infusion. Ask the patient if experiencing any pain or discomfort related to the IV infusion.

Seeing a video or observing, it live in ward or causality will give a better picture as how to perform the above procedures:

Priming IV tubing: Primary and secondary IV tubing must be primed with IV solution to remove air from the tubing. Priming refers to placing IV fluid in IV tubing to remove all air prior to attaching the IV tube to the patient. IV tubing is primed to prevent air from entering the circulatory system. An air embolism is a potential complication of IV therapy and can enter a patient's blood system

Spiking: It is to attach a tubing to the IV bag in order to infuse your solution or medication.

Index

Page numbers followed by *b* refer to box, *f* refer to figure, and *t* refer to table.

B

C

E

F

G

H

N

O

Q

R

U

V

W

X

Y

Z